21st CENTURY OBSTETRICS NOW!

VOL 2

Cover Photo Caption . .

ENGROSSMENT

So proud.
This mother.
This boy barely born.
Pairs of peering eyes, probe,
    Penetrate,
    Locked in love.
"He's so beautiful...So perfect...
    So bright...my boy..."
"My mom...my mom...my mom..."

D. Stewart

National
Association of
Parents & Professionals for
Safe
Alternatives in
Childbirth

21st CENTURY OBSTETRICS NOW!

VOL 2

DAVID STEWART, PHD, & LEE STEWART, CCE
EDITORS

AUTHORS

George J. Annas, JD, MPH
Tom Brewer, MD
Mayer Eisenstein, MD
Janet L. Epstein, CNM
Fremont Birth Collective
Doris B. Haire, DMS
Michelle Harrison, MD
Jay Hodin
Myrtle E. Hosford, CNM, MA

Cedar Koons
Thya Merz
Ashley Montagu, PHD
Ruth D. Rice, PHD
Merilyn Salomon, MA
Victoria Schauf, MD
Anne Seiden, MD
David Stewart, PHD
Gregory White, MD

Indexed By
JAMY BRAUN, RN

Published by NAPSAC, Inc.
Chapel Hill, NC

First Edition, July 1977, 2000 copies
Second Edition, February 1978, 5000 copies

Library of Congress Catalogue Number: 77-72854
ISBN 0-917314-07-7   (Vol. 1 only)
ISBN 0-917314-08-5   (Vol. 2 only)
ISBN 0-917314-09-3   (Both Vols. Together as a Set)

Available from: NAPSAC, P.O. Box 267, Marble Hill, MO 63764
Price: $6.50 per single volume/$11 per two-volume set
      (Add 75¢ shipping if ordered direct from publisher.)

All proceeds from this book go toward the accomplishment of the
goals of NAPSAC (see pages 613-615), a non-profit, tax exempt
service corporation. None of the authors receive royalties. All
have generously contributed their time, insight, expertise, and
work to produce this anthology. Among other things, these books
are a monument to their dedication to the betterment of our society through more humane maternity care.

Book Printed by Carolina Copy Center, Chapel Hill, NC, USA
     Master Printer: Ken Cash
     Assistant Printers: Jessie Robinson, Risden Hill, Don Rich
Cover Printed by Creative Printers, Inc., Chapel Hill, NC, USA
     Cover Design by David Stewart
     With Technical Assistance from Karen Simon
Book Binding by Wake Trade Bindery, Cary, NC, USA
     Master Binder: Margaret L. Jones

* CONTRIBUTIONS TO NAPSAC ARE TAX DEDUCTIBLE

21st CENTURY OBSTETRICS NOW! V. 2

TABLE OF CONTENTS - VOL. 2

TABLE OF CONTENTS CONT'D

DEDICATION

These volumes are dedicated to our children: Jonathan, Lora Lee, Keith, Ben, and Anthony (ages 14, 10, 7, 4, and 1 respectively). Were it not for their ability to be flexible and share our time, as well as a certain amount of our work around the house, this book would never have been published.

As we have watched them grow we have become convinced more than ever of the importance of the choices we make in childbirth. The long-term benefits of drugless pregnancy and of family bonding at birth are daily demonstrated by the health, harmony, and happiness of our own home.

In a broader sense, we also dedicate these volumes to the children and parents everywhere, today and yet to come. We wish for everyone to have the opportunity and the freedom to make the choices we were able to make for our own family and to reap the rewards we continuously receive through our own children.

ACKNOWLEDGEMENT

We wish to express our appreciation to the many persons who offered helpful suggestions for the second edition.

In particular, we appreciate the work of MARIE FOXTON who carefully proofread the entire two-volume set. As a result, this edition is considerably improved. Thank you Marie, for your willing patience in this task.

FOREWORD AND INTRODUCTION
20TH & 21ST CENTURY OBSTETRICS: HOW & WHY THIS BOOK

Childbirth of the future will not primarily be in hospitals, but in the home, and the primary health professional for most women will not be the physician, but the midwife. Furthermore, the primary rights and responsibilities for childbirth will not be upon the professional, but upon the parents, because it is they who must bear the responsibilities of raising the child.

Present-day obstetrics is interventive and aggressive, and it reflects an attitude of technologic arrogance. It focuses upon the expectation of high-risk while not seeming to recognize the normality of most mothers. While sometimes benefiting the truly high-risk patient, this approach often damages the physical and/or mental health of low-risk mothers and babies. Its philosophy seems to be one of salvage after problems occur, and, to that end, an impressive technology has been developed. (For a view of prevailing attitudes, read Chapter 33, Vol. 2, by Michelle Harrison.)

21st Century Obstetrics will be non-interventive and stand-by, and its attitude will be one of reverence for natural process. It will focus upon the vast majority of normal mothers to preserve and enhance their health while still providing the best of medical technology when problems occur. More than mere physical survival from the delivery room, the goal of 21st Century Obstetrics will be total integration of the birth experience -- mentally, physically, emotionally, and spiritually -- for the optimization of the entire family -- baby, mother, father, siblings, grandparents, and friends. The philosophy will be one of prevention and, to that end, nutrition will be recognized as one of the single most important factors in prenatal care because, as Tom Brewer has so aptly said, "There are no safe alternatives in childbirth without adequate nutrition." (For a view of what birth could and should mean to the family, read Chapter 18, Vol. 1, by the Tompson Family.)

These volumes are the result of a major conference entitled "21st Century Obstetrics Now!" held March 11-13, 1977, in Chicago, Illinois -- medical mecca of the nation wherein resides the national headquarters of a number of major professional organizations. It was the Second American Conference to be sponsored by NAPSAC -- the National Association of Parents and Professionals for Safe Alternatives in Childbirth.

The conference was attended by more than 1,100 persons from nearly 40 states, Canada and Mexico -- more than double the attendance at the first NAPSAC Conference near Washington, D.C., in May of 1976. Representatives from a large spectrum of population were there -- parents, physicians, lay midwives, nurse-midwives obstetricians, psychiatrists, feminists, osteopaths, social workers, chiropractors, government officials, major medical associations, authors, journalists, lawyers, anthropologists, home birth groups, ICEA groups, La Leche League parents, children and babies. The breakdown was approximately 15% nurses, 10% certified nurse-midwives, 10% physicians, 15% lay midwives, with the bulk of the remaining 50% being parents with an unknown number of childbirth educators, students, and others. It was truly a gathering of "parents and professionals."

While based upon the conference and the presentations there, this book is much more. Of the 34 chapters, 10 of them are of titles not presented at the conference. Furthermore, of the 24 titles that were presented as part of the conference program, most are considerably more extensively treated here than was possible in the brief speaking times allotted in Chicago. Many of the presentations are also thoroughly documented by references to the journals of scientific medicine. Many of the chapters are completely in a written format and, as such, the reader would not be able to know that they were first presented orally. Others maintain the spontaneous flavor of the spoken word.

In a number of the chapters, selections from the author's thoughts were chosen by the editors and featured on the page in bold-faced type. In all instances, they were taken from the chapters in which they appear. Usually, there are direct quotes taken from the author's text, but in some instances they are concise paraphrases by the editors taken from a larger body of text by the author.

Written for the educated consumer, yet documented for the professional, in the spirit of NAPSAC philosophy, this book is truly for both parents and professionals. Some articles contain original research never before published. Others are based upon extensive research into the available scientific literature -- there being literally hundreds of citings in the bibliographies of these volumes. Others are empirical -- based on actual experience and practice. In yet another category are the articles of insight and inspiration. A cornucopia of information and guidance to the consumer, the book is also suitable as text material for the student of medicine, public health, midwifery, or nursing. For example, there are two chapters on nutrition: Chapter 25 is thoroughly documented with over

100 technical references and will be useful to those who want to dig into the scientific facts, while Chapter 26 is brief and goes directly to the specifics of diet for an expectant mother.

Also in the spirit of NAPSAC is the presentation of alternatives to the reader. Hence, differences and variations of viewpoint are presented here within a single publication. Some of these viewpoints are diametrically opposite. In some instances the viewpoints, such as those that would bring all birth into the hospital, are even counter to the ideals of NAPSAC, which is one of freedom of choice. We of NAPSAC can accept the hospital-based, technologic view as an alternative, but not as the only alternative.

We recognize the profound benefits the advances of modern medicine have brought our society. With technology and humanity combined, childbirth can now become safer than ever before in history, while at the same time play a greater role in the establishment of wholesome family ties than ever before possible.

These volumes are unique in many respects. One of the most profound chapters, in the view of the editors, is the one on Family Bonding (Chapter 18) which is an informal presentation of the home birth experiences of the Tompson Family. While not a scientific paper, it yet presents in irrefutable terms the truth of the phenomena of family bonding that can take place at birth if unimpeded by unnecessary intervention. Among all the chapters, this one stands out as one of the most original, inspiring, and most reflects the ideal of what true "family-centered maternity care" can and should be.

Although in our view, all of the chapters of these volumes are distinctively noteworthy and it is tempting to comment upon them all in this forward, the chapter by Herbert Ratner, however, on "The History of the Dehumanization of American Obstetrical Practice," is truly unique in the published annals of childbirth. Documented with references dating from the 1800's to the 1970's, this work places our current state of affairs in obstetrics into a perspective that both explains the past and warns for the future.

One of the most powerful chapters is the original research of Lewis Mehl published in Chapter 16. The import of this study is summarized on p. 199. No longer can there be any doubt that hospitals pose hazards unique to the hospital.

One of the most encouraging elements of this book is the beginning of genuine dialogue between the community of obstetricians and consumers and others of the medical community. Chapters 3 and 5 present views of the American College of Obstetricians and Gynecologists (ACOG), certifying agency for the nation's obstetricians, while Chapters 4, 6, and 7 present alternative views in direct

reply to the views of ACOG. As a reader you can witness this exchange and decide for yourself. Most encouraging is the statement
within the ACOG view itself (Chapter 3) that espouses family-centered
concepts in hospital maternity care and endorses the participation
of consumers in the implementation of hospital practices and policies.
This is an unprecedented stand for the ACOG. It is hopeful that this
endorsement will hasten family-centered care in all hospitals and for
all patients. Family-centered maternity care is not flowered wallpaper in the labor rooms or "letting" fathers be present at birth.
Family-centered care is an attitude of respect for the birthing family.

To quote the words of Ruth Wilf (Chapter 8), "good hospitals
will always be needed," and "if you need a hospital for birth you
have a right to have one close to your home that will be family-
centered and people-oriented and give quality care." But in 21st
Century Obstetrics, family-centered maternity care in hospitals
will not be good enough in itself. As was stated in the opening lines
of the book, Safe Alternatives in Childbirth, "Hospitals have never
been proven to be the safest place for most mothers to give birth."
What is needed is a concept of maternity care that offers the appropriate degrees of medical care for all, not just the mothers in trouble.

What is needed are family-centered hospitals for the very few
who actually need or desire them, and out-of-hospital choices for
the vast majority. It should not be, as it now is, "hospitals over
here and home births over there," as if they are somehow in competition and represent different goals. The goal is one: optimal
outcomes for the entire family, physically, mentally, emotionally,
and spiritually. What is needed are hospitals working in harmony
with birth centers working in harmony with home birth programs.
What is needed are programs where parents needn't necessarily
choose one option to the exclusion of another but remain flexible
throughout, shifting to and from home or birth center or hospital
smoothly, at will, as developing circumstances indicate, and always
with continuity of personnel. What is needed are comprehensive
programs offering all of these options under a well-coordinated,
cooperative plan. This is 21st Century Obstetrics -- sane in the use
of technology, yet humane, responsible, and family-oriented.

We who are having our babies now cannot wait for these ideals
to materialize in full. We must have 21st Century Obstetrics Now!
That's what these volumes are all about.

David & Lee Stewart, Editors
Hillsborough, NC
July 1977

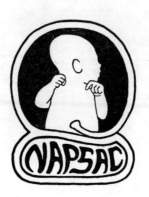

CHAPTER TWENTY

THE LIMITS OF SCIENCE IN CHILDBIRTH

David Stewart, Ph.D.

Science has lifted us from the ignorance of the dark ages into the understanding we hold today. It has increased our standards of living, lengthened our longevity, and enriched our lives in every way. Music, the arts, our governments, our social customs, our religious beliefs, our educational institutions, our recreation, our working, our eating, our sleeping -- all aspects of our culture have been transformed by the touch of technology. It is little wonder, then, that we have become conditioned to look to science for the solutions of all our problems and for the answers to life's questions.

But science, powerful as it is, is a false god. Awed by the spectacular material advancements science has brought us, we have come to expect more of science than it is capable of delivering. Many individuals, not recognizing the limitations of science, stand in expectation of results that will never come. Science does not have all the solutions. It does not have all the answers. It never has and it never will.

The purpose of this presentation is to present science for what it is -- no more and no less -- and to explore the extent to which answers to childbearing, child-rearing, and family relations can be obtained by the scientific method. As we shall see, many answers can be obtained by the scientific method. But most cannot.

It is not my intent to destroy your faith in science. I am a professional scientist myself and am duly respectful of its potential. I am also fully aware of its limitations. When it comes to consideration of life in its fullness, these limitations are very great. Therefore it is my intent to disturb your faith in science and to encourage you to question its validity as an approach to living.

DAVID STEWART is Director, MacCarthy Geophysics Laboratory, University of North Carolina; Executive Director, NAPSAC; Author of over 50 publications in the physical sciences and other topics including childbirth; Member, American Public Health Association, Committee on Alternatives in Maternity Care.

While the essence of science is characterized by its inherent lack of mysticism, to the non-scientist, it often bears a veil of the mystical. One of the most common persuasive devices of the advertiser is to cloak its advocacy in the jargon of science: 'If it sounds scientific, it must be right," so goes the unspoken implication. And people buy it. It is my hope that this presentation will serve to demystify science for those unfamiliar with its inner workings, for it is not in our best interest, as human beings, to hold science in a degree of esteem that exceeds its capabilities.

Science is not the only approach to inquiry into the nature of life. In fact, it is an approach that fails in most of life's situations. While it has great capabilities, it can only do so much and no more. It is my hope that this presentation will assist you in obtaining a realistic expectation of science because without a realistic expectation you will not be able to rely upon it when appropriate and you will be disappointed when it fails.

Science may be a high-speed aircraft in some ways, but an airplane cannot get you everywhere. If you want to walk about your home, visit a neighbor, enjoy a stroll through the woods, climb the heights of a rocky mountain, or travel to places without airports, you cannot do it with an aircraft. Modes of locomotion must be appropriate to the circumstances. Likewise, modes of inquiry must be appropriate to the subject matter and in the case of the scientific mode of inquiry, it is inappropriate to most of life's matters.

In order to clearly understand the limitations of science, one must first have a clear picture of what science is. Interestingly enough, there is a large fraction of even scientists, themselves, that do not have an accurate and complete picture of the potentialities and limitations of science. This might sound hard to believe, but it is true. It is entirely possible to practice science, even being quite successful in obtaining useful, valid results, while at the same time never being fully aware of the limits of science.

 THE PRACTICE OF MEDICINE IS NOT A SCIENCE. IT IS A DISCIPLINE OF OPINION WHERE "ACCEPTED PRACTICE" IS DETERMINED BY MAJORITY VOTE OF THE PROFESSIONALS, NOT BY THE SCIENTIFIC METHOD.

In an analogous way, it is entirely possible, if not common, for doctors to practice medicine without being aware of its limits. In fact, it is not at all uncommon for people to confuse medicine with science. But the practice of medicine is not a science. While medicine bases some of its practices on scientifically derived data, the practice of medicine is not, itself, a science. Medicine is a discipline of opinion where "accepted practice" is determined by a majority professional vote, not by the scientific method.

The reason this is not widely recognized and understood lies in our educational systems that train scientists and doctors in how to exercise the methods but do not, as a rule, stimulate and encourage questioning of the fundamental methods themselves in order to discover their limits.

The Limits of Science in a Nutshell

The limits of science can be condensed into the following 16 statements. First, I shall state them all and then explain why they are true. Then I shall discuss their implications with respect to childbirth. The statements are as follows:

1. Science explains nothing; it can only describe.
2. Science proves nothing; it can only verify or disprove.
3. Science cannot deal directly with subjective experience; it can only deal with the objective.
4. "Scientific" does not necessarily mean right, valid, or best; it only means that a certain method was followed.
5. "Objective" does not necessarily mean right, valid or best; it only means that observations are independent of the observer and can be measured scientifically.
6. "Subjective" does not mean invalid or irrelevant; it only means that observations are dependent upon the observer and cannot be measured scientifically.
7. Most of the things we experience and value in life are subjective and are, therefore, beyond science.
8. Belief in science is an act of faith and is, in itself, a choice made subjectively and personally, not scientifically.
9. Science is limited by time; tomorrow's research cannot help us today.
10. Science is limited in space; there will always remain portions of the universe beyond its reach because of distance.
11. Science is limited in its ability to observe natural living processes because the effect of the observer usually changes, if not halts, the process.
12. Science is limited by experimental error; its results can be no better than the reliability of its data.
13. Science is limited by human bias in the application of the scientific method itself.

14. Science is limited by human bias in the choices of topics upon which the method is applied.
15. Science is limited in its impact upon society in that people generally do not follow facts unless the facts agree with their feelings.
16. The scientific method is not the only valid method of inquiry into the nature of things -- there are others, and when it comes to practical inquiry into the subjective, other methods must be used because, in such experiences, science fails.

Realization of the above 16 statements leads me to conclude the following two points:

1. Science cannot tell you what is optimal for your particular pregnancy or your own personal labor and birth; and
2. While using science as a guide where appropriate, optimal birth is assured by assuming that nature knows best and going along with it, allowing no unnecessary interference, and making decisions during labor by calm, intuitive judgment on the parts of the mother, the father, and a sympathetic, educated, thoroughly experienced birth attendant who stands by as a consultant and, if need be, a technician.

In order to see how one can be led to these conclusions, let us begin with a thorough and accurate description of what science is and what it is not.

 THE FIRST HOPE WE MUST GIVE UP FOR THE SCIENTIFIC METHOD IS THAT IT WILL LEAD US TO ABSOLUTE ANSWERS ABOUT LIFE AND THE UNIVERSE. IT CANNOT.

What is Science?

Science is an approach to the study of the universe around us -- both living and inanimate. It is only one of several approaches. The purpose of science is to discover and describe the details of the universe. It does not attempt to explain, in an ultimate sense, why things are the way they are. Science merely observes and describes. For example, Newton's Second Law states that Force is equal to Mass times Acceleration: $F = MA$. The law does not explain why force, mass, and acceleration are so related. It merely states that between these three quantities, that is the way it is. It is only a description o f what scientific observations h a v e seen time and time again.

The law is no different than stating that "average human pregnancies last 8-10 months." If you ask a medical scientist, "why pregnancies last this long," they may reply, "because this is how long it takes the fetus to develop into a stage where it is able to live outside the womb and yet is not too large to pass through the birth canal." But this is not really "why" in an ultimate sense. To really answer the question of "why?" one would have to explain why fetal development progresses at the rate that it does. A medical scientist might be tempted to answer this by going into the chemistry and embryology of fetal processes and how these occur in a certain sequence over a certain period resulting in an 8-10 month average gestation. But here, again, one would merely have explained "how" the growth rates resulted, not "why?" At this point we could ask "why these chemical and biological processes proceed at the rates and in the manners in which they do?" Trying to track down an ultimate "why" in this manner is endless. This is the reason that science does not concern itself with such considerations.

Therefore, one of the principle features that distinguishes science from other approaches to life's problems is the problems to which science limits itself. In other words, science is concerned only with "what, when, and how." When we ask, "why?", and require an ultimate answer, we have left science a n d have entered realms that are more properly designated to philosophy, religion, and personal subjective judgment.

Consequently, the first limitation of science is that it does not deal with absolutes. It does not deal with "truth." It deals with facts, as perceived, but not with absolute truth. Hence, the first hope we must give up for the scientific method is that it will lead us to absolute answers about life and the universe. It cannot.

In addition to being restricted only to certain questions, science is further restricted by the approach it takes to finding answers to those questions. This approach is called the "scientific method." We shall describe this a bit later, but first, let us further pursue the degree to which science is capable of dealing with "truth." In particular, let us explore the real meaning of the term, "scientific proof."

 TRUTH IS NOT PROVEN BY MAJORITY VOTE. TRUTH IS TRUTH AND HAS NOTHING TO DO WITH PREVAILING OPINIONS NOR OUR PERCEPTION OF IT OR LACK THEREOF.

What is Proof?

Absolute proof is strictly the domain of logicians. In mathematics, for example, once a theorem is proven it is proven for all time and all circumstances. Mathematical proof is absolute. Mathematics, however, is not science. This is a point about which many are confused. Mathematics is a language used by science, but is not itself, a science. Mathematical proof and scientific proof are not the same thing at all.

In order to see this point clearly, consider the Pythagorean Theorem -- a mathematical proof that relates the sides of a right triangle to the hypotenuse. It was proven thousands of years ago once and for all time. We needn't worry that tomorrow a right triangle may be discovered that disproves the theorem. Neither should we be concerned that the theorem was proven in Greece and, therefore, may or may not apply to the United States or to astronauts on another planet. Proof of the Pythagorean Theorem is absolute -- valid for all times and places. In mathematics, once proven is always proven. This is not so in science.

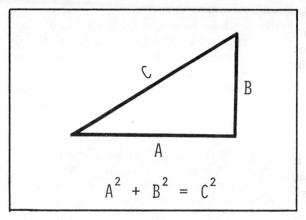

$$A^2 + B^2 = C^2$$

THE PYTHAGOREAN THEOREM

The reason that mathematicians can prove their theorems absolutely is because their universe of mathematics is a complete fabrication of the human mind. The elements of this universe (numbers, functions, vectors, etc.) were all made up by mathematicians themselves. Therefore, since they created their own universe and, in principle, have knowledge of all of its parts, when they prove a theorem they are assured that the proof will stand for all time and in all places because in making the proof they were able to consider their entire universe whose complete past, present, and future they know.

To think of it another way, mathematics, as are all systems of logic, is exactly like a game with certain elements and rules devised by somebody in an arbitrary, but definite and orderly fashion. Once the game is established, the elements and the rules are not changed. If you change anything, you have a different game. When you prove a mathematical theorem, you are merely playing the game and, by agreement with other mathematicians, you must make your proof using only the elements and rules laid down for the particular mathematical system in which you are working. If you change the rules then you are not playing the game -- you are inventing a new game.

Take baseball, for example. The elements of the game are the ball, the bat, the bases, the field, and the players. Among the established rules is that three outs constitutes the end of a team's time up to bat for that inning. Now this is a completely arbitrary rule. It could have been decided that two outs would do it, or five, or seven. But for some reason, three was chosen. If we want to make it something different, then we cannot call it baseball. In any case, once the game begins, the rules remain fixed. In a mathematical sense, you could prove that if one member of your team strikes out, another pops a fly to shortstop, and a third is thrown out on first, your team is finished batting for that inning. This proof would be absolute because it is based upon a finite set of elements and rules that were invented by man. Even if afterwards someone changes the rules and elements so that three outs no longer retires the side up to bat, they will have only changed the game to something else. They will not have affected the absoluteness of your former proof since now, in effect, they are talking about a different game than the one in which you made your proof.

Just as there are many kinds of games, there are many systems of mathematics. In Euclidian Geometry the shortest distance between two points is a straight line. This follows from the manner in which the elements and rules of Euclidian Geometry are defined. In some other systems of geometry the shortest distance between two points is not a straight line. This does not disprove the Euclidian notion any more than citing the case of bowling, where the high score wins, can be used to disprove that the low score wins in golf. The two systems of geometry are entirely different games. All they have in common is that both were arbitrarily fashioned by the human mind.

 To STATE THAT YOU BELIEVE IN A TENET OF SCIENCE IS AN ACT OF FAITH.

What is Scientific Proof?

Scientific proof is not really proof at all, in the mathematical sense, but is either verification or disproof. Since scientists deal with a universe that is not of their own creation, they cannot prove their laws absolutely as can mathematicians. Scientists can never know for a certainty that the laws seemingly in effect today were always so or that they will be in effect at all future times. Neither can they know that their laws, as observed to date within the limits of current observations, will continue to be upheld by future observations.

The universe in which we live is limitless in two opposing directions: expansively outward into the farthest reaches of unplumbed space and infinitesmally inward into the fundamental e s s e n c e of things. Human bodies, for example, are so complex the more we learn the more we realize we do not know. So vast is the number of bodily parts and functions, each individual person's body is itself a limitless universe. Furthermore, in the study of living processes, most are beyond observation because any attempt to observe would so interrupt and perturb the process that what might be perceived would not represent the way things were naturally. In fact, the bulk of what is believed biologically has been deduced from dissection of dead tissue or by experiments that result in the destruction of the living. With regard to childbirth, no one has even so much as been able to observe the living development of a human fetus from the fertilization of the egg to its emergence at birth months later. What we are able to perceive scientifically of life's secrets is but a hint of what is really there.

The point is that scientists, both medical and non-medical, can never know all the elements and rules of their universe because not only did they not create it, but at least a portion of it will always remain beyond them in time and/or space -- where the term, "space," is used here to designate the limitlessness of both the inner and the outer universes.

Unlike mathematics, the tenets of science are forever in jeopardy of ambush by a new set of facts. How many ideas formerly considered scientifically sound are now considered disproven? How many times has medical science reversed itself? Man-made formula was once thought by scientists to be an adequate substitute for human breast milk. Now science has demonstrated that this is not so.[10] Many physicians used to think (and some still do) that prescribing diuretics, limiting weight gain, and restricting salt were all scientifically proven beneficial to pregnant mothers. Now science tells us that the opposite is true (see Chapters 25 & 26, Vol. 2). Science once recommended large doses of oxygen for certain cases of prematurity, but now doctors are being sued for causing blindness (retrolental fibroplasia) in young adults for oxygen they administered at birth 20 years ago.

 THE TENETS OF SCIENCE ARE FOREVER IN JEOPARDY OF AMBUSH BY A NEW SET OF FACTS. HOW MANY IDEAS FORMERLY CONSIDERED SCIENTIFIC ARE NOW CONSIDERED DISPROVEN? HOW MANY TIMES HAS MEDICAL SCIENCE REVERSED ITSELF?

How much of present-day medical practice, deemed scientific and beneficial today will, in a few years, be demonstrated unscientific and harmful? Think of all the technologic interventions in current maternity practice: fetal monitors, cesarean sections for breech, episiotomy, drugged labor, ultrasound, oxytocin challenge tests, elective induction, artificial rupture of membranes, amniocentesis, perinatal regionalization of hospital services, etc. I even question the wisdom of vaginal exams during labor. Who knows which, if any, of these will turn out to be more beneficial than harmful when all the data are in? How many of these practices and ideas will survive the scientific test of time? For all we know, science may eventually invalidate them all. Bleeding patients with leeches sounds absurd to us now, but at the time it was considered good medical practice and within the framework of the scientific understanding of the time it seemed most reasonable.

In this modern age when we know so much, and yet still know so little, optimal outcome in birth can only be obtained by couples who question everything, who expend a lot of contientious effort to educate themselves, and who accept the bulk of responsibility for their own births themselves -- and this applies to all couples whether they choose to give birth in a hospital, a birth center, or home -- whether with a physician, a midwife, or no medical attendant.

The humanly derived tenets of the life sciences suffer more frequent mortality than the tenets of physical sciences because the processes of physics are so much more simple than those of biology. We have no assurances, however, even in physics. We cannot be certain that even Newton's simple laws of inanimate forces will stand forever. Though verified countless times, how do we know they apply in the farthest reaches of inner or outer space? We cannot even be sure they were followed on earth a few billion years ago or that they will continue to be followed indefinitely into the future.

BLEEDING PATIENTS WITH LEECHES SOUNDS ABSURD TO US NOW, BUT AT THE TIME IT WAS CONSIDERED GOOD MEDICAL PRACTICE AND WITHIN THE FRAMEWORK OF THE SCIENTIFIC UNDERSTANDING OF THE TIME, IT SEEMED MOST REASONABLE.

All scientific laws only describe what we see here and now within the limits of our history and of our restricted vision. No matter how much data has been accumulated on however many mothers, we can never know scientifically exactly what will happen in the next birth.

Science, at best, can only provide us with a set of likely probabilities based upon and limited by current data. Some sciences can offer more certainty than others. Physics, as mentioned above, is one of the more certain sciences. Medical science, by contrast, is one whose probabilities are possibly among the least certain because of the unimaginable complexity of life processes and their unknown interactions with the human mind coupled with the impossibility of objective and complete measure. Because of this doctors resort to statistics and this is one of the greatest fallacies of the practicing physician -- the application of statistical probabilities to individuals. Just because something is average doesn't mean it is normal, common, or necessarily desirable. Yet doctors continually fall into the logical trap of assuming that average is normal, etc. Because the average human gestation is 272 days does not mean that 272 days is best for you and your pregnancy. 272 days may be premature for your baby. Yet doctors induce and do cesarean sections based upon this fallacy. As a consequence, such practices are a leading cause of prematurity in the U.S. today.

In the end, scientists can only do two things: verify or disprove. Disproof of a hypothesis is easy. All you need is one exception. To verify means that you have observed that the physical or biological law under question has been followed. You may verify again and again, but never prove, because to prove means that you have investigated every possible situation, past, present, and future throughout the entire universe -- within and without. This is, of course, impossible. It is impossible now and it always will be within the scope of the scientific method. Hence, when scientists say they have "proven" something, they really only mean that they have verified it enough times to be confident that if they try again, it will work, according to the stated limits, and if anyone else tries it they, too, will make the same observations.

To state that you believe in a tenet of physical or biological science is actually an act of faith based on your experience or on the experience of other scientists in whom you hold confidence. How many people have personally verified Mendel's Laws of dominant and recessive genes in genetics? Even if you have verified it for some traits in some species, how can you be absolutely certain, without taking a leap of faith, that the laws will apply in any future specific instance?

 IN THIS MODERN AGE WHEN WE KNOW SO MUCH, AND YET STILL KNOW SO LITTLE, OPTIMAL OUTCOME IN BIRTH CAN ONLY BE OBTAINED BY COUPLES WHO QUESTION EVERYTHING.

To more clearly delineate the difference between "proof" and "verification" consider the Pythagorean Theorem again. One may verify the theorem quite easily by carefully drawing a right triangle, measuring the lengths of the sides, squaring the lengths, adding the results, and comparing the sum to the square of the measured length of the hypotenuse. Even if you drew a million different right triangles and verified the theorem for all of them, no mathematician would consider this a proof. To prove it you must, somehow, deal with all right triangles, past, present, and future, all at once. Only this would constitute absolute proof. Fortunately for mathematicians, this is possible. Since the idea of a triangle is an abstract creation of the mind (what we draw on paper is merely a representation of that abstract idea) all right triangles can be dealt with simultaneously so that within the realm of mathematics, absolute proof can be accomplished. Unfortunately, for scientists, such accomplishments are not possible.

Therefore, it is a fallacy to assume that because something is "scientific" it is true, in an absolute sense, or that it is even better than something arrived at non-scientifically. "Scientific" only means that a certain approach has been taken (i.e. the scientific method). One can apply the method perfectly well and obtain truly "scientific" results whose application may not only rest upon an ultimately false foundation, but could, if put into practice, eventually prove to be harmful. Conversely, a "non-scientific" approach is often the best. There is a place for both science and non-science and both must be used only in the right circumstances and with discretion.

Hence, only mathematicians and other types of logicians can prove things. Scientists must content themselves with verification or disproof. While mathematicians live in a comfortable realm of

certainty within the universe of their own minds, scientists, coura-
geously exploring the universe around, live in perpetual uncertainty.
In order to make the most effective use of science, we must recognize these intrinsic limitations.

IT IS A FALLACY TO ASSUME THAT BECAUSE SOMETHING IS
"SCIENTIFIC" IT IS TRUE OR THAT IT IS BETTER THAN
SOMETHING ARRIVED AT NON-SCIENTIFICALLY. "SCIENTIFIC" ONLY
MEANS THAT A CERTAIN METHOD HAS BEEN APPLIED.

What is the Scientific Method?

A scientist's task is to invent a story to explain his observations
and then to decide just how likely the story is. Organizing this process into steps, we arrive at the "scientific method" consisting of
three parts: (1) Observation; (2) Hypothesis; and (3) Experimentation.
These three steps may occur in any order during the scientific process, but usually a scientist first observes something that suggests
a certain explanation. They then set up experiments and make further objective observations to test their hypothesis. In the beginning
they may modify their hypothesis from time to time, refining it to
more closely fit the data. Eventually, they may reach the point
where the hypothesis fits most, if not all, observations and they feel
it can be refined no more. If they have verified it repeatedly and
have a great deal of confidence in the hypothesis, they may then call
it a "theory." If many other scientists also verify the theory, it may
become elevated to the status of a "law." A "law of nature" or a "law
of physics" is merely an accurate description of how certain para-
meters are related verified over a period of time by many scientists.
This is the scientific method.

When scientists have several theories, each of which partially
describe a situation, but none completely, they may choose the theory
with the fewest inconsistencies as being the "best theory." It is not
unscientific to apply a theory that has not been shown to be completely
accurate if it is the theory that seems to account for more observations than any other. As a scientist you never deal with absolutes.
You must continually apply theories and ideas that, although not
necessarily shown to be completely correct, are still workable and
seem to yield acceptable results. Here, again, the idea of absolutes
is one that only mathematicians can enjoy.

This lack of exactness in science is readily apparent in the
life sciences where processes are so complex that precisely repro-

ducible results are never obtained. In the limit, this lack of exactness is present even in the sciences of physics or chemistry which deal with the simpler inanimate world. The truth is that there is no such thing as an "exact" science. No science is exact. In the real world, we must always accept approximations and make choices between theories, none of which are perfect. If it were considered unscientific to use a theory that is not perfect, there would be no science. Choosing the lesser of two imperfects must be considered one of the most important aspects of the scientific method.

 No matter how much data has been accumulated on however many mothers, we can never know scientifically exactly what will happen in the next birth.

The last consideration leads us to the relative roles of objectivity and subjectivity in science because, as it turns out, the "choice" of one theory over another is primarily subjective and depends a great deal upon the personal bias of the scientist.

For example, infant and maternal mortalities have become less in the U.S. over the past 25 years. Several theories could account for this. The American College of Obstetricians and Gynecologists (ACOG) was founded in 1951 (see Chapter 3, Vol. 1). This is the organization that determines the training requirements for obstetricians and gynecologists in the U.S. and acts as the official certifying agency. Their theory to explain this reduction in mortalities is that it is largely due to the efforts of the ACOG, the increased use of obstetricians (as opposed to general practitioners, midwives, etc.), and to the increased use of the hospital with its available armamentia of technology. Another theory is that the improvement in pregnancy outcomes has been due to improved living conditions, greater public awareness and education, prenatal care, better public health such as antibiotics and immunizations, etc., and better nutrition. Which theory is the "best" theory. Ask an obstetrician of the ACOG and his answer is fairly predictable. But has the ACOG theory been verified by science? The answer is "no, it has not." The only study of which I am aware that has attempted to statistically correlate improved pregnancy outcomes with the various possible theoretical causes showed no better correlation with hospitals and obstetricians than with the increased sales of televisions over the past two decades.[1,2,3,4] The suggestion is that the important factors are the other aspects listed above -- none of which require a hospital or obstetrician. To my knowledge, no conclusive nor definitive study has been made at this time to resolve the issue of "which theory is best" once and for all. The tentative scientific conclusion I draw from available data is that the whole question is open to discussion, and that further studies are called for. Until then, each of us is entitled to make our own "subjective" choice as to which theory we prefer.

The important thing for parents to realize is that if their physician says that "hospitals are safer than homebirth or birth in a birth center" this is a purely subjective opinion based on his own limited experience and the traditions of his profession. It is not based on science. To back up their claims, doctors favoring hospitals usually cite the extreme cases of the "baby who did not breathe" or the "mother who would have bled to death had she not been in the hospital," etc. The point is that however valid these claims may be in the individual cases involved, the statistical evidence does not support them in general.[1] Placing 90-100% of mothers in hospitals in an attempt to save the small percent of mothers and babies genuinely falling into the high-risk categories through natural causes increases the risk for the many.[1, 2, 3] According to the recent research of Tew [1], a medical statistician, "The statistics show that an increased rate of hospitalization does not promote the objective of reducing overall mortality."

However, the object of this chapter is not to debate such issues as homebirth versus hospital birth. The object is to delineate the limits of science. The above is only intended to illustrate the role of subjective choices in science in general, and in childbirth in particular, as opposed to choices based upon acceptance of genuinely objective fact.

 SUBJECTIVITY, PER SE, IS NEITHER GOOD NOR BAD; SCIENCE, PER SE, IS NEITHER GOOD NOR BAD. INAPPROPRIATELY APPLIED, BOTH ARE BAD, BUT APPROPRIATELY APPLIED, BOTH ARE ESSENTIAL, IN COMBINATION, TO OPTIMIZE CHILDBIRTH.

Objectivity and Subjectivity in Science

The rules of the scientific method require that observations be objective. This means that, theoretically, regardless of who makes the observations, the account should be the same, within limits, of course. For example, if ten technicians analyzed the same blood sample, they should all get about the same results. Such data would be considered to be "scientific."

It is from objectivity that science gains its power. It is from objectivity that science obtains its universal appeal that cuts across the barriers of language and nationality. But paradoxically, while objectivity is its greatest strength, it is also its greatest weakness, because it is also objectivity that makes science incapable of dealing with most of the important aspects of human life -- the aspects that bring us warmth, affection, pleasure, and happiness. Science cannot cope with the subjective. Where subjective experience has objective consequences, these consequences can be studied scientifically, but not the experiences themselves.

A perfect example of a subjective experience is that of childbirth. Only the mother can know what it is truly like. There are objective aspects, too, of course. A new baby enters the world for all to see. That is objectively verifiable. But the greater portion of the process of birth is beyond the scope of objective measurement.

Can birth be adequately described in terms of a meager sample of measurements of such things as cervical dilation, maternal blood pressure, periodicity of contractions, or fetal heart rate? I think not. When literally thousands of processes are taking place in birth simultaneously and synergistically, how can a dozen or so physical measurements, however objective, really tell the complete story, or even the essential parts? I cannot believe that the complexities of childbirth can be reduced to a few wiggle traces from a monitor on a strip of paper.' When science cannot so much as even tell a pregnant mother exactly when her baby will be born, or what will be the sex of her unborn child, how can we expect science to provide reliable guidance to a mother in the midst of labor? The answer is simple. It cannot.

 I CANNOT BELIEVE THAT THE COMPLEXITIES OF CHILDBIRTH CAN BE REDUCED TO A FEW MONITOR WIGGLES ON A STRIP OF PAPER.

I do believe that the complexities of childbirth, for each unique individual mother and child, can be comprehended by an intuitive, experienced birth attendant who is attuned and present throughout the birth -- not just in and out every few hours to "do an exam," but really there. Now what I have just stated is non-scientific to be sure. But I figure that this sort of non-science has as least as much validity as the needless non-science applied to normal birth in most hospitals. Let's face it: There is no scientific way to completely describe childbirth, and we fool ourselves to think that limiting ourselves to objective data only is in the best interest of mothers and babies in need of assistance at birth. Properly exercised and combined with objective data, subjective judgment on the part of an experienced birth attendant can be as consistently reliable as anything we now know.

As already mentioned, "scientific" is not necessarily right. Conversely, "subjective" is not necessarily wrong. We have become conditioned in our modern society to think that if something is scientific, it must be true. But don't be intimidated by science. And don't be intimidated by professionals who hide their subjectivity behind a cloak of what seems to be science. The scientific method is merely one of several approaches to establish an understanding of the nature of things and is not the most effective approach most of the time. It is extremely limited and excludes, among other things, the whole universe of subjective experiences and value judgments. It does not and cannot cope with such things.

To attempt to apply the scientific method to subjective experience is invalid. It would be like attempting to take one's blood pressure with a thermometer, or to time the contractions of labor with a pair of scissors. It is simply the wrong tool. What we have to realize is that just because the application of the method to subjective experiences is invalid does not mean that subjective experiences are, themselves, invalid. Because an experience is subjective does not make it less real.

LIMITING OURSELVES TO OBJECTIVE DATA ALONE IS NOT IN THE BEST INTEREST OF MOTHERS AND BABIES AT BIRTH. PROPERLY EXERCISED, AND IN COMBINATION WITH OBJECTIVE DATA, SUBJECTIVE JUDGEMENT ON THE PART OF AN EXPERIENCED, INTUITIVE, AND ATTUNED BIRTH ATTENDANT IS AS CONSISTENTLY RELIABLE AS ANYTHING WE KNOW.

On the Nature of Subjectivity

"Subjective" merely means that the experience has meaning only to the person involved and is beyond scientific measurement. Take eating, for example. It is almost purely a subjective experience. The way foods taste to you is your own unique experience. No one will ever quite have your experience. Tasting food can be more or less objective to the extent that given a thousand people eating lemons, they would probably universally agree that they tasted sour. However, there would be many opinions as to whether they tasted good or not.

Subjective experiences are essentially yours and, as such, cannot really be shared with others. If you smell a rose, that experience is yours. You can tell it to me in words, but until I smell it for myself, I cannot know what the smell of a rose is all about. Even after we have both smelled it, we can never know just how much each of our sensations was like the others. If it turns out that you don't like the smell of the rose while I do, your experience does not make my experience any less pleasant or real. Contradictory subjective experiences on the part of two people cannot invalidate the experience of either.

 SINCE IT IS YOUR LIFE AND YOUR BODY, YOU HAVE RIGHTS THAT THE PHYSICIAN DOES NOT HAVE UNLESS YOU HAVE GIVEN THEM UP.

Applying these concepts to your relationship with your physician regarding your own body or your own birth experience, we see that if you feel one way and your doctor feels another, that does not make either of you right or either of you wrong. As an individual, however, and since it is your life and body, you have rights that the physician does not have unless you give them up. Hence, when there is a conflict of feeling between you and your physician, you have the right to believe in yourself first. There is a price to be paid for this freedom, however. If you do not follow the doctor's word or the hospital policies, you must also assume the responsibility for the consequences. All I am trying to say here is that considering the subjective nature of many of the judgments that need to be made in a childbirth experience, your subjectivity may be as good or better than the doctor's or the hospital's. You have a right as a parent to make, what may seem to the medical community, a wrong decision in childbirth. In a way, you would be assuming more responsibility by following your own inclinations when they differ from your doctor's. But in reality, the responsibility for raising your child is totally yours regardless of who makes the decisions at birth. If your child is damaged by some medical procedure, the hospital will not raise your child.

Since the scientific method is inapplicable to all subjective experiences, this means that scientifically you cannot so much as prove that you love your spouse or that your spouse loves you. Scientifically you cannot prove to your doctor that you did or did not have a good childbirth experience. But whatever your experience, you know it was real even without scientific verification.

THE MOTHER IS IN THE BEST POSITION TO KNOW WHAT IS HAPPENING DURING LABOR. IT IS HER BODY AND HER BABY AND ONLY SHE CAN KNOW THE SENSATIONS AND THE EXPERIENCE FIRST HAND. FROM A SCIENTIFIC VIEWPOINT, TO IGNORE THE MOTHER'S INPUT IS TO IGNORE WHAT, PERHAPS MAY BE THE MOST VALID AND USEFUL DATA OF ALL.

In the midst of a birth experience, the mother is theoretically in the best position to know what is going on. It is her body and her baby, and only she can know the sensations and the experience first hand. Birth attendants must learn how to listen to the mother, to tune in, to understand and respect what she can tell them. She is in the best position to sense when danger is imminent and when intervention may be needed. She is also in the best position to sense when things are all right, too. From a scientific viewpoint, to ignore the mother's input is to ignore what perhaps may be the most valid and useful data of all. (cf. Arms, Chapter 10, Vol. 1, p.75)

The reason many mothers do not know what is going on in their births and are apparently unable to handle it themselves probably lies in the fact that our culture has systematically undermined their confidence. Furthermore, the very act of going into the overbearing environment of a hospital is enough to cloud most women's abilities to tune in with their own bodies in birth. It is still the exception for women to take childbirth education classes to learn how to give birth. The removal of birth from the home to the hospital has also prevented most women to have the opportunity to witness a birth before experiencing their own. In addition to these complicating factors, medical professionals have given society the erroneous impression that a woman can obtain what is best by just "leaving it all up to the doctor and hospital." But this simply isn't true. The best is not possible without a knowledgeable, cooperative mother and father. Furthermore, women entering a hospital are often treated in such a humiliating and dehumanizing way, it is no wonder their intuitive judgment is not functioning up to par during birth.

The final blow to preventing women from exercising the potential wisdom of her unique place in her own birth, however, consists of the fact that even if a woman is educated, attuned to her body, and in good control -- remaining calm and knowing what is best throughout her labor -- doctors and hospitals are not accustomed to permitting the parents to be the ones to decide on how labor should be handled. As a culture and as health professionals, we must help mothers restore their confidence in their own bodies and judgment so that they may take charge of their own births.

In summary to this point, we can say that science, alone, is not adequate to handle birth. It takes subjectivity, too -- intelligent, calm, intuitive subjectivity -- upon the parts of the mother, the father, and a sympathetic birth attendant attuned to the "feminine principle" (see Chapter 10, Vol. 1).

Subjectivity, per se, is neither good nor bad. Science, per se, is neither good nor bad. It all depends on how they are each applied. Inappropriately applied, they are both bad; but in the right circumstances and with an accurate concept of their limitations, both are essential, in combination, to optimize childbirth.

 ONE CAN APPLY THE SCIENTIFIC METHOD PERFECTLY WELL AND OBTAIN TRULY "SCIENTIFIC" RESULTS WHOSE APPLICATION MAY NOT ONLY REST UPON AN ULTIMATELY FALSE FOUNDATION, BUT COULD, IF PUT INTO PRACTICE, EVENTUALLY PROVE TO BE HARMFUL.

The Intrinsic Limitations of Science

The preceding discussion reveals the inherent limitations of the scientific method itself -- independent of the human element. That is, no matter how rigorously applied or how much research money is spent, the method can only do so much. It cannot provide ultimate answers. It cannot explain or prove. Although it can deal with objective results from subjective causes, it cannot deal with subjective processes themselves. Furthermore, because of the awesome complexity and subtlety of bodily processes and because statistical data derived from populations cannot predict outcomes of particular pregnancies, science alone cannot provide adequate support for decision making during actual labor. This means that objective data in childbirth such as length of labor, etc., may or may not be useful.

But the intrinsic limitations of science are not the only ones. There are others, perhaps even more restrictive.

 WHEN SCIENCE CANNOT SO MUCH AS EVEN TELL A PREGNANT MOTHER EXACTLY WHEN HER BABY WILL BE BORN OR WHAT WILL BE THE SEX OF HER UNBORN CHILD, HOW CAN WE EXPECT SCIENCE TO PROVIDE RELIABLE GUIDANCE TO A MOTHER IN THE MIDST OF LABOR? THE ANSWER IS SIMPLE: IT CANNOT.

Limitations of Science in Time

One of the severest restrictions of science is that of time. Tomorrow's research cannot benefit today. Furthermore, we can never know what scientific principles applied now will be disproven in the near future. While some scientific conclusions are more enduring that others, in the end all scientific conclusions are tentative pending the discovery of additional data. Life, the universe, and their ramifications are infinite. Science can never get around to all of it. So when it comes down to the problems of your own personal concern now, scientific answers may or may not be there when you need them.

If you are pregnant now, you cannot wait for science to tell you what birth method is best. If you are raising your family now, you cannot wait for science to tell you how to deal with your children. You must act now, making dozens of decisions daily, with or without the help of science. Science is a good method for research, but it is not a good method for living.

No matter how much science studies and resolves, there will always be more that it has not studied and resolved. Science deals only with the known which, for all we can tell, will always be relatively infinitesmal when compared with the unknown.

In so far as what you should decide now in your own birth, here are some considerations you can make, consistent with currently available scientific fact: First, science has never proven that hospitals are the safest place for most mothers to give birth; second, science has never proven that obstetricians are the safest birth attendants; third, no study has been made over an adequately long term and large cross-section to scientifically establish where the safest place or who the safest birth attendant would be; and four, what scientific evidence currently does exist (see [6] and Chapter 16, Vol. 1) is more that sufficient to justify a contientious couple, midwife, or doctor to conclude that for normal mothers, home may be as safe or safer than hospitals. Right now there is not enough data to scientifically prove home is a safe alternative, but neither is there enough scientific data to prove hospitals are a safe alternative either. The American College of Obstetricians and Gynecologists (ACOG) has an official stand against out-of-hospital birth. Your physician may also be against out-of-hospital birth. But don't confuse professional concensus with science. At this point in time, sufficient data are just not there either way.

Therefore, no matter who or how many say birth at home is not as safe as the hospital, they cannot be speaking scientifically or objectively. They are only stating their beliefs, not facts (see Chapter 19, Vol. 1, for a discussion of belief versus fact). Only time will settle the issue by the scientific method, and I mean time measured in years. Until then, if you are a parent, consider your judgment as medically valid as your doctor's on this point. Or if you are a professional, consider your judgment as medically valid as any other in your field, even though for the time being your view may be a minority one within the profession. Truth, you must remember, is not proven by a majority vote. Truth is truth and has nothing to do with prevailing opinions nor our perception or lack of perception of it.

Experimental Error

Most of us have heard of instances of needless hysterectomies or mastectomies from erroneous lab results, the inducing of premature babies because of inaccurately determined due dates or faulty fetal maturity tests, or unnecessary cesarean sections based on malfunctioning fetal monitors. That science is limited by the accuracy of its data is obvious and need not be discussed at length.

Technologic failure and unintentional human error are problems we shall always have. But human bias is another matter altogether.

Human Bias in Science

While the ideals of science presume freedom from human bias and prejudice, the actual practice of science is not free of this human element. Scientists are people, and people always have their preferences. No matter how hard we try, it is impossible to completely eliminate bias from science.

Human bias enters the scientific method in several ways. It can creep into the scientific method itself in the gathering and the interpretation of data. Medical journals are full of this kind of bias. For example, when you read a technical paper on the topic of, let's say, "high risk pregnancy," the whole paper and its conclusions will depend on how the author defined "high risk."[8] Some experts say that factors such as the number of births, the number of miscarriages, whether there was use of "the pill" or an IUD prior to conception, and the mother's socioeconomic status are the main determinants of high risk. Others say it is mainly determined by nutritional habits and general state of physical fitness of the mother. It seems that every doctor has his or her own criteria, and one doctor's criteria may contradict another's. The point is that the conclusions drawn by such papers on "high risk" are dependent upon the subjective choices of how to define "high risk." With one set of definitions, a certain conclusion may be drawn while if another set had been used, the opposite conclusion may have been drawn. The bias of the matter lies in that if one believes in hospitals for birth, the tendency is to define "high risk" to include as many mothers as possible which, of course, justifies the view that most, if not all, mothers should go to hospitals.

 DON'T BE INTIMIDATED BY SCIENCE. AND DON'T BE INTIMIDATED BY PROFESSIONALS WHO HIDE THEIR SUBJECTIVITY BEHIND A CLOAK OF PSEUDOSCIENCE.

Even when the scientific method is <u>applied</u> completely without bias within a given research project, and I am not sure it can, our <u>choices</u> of projects to which to apply the method is always biased. If a medical researcher chooses to do research on the relative merits of drug therapy, the data are not likely to produce conclusions on the relative merits of therapy by nutrition or exercise. Likewise, if an obstetrician chooses to spend years of research on hospital maternity care, his or her data are not likely to produce conclusions favoring birth centers or homebirth programs. The outcome, however scientifically obtained, is going to be biased.

Therefore, when District II of the ACOG published a statement (see Chapter 5, Vol. 1) against out-of-hospital birth it was not surprising. It was completely predictable. What else could they conclude? Hospitals are all they know. Although the contributors to the ACOG position paper may be competent medical scientists, they are scientists who have chosen to make their scientific careers within the hospital. Therefore, their conslusions were predetermined from the outset by limiting their vision to the confines of the hospital. If you don't apply the scientific method to the right things you are not going to get the right answers no matter how rigorous your technique.

It is interesting to note that even though, by their own admission (see first paragraph, Chapter 4, Vol. 1), the ACOG push toward increased hospitalization has not resulted in the desired reductions in perinatal mortality and morbidity, they still cling to their faith that hospitals are the answer. What they recommend is that the hospitals just need to be bigger and more expensively equipped, i.e., we should eliminate all the small hospitals from maternity services and concentrate on a few really big regional centers. Not only would they force all mothers into hospitals, but now they want to tell mothers which hospitals they are to use and which not. This is the perinatal regionalization concept.[8, 11] This is concluded by the ACOG despite the fact that their own data, which NAPSAC has published on pages 89-91 of the second edition of Safe Alternatives in Childbirth [7], show that bigger is not better; it may even be worse.

Another interesting note on the District II ACOG position paper is their ready willingness to take credit for the improvement in maternal mortality in the past decades (see paragraph 1, Chapter 5, Vol. 1). They fail to recognize that this reduction in maternal mortality has not been proven to be due to obstetricians or to hospitals and may be largely due to other factors such as prenatal care, better nutrition, improved living conditions, etc.[1, 2, 3, 4] The medical profession also fails to take the appropriate blame for having been the cause of a large portion of the maternal mortality in times past by practices such as the infecting of healthy mothers by vaginal exams with unwashed hands or the administration of drugs during labor.

Another element in the reduction of maternal mortality for which ACOG can rightfully take the major credit is the modern, refined state of their "patch-up technology." Their philosophy seems to be that these days they needn't worry so much if they introduce an infection by a pelvic exam because today they have antibiotics. And if they cause a woman to hemorrhage from their drugs or by their hasty pulling on the cord, they can save her with the hospital blood supply.

But is patch-up medicine really in the best interest of health? What about the doctor-infected mother who has to be hospitalized and separated from her new baby and family for the first crucial days or weeks of her newborn's life? The six million dollar man we see on TV is a fiction, yet it represents a type of belief found among some obstetricians and others that such things as "surgical birth" are as good or better than natural birth because "technology can fix anything and even make it better." But can technology really fix an episiotomy-cut perineum or an incised cesarean-sectioned abdomen and restore it to its former wholeness? I think not.

When a scientifically based medical innovation results in better outcomes, one must always ask, "Better that What?" Often, in the history of medical evolution, the innovation was merely the substitution of a less harmful practice for one that had been more harmful. It is simple to show, by science, that one set of practices obtains better results than some other. This is what science is best suited to do. But the question is always, "Are these 'better results' optimal?" Science, you must always remember, cannot offer absolute answers, only relative ones.

As an illustration of this point, the current debate over fetal monitors is a classic. No scientific study has shown that fetal monitors produce <u>optimal</u> results, and no scientific study ever will because this is beyond the capability of science. All that monitor research can do is to show that fetal monitors can produce <u>relatively better</u> results. But we must ask, "Relative to What?" No research has shown that better results are obtained relative to adequate maternity care and good obstetrics where, by this, I mean "effective nutritional assistance in pregnancy, education for natural childbirth, non-interventive obstetrics, and truly sympathetic, caring support during labor." What has been shown is that inadequate maternity care and aggressive, impersonal obstetrics <u>plus</u> fetal monitoring is better than inadequate maternity care and aggressive, impersonal obstetrics alone.

SCIENCE IS A GOOD METHOD FOR RESEARCH, BUT IT IS NOT A GOOD METHOD FOR LIVING.

Of What Impact, Science?

Science is a powerful tool. And despite what I have been saying, I believe in it within its limits, just as I believe in hospitals within their limits. Obviously, science cannot solve all our problems, but it could solve a lot more than it is <u>allowed</u> to do. The greatest limitation of the scientific method is not that it has inherent weaknesses or that it is sometimes used invalidly or inappropriately. The greatest limitation is t h a t it is <u>not used</u> where it could and should be used.

The problem is that as humans we are basically not scientific. Socially, financially, culturally, emotionally, psychologically, and spiritually we don't live by science. The scientific attitude is a mental discipline most of us have to practice to acquire. Given a choice between facts and feelings, we almost always choose feelings. As a rule, it is only when we find the facts in line with our feelings do we follow facts.

Because of this human propensity to ignore fact, countless valid scientific studies have been published in the journals of medicine crying for changes in maternity care, and yet obstetricians and the ACOG continue on their apparently immutable technologic course (see, for example, the hundreds of scientific citations after the chapters of these two volumes, many from journals of OB/GYN). Why, for example, do physicians continue the indiscriminate use of drugs in pregnancy and birth when their association with birth defects could hardly be more clearly indicated (see [4,5,9] and Chapters 25 and 32, Vol. 2)? Why do physicians still fail to recognize breast-feeding as the best possible nutrition for babies when the scientific evidence is so overwhelming?[10]

This tendency is true for both scientists and non-scientists, both in the practice of science and in the living of life. The tendency is as true for physicians as it is for patients, as true for obstetricians as for mothers.

We have discussed the limitations of the scientific method at length in this chapter and have pointed out that science alone cannot lead one to optimal outcomes in birth. We have tended to concentrate on the areas where science is not the appropriate approach. But there are many circumstances where science is the answer. The sad thing is that so often, in the very circumstances most suited to the capabilities of the scientific method, it is not used.

For example, when it comes to evaluating and comparing the objective outcomes of birth between hospital and out-of-hospital alternatives, the scientific method would be most appropriate and should be used. But political hospital-based organizations such as the ACOG have not shown a willingness to apply the scientific method to this unanswered question. Instead, they express their professional concensus against out-of-hospital birth in dogmatic official statements and cite no valid scientific basis for their stand (see Chapters 3-7, Vol. 1). The reason they cite no carefully controlled scientific studies is because none have been made that support their view (see Chapter 23, Vol. 2, for reference to a massive study in New York State in the 1930's). The only modern studies comparing in- and out-of-hospital birth do not support their view (see [6] and Chapter 16, Vol. 1).

The ACOG was given the opportunity to document and present their views in this very book (see Chapters 3 and 5, Vol. 1). They were encouraged to present data in a valid and scientific fashion, yet they did not. The only data they cite to support their view has alternate interpretations counter to their own, and in one instance, the presentation of the raw vital statistics from Oregon (see Chapters 3 and 4, Vol. 1), they presented data in a biased and incomplete manner that contradicts the very spirit of the scientific method.

If the ACOG wanted to be scientific in their approach, the District II ACOG position paper and the ACOG position stated in

Chapter 3 would have acknowledged the lack of adequate data and would have proposed some long-term (5-10 years) scientific studies to obtain the missing data by comparing the objective outcomes of good homebirth programs and birth centers with the objective outcomes of hospitals. Instead, they assume, without such data, that hospitals are safer and in the closing lines of their position paper they propose a set of political objectives (not scientific, but political) designed to inhibit, if not outright prohibit, out-of-hospital birth. Instead of proposing a means of filling the need for more scientific data, they propose a plan of preventing that the data be obtained at all. If you outlaw homebirth, the research becomes impossible. If the ACOG is so confident in their hospitals, why are they so afraid to expose themselves to the impersonal scrutiny of scientific objectivity?

It is sometimes difficult to communicate with obstetricians about alternatives in childbirth. They seem to feel no obligation to justify their views to the parent-consumer by research. But if you don't cite research to support your view they say, 'Where is your data?' Then when you do cite studies you know to be as good or better as most of the studies in which they believe and carefully try to draw sensible conclusions that neither underrate nor overextend the data, they respond by belittling data in general with comments like, "Well, you can prove anything with statistics," etc. If they think the study you cite may have some obvious scientific merit they cannot superficially discredit, they then try to evade it geographically with such comments as, "The study may be okay, but it was made in California or in Sweden and doesn't really apply in our area. What is needed," they will say, "is another study with data from several areas." But even if you would then quote such a study, they would probably dismiss it on the grounds that "comparison of birth populations in different areas is not valid," and so on and so on it goes -- ad infinitum.

You eventually realize that no matter what data you produce, however rigorous and comprehensive, if the doctor doesn't want to accept it, he won't. In the end, "science be damned" -- they will follow their feelings whether verified by fact or not.

And as for requesting that the obstetrician produce data to support his practices, for the most part, forget it. Since obstetricians operate basically by tradition rather than by science, you would be asking for something that cannot be produced, because it probably does not exist. What you may well receive for your request, unless you are fortunate enough to have a humble and confident physician, is a defensive emotional outburst. Such an emotional response would be, in a way, at least an honest expression of the basis of their practice, which is feeling -- not science.

Now I believe feeling is okay -- if it is the right kind. Calm, intuitive feeling based on the right kind of professional experience and based on true concern for the optimal benefits to mothers and babies as persons is essential to good maternity care. But egotistic reactions to save face are not the right kind of feelings and can only lead to harm.

Please do not misinterpret my thoughts here. The above comments are not intended to be applied to all physicians or to all medical professionals. There are many well-informed, sensitive professionals who, in league with well-informed parents, are the courageous pioneers that are bringing about the needed reform in maternity care today. Some, as well, are members of ACOG. I also recognize that there is an influential element in the medical professions that is misguided and miseducated and which has not shown the proper sensitivities to consumer needs. My comments are directed at them.

 YOU HAVE A RIGHT AS A PARENT TO MAKE, WHAT MAY SEEM TO THE MEDICAL COMMUNITY, A WRONG DECISION IN BIRTH.

So What is the Answer?

We have shown that science is limited inherently, limited in time, limited by experimental error, limited by human bias, and limited in the extent that it is actually put to use. It is clear from all of this that science cannot have all the answers and never will. Science alone cannot offer you optimal guidance through your pregnancy, your birth, and your parenting. What do we do, then, when we must make decisions regarding our babies, our bodies, and our births now?

First, let us look to nature, the master scientist who has perfected her processes in the laboratory of life through eons of evolutionary experiment on countless subjects. Let us assume that nature knows best, learn her ways, and harmonize with her in a conscious, intelligent way.

Let us foster good training programs for professional birth attendants that subscribe to the philosophy of natural, non-interventive obstetrics.

Let us also follow science when good data are available and let us apply the scientific method wherever possible to test the relative merits of alternatives in childbirth. But let us realize that science cannot lead us to the right answers unless we lead science to the right topics for research.

Therefore, we must allow and encourage homebirth programs and birth centers to flourish freely according to public demand and apply the scientific method to determine the objectively optimal outcomes. Data does count in our technologic culture, like it or not, and we who are proposing alternatives to hospital birth must do all we can to get such data. We who believe in alternatives in childbirth are eager to put our views to a genuine scientific test. And we feel we have a right to insist that groups such as the ACOG do the same with their ideas.

But let us also understand and recognize where the effacacy of science ceases and rely on other means to also base our judgments. Let us assume that what mothers' inclinations have been saying for centuries is correct until proven otherwise.

Let us openly restore and practice our faith in our feelings and our common sense. Let us not be afraid to depend upon our intuition. And let us learn how to refine and develop that intuition by practice, experience, and association with others that use it.

For it will not be through science, alone, that we will realize the optimization of maternity care. Science is a powerful ally. But its fullest potential can only be realized in combination with the full and proper application of all our faculties -- both objective and otherwise.

 SCIENCE CANNOT LEAD US TO THE RIGHT ANSWERS UNLESS WE LEAD SCIENCE TO THE RIGHT TOPICS FOR RESEARCH.

CITED REFERENCES

1. Tew, M., Where to be born?, New Society, pp. 120-121, January 20, 1977.

2. Bradshaw, J., Babes in the Ward, Undercurrents, London, January 1977.

3. Watkin, Brian, Back to home deliveries?, Nursing Mirror & Midwives J., p. 42, February 3, 1977.

4. Haire, D., The cultural warping of childbirth, 2nd ed., Hillside, NJ: Int'l Childbirth Education Assoc., 1975.

5. Haire, D., Maternity practices around the world: how do we measure up?, in Stewart, D., and Stewart, L., (eds.), Safe Alternatives in Childbirth, 2nd ed., pp. 13-22, Chapel Hill, NC: NAPSAC, 1977.

6. Mehl, L., Statistical outcomes of home births in the U.S.: The current status, in Stewart, D., and Stewart, L., (eds.), Safe Alternatives in Childbirth, 2nd ed., pp. 73-100, Chapel Hill, NC: NAPSAC, 1977.

7. Haire, D., Birth related mortality rates by size and type of hospital, in Stewart, D., and Stewart, L., (eds.), Safe Alternatives in Childbirth, 2nd ed., pp. 89-90, Chapel Hill, NC: NAPSAC, 1977.

8. Aubry, R., and Pennington, J., Identification and evaluation of high-risk pregnancy: The perinatal concept, Clin. Ob. Gyn. 16:3-27, 1973.

9. Maugh, T., Irrational drug prescribing and birth defects, Science 194:926, 1976.

10. La Leche League International, for access to dozens of studies confirming the benefits of breastfeeding contact LLLI directly at 9616 Minneapolis Ave., Franklin Park, IL 60131, phone: (312) 455-7730.

11. Sugarman, M., Regionalization--update on consumer involvement, ICEA News 16:1, 8, Spring 1977.

310

CHAPTER TWENTY ONE

IMPLEMENTING A MEDICALLY SOUND CHILDBEARING CENTER:
PROBLEMS AND SOLUTIONS

Myrtle E. Hosford, C.N.M., M.A.

In this presentation I shall share with you the highlights of our experience to date in implementing a relatively new alternative -- namely, THE CHILDBEARING CENTER. The Childbearing Center is one of the most recent projects of Maternity Center Association in New York City -- a voluntary organization with a history of six decades of pioneering efforts in behalf of improved maternal and newborn care.

The Childbearing Center marked the first 12 months of operation on September 30, 1976. Two years in the planning, the project was envisioned and designed in response to the needs of a growing number of parents who were bypassing traditional hospital maternity care and turning to their own resources to attain the joy and long term advantages of welcoming babies at home.[4] The project was set up to serve families at low medical risk who were interested in assuming a more active role in their own health care. It has included highly personalized and educational antepartal care, birth in a home-like setting, and careful postpartal follow-up care. The Center is staffed by an obstetrician and nurse-midwife team assisted by a pediatrician, nurse-midwife assistants, and public health nurses. The input of families themselves is the sine qua non of the team's functioning.

On January 16, 1977, Maternity Center Association held a birthday party to celebrate the first year of functioning of the Childbearing Center, and the occasion of the first birthday of the first baby born at the Center, Ian, who arrived in January, 1976.

The party was a gala affair, in spite of snow and wind and Ian's not being able to attend. (He had to give priority to a large family celebration in Albany). Over 200 people did come --babies, mothers, fathers, brothers, sisters, grandparents and aunts. The party

MYRTLE E. HOSFORD is coordinator, Maternity Center Association, Childbearing Center, New York City; former Educational Director, Nurse-Midwifery Internship, Downstate Medical Center, Brooklyn; and coauthor of "Childbearing Centers as Alternatives to Home Birth and Hospital."

proved to be a warm and happy reunion. Perhaps, most of all, it was a testimony to the philosophy of care embodied in the Childbearing Center.

There were babies of various weeks and months of age, and rarely a peep of distress. Mothers and fathers were sharing childcare activities, lovingly, joyously. Brothers and sisters were sharing equal time -- their needs, too, obviously being met. In vivid living drama were the fruits of the bonding [3] we had so thrillingly observed at the Center where family togetherness during labor, birth, and the magic early postpartal period has taken precedence over procedures and routines from the earliest birth -- always within the limits of safety.

There were families who had needed to transfer during pregnancy or labor who expressed appreciation for the care and preparation they had received up to the point of transfer. Their enrollment in the program had enabled them to attain much the same philosophy of care inherent in the Childbearing Center. This was particularly true of those who were followed in hospital by an obstetrician associated with the Center.

Of particular personal satisfaction was seeing one of my early "first" babies, at nine months walking all over the large ballroom, confident, friendly, and completely intrigued with the whole affair. I must admit, he was a bit of a scavenger and could spot pieces of cookies under chairs and retrieve them like a pro -- germs notwithstanding!

One thought recurred throughout the festivities of that afternoon -- a thought which in essence became a commitment to those of us intimately involved in the Project: "This is worth fighting for! Fighting, in the sense of working tirelessly, perseveringly, aspiring for quality in all that is done, and striving to communicate what we have heard, and seen and felt. As you may have guessed, the first pioneering year was a challenging one.

The First Year -- A Test For Safety and Viability

The Childbearing Center Project was launched to meet the needs of families seeking out-of-hospital birth. The plan for a carefully staffed and well-equipped birth center was implemented to learn: (1) if indeed such a center might be a safe and viable alternative to unsupervised home birth, and (2) to identify needs and problems related to establishing this kind of alternative.

In November, 1976, members of Maternity Center Association's Research Advisory Committee and Medical Advisory Board, discussed data gathered during the Childbearing Center's first year of operation. During the inaugural year, 221 families were enrolled in the program after initial prenatal screening. 89 were awaiting delivery. 53 had delivered at the Center.

Of 256 families who initially registered, 1/4 were ineligible for care or became ineligible during the antepartal period. At the time of labor, about 33% of the nulliparas transferred to hospital medical care. There were no multipara transfers during the intrapartal period. In part this might have been due to the fact that twice as many nulliparas as multiparas were enrolled in the program. There were, in fact, many successful nulliparous births at the Center. There were no infant or maternal mortalities.

Transfers during the antepartal period included medical conditions such as gestational diabetes, hypertension, breech presentation up to the 37th week, premature labor, premature rupture of membranes, and others. Intrapartal transfers were made largely for slow progress, prolonged first or second stages, hypertension, and meconium staining. Three babies were transferred, two for observation of mild transitory respiratory distress, and one for signs of postmaturity. All three were discharged from the hospital in good condition within a few days. One mother was transferred postpartum for a prolonged third stage of labor. There were no emergency transfers.

Details of the first year's statistics will be published in report form in a forthcoming article.[6] In a second phase of evaluation, Maternity Center will conduct a matched-pair sample study, comparing pregnancy outcomes among families at the Childbearing Center with outcomes in a group of mothers at a large hospital.

". . . AFTER A YEAR'S EXPERIENCE, THE PROGRAM (MCA'S CHILDBEARING CENTER) HAS UNEQUIVOCALLY ESTABLISHED THE FACT THAT SAFE, MORE PERSONAL, COMPASSIONATE MATERNITY CARE CAN BE OFFERED MORE ECONOMICALLY THAN IN THE HOSPITAL . . ."

SEYMOUR ROMNEY, M.D.
DEPARTMENT OF OB/GYN
ALBERT EINSTEIN COLLEGE OF MEDICINE

When all facts were in, the consensus of the Center's medical advisors was reflected in a statement by Dr. Seymour Romney, of the Albert Einstein College of Medicine's Department of Obstetrics and Gynecology, when he wrote: ". . . After a year's experience, the program has unequivocally established the fact that safe, more personal, compassionate maternity care can be offered more economically than in the hospital . . . ".

Viability of the Birth Center as an alternative seems assured if one considers the interest expressed by the increasing numbers of parents, prospective parents, professionals, and representatives from the media who are attending the Childbearing Center's orientation sessions.[7] Families who have birthed at the Center are spreading the word to friends and neighbors. Various health agencies and organizations have come to learn and, in turn, refer families for care. Already families are returning for second experiences. The Childbearing Center seems welcomed as a new alternative on the obstetrical scene by consumers and professionals. It is especially valued for: (1) Providing care in a setting which enables parents to maintain control of their childbearing experiences as active and informed members of the team; (2) Its provision of highly personalized care; (3) Its provision of a truly home-like setting with, at the same time, equipment for obstetrical and neonatal first aid and channels for transfer to a hospital setting should either or both be required; and (4) By making available maternity care which is priced within the realm of financial survival.

 IN ALMOST A YEAR AND A HALF OF THE PROGRAM, THERE HAS BEEN NO EMERGENCY TRANSFERS TO THE HOSPITAL.

Problems and Solutions

As I intimated earlier, the first year of operating the Childbearing Center has been both rewarding and challenging. However, one of the purposes of the demonstration has been to identify problems. We have been most successful in identifying problems -- dozens of them! Internal and external problems. Some of them are more relative to the metropolitan area in which the Childbearing Center is located. In that sense the Center is unique. On the other hand, some of the most important major problem areas to which we have given attention might also be major concerns in the establishment of birth centers in other areas. It is to these I would like to draw your attention. The approaches we have arrived at to date in meeting the problems are just that, rather than solutions with which we are completely satisfied. The problem areas are inter-related. Hopefully, our experience will prove to be of help and interest to others.

The following have been major concerns in developing the program of care in which safety, satisfaction and economy are the main goals:

Identifying Families Who are at Low Medical Risk.

Basic to selection of families eligible for care at the Center are the screening criteria developed by a committee of experts in the maternal and child health field. Experience to date has enabled us to further refine these so-called "transfer criteria." Families accepted for care are monitored throughout pregnancy, labor, and the postpartal period. Potential problems are identified at an early stage so that transfer of the family at "medium risk" to direct medical care and hospital facilities when needed can be made smoothly and at a favorable time.

Our transfer criteria are stringent but must be considered effective to the degree that in almost a year and a half of the program's functioning there has been no emergency transfers. But having transfer criteria and making them work are two separate entities. We think we have some answers to the latter. Basic is an inclusive medical health history. Parents fill out three pages of details. These are discussed with the parents by the physician who conducts the first visit and complete physical examination. Return visits are comprehensive in scope with painstaking assessment and followup of any discernable problems. Before every subsequent visit the mother's record is completely reviewed by a staff member who notes all details for which followup is indicated. Maximum use is made of laboratory and technological aids to ascertain that all is well. This may include attention to everything from accelerated uterine enlargement to the existence of an indoor/outdoor family cat!

Of no minor importance is the informed participation of parents themselves in the whole screening process. These parents from their earliest contact with the Center are made aware of the Center's functions and limitations, the significance of maintaining optimal health, and the management of normal pregnancy. They are highly motivated and effective co-monitors on the team.

I BELIEVE I SPEAK FOR MY NURSE-MIDWIFE COLLEAGUES AS WELL AS MYSELF IN SAYING THAT THE EXPERIENCE AT THE CHILDBEARING CENTER HAS BEEN THE MOST REWARDING PROFESSIONAL EXPERIENCE WE HAVE KNOWN.

IT IS NOT ENOUGH TO MERELY MONITOR LABOR AND SAFEGUARD ITS COURSE. CREATING A PHYSICAL AND EMOTIONAL ATMO-SPHERE IN WHICH SENSITIVITY TO NEEDS AND INTIMACY PREVAIL MAY BE MORE IMPORTANT TO THE PROGRESS OF LABOR AND ITS ULTIMATE OUTCOME THAN ANY OTHER SINGLE FACTOR.

Striving for Excellence of Maternal and Newborn Care

Continuously working to provide the highest possible quality care is central to all other concerns related to the Childbearing Center. Attention is focused on refinement of all aspects of care -- physical, emotional, and educational. The goal is preventive health care. The common denominator is safety. However safety in terms of physical survival alone falls short of the goal. We are committed to safeguarding families by promoting optimal health of mothers and babies; by protecting and enhancing delicate family relationships which are so critical to long term health and happiness of parents and children; and by promoting health through in-depth education which enables the childbearing couple to move into parenting with confidence and readiness to assume a more independent role in their own health care. It is our belief that parents in general, and mothers in particular are the primary health care providers of families.

We are moving in a number of directions on this major concern:

(1) Medical, technical, and physical aspects of care are constantly re-examined. Protocols and procedures are subjected to review in terms of latest research findings. Management of families who require transfer as well as management of families with relatively few problems is discussed and evaluated. All of this is done on a continuing periodic basis by an obstetrician, pediatrician, and nurse-midwife staff team.

(2) Educational aspects of the program are likewise given continuing priority in the Center's prevention-oriented program of care. Over twenty hours of parents classes are complimented by many more individual teaching sessions during antepartal visits. Nutrition is stressed as basic health insurance. Health, pregnancy, birth, and parenting are primary concerns. During visits parents learn how to monitor pregnancy. Families check their own charts. Mothers help to keep their records in regard to weight, urinalysis and how they are feeling. Parents can learn how to take a blood

pressure, use a stethoscope, take a temperature, examine a throat. It's not that we expect to make physical assessment experts of them. The aim is to r e m o v e some of the mystique and increase their awareness of their own observational capabilities. Children enjoy some of this, too. We have had a 5-year-old who regularly tested his mother's urine with a dipstick and a 2-year-old who insisted upon checking on the nurse-midwife's measurement of his mother's fundal height -- even six weeks after his sister was born!

Nothing is static. We're learning! Most recently we have begun meeting with a group of alumni of the program who will be guiding us in further development of the educational aspects.

(3) Providing increasingly m o r e effective emotional support has been another challenging area. I believe I speak for my nurse-midwife colleagues as well as myself in saying that the experience at the Childbearing Center has been the most rewarding professional experience we have k n o w n. We have observed, not only what a minimum of stress can mean, but what actual joy can mean to the progress of labor and the protection of the unborn baby. We've seen the "bonding" of mothers and fathers to each other as well a s t o their babies -- interactions and effects which the slightest negative note may distort or destroy. We're learning that it is not enough to merely monitor labor and safeguard its course. Creating a physical and emotional atmosphere in which sensitivity to needs and intimacy prevail may be m o r e important to the progress of labor and its ultimate outcome than any other single factor.

Likewise, it is no longer enough to assist the mother safely through birth. The true professional challenge is to help parents achieve the kind of birth experience they desire and to appreciate ever more sensitively and opportunistically the critical nature o f the early minutes, hours, and days following t h e baby's arrival. This can mean standing by breathlessly, as we did the other evening while a 5-minute-old baby girl gazed intently into her father's eyes, and helping him to absorb the impact of that moment!

As one steps back and contemplates responsibility here, it is awesome. It is quite likely that in the provision of truly supportive care and attention to significant emotional factors we are just beginning to touch the surface.

 RECLINING CHAIRS FOR FATHERS TO REST IN HAVE BEEN USE-FUL, BUT WE HAVE LEARNED THT DOUBLE BEDS WOULD BE BETTER STILL!

SAFETY IN TERMS OF PHYSICAL SURVIVAL ALONE FALLS SHORT OF THE GOAL. WE ARE COMMITTED TO SAFEGUARDING FAMILIES, PROMOTING OPTIMAL HEALTH OF MOTHERS AND BABIES, PROTECTING AND ENHANCING DELICATE FAMILY RELATIONSHIPS, AND ENABLING COUPLES TO MOVE INTO PARENTING WITH CONFIDENCE AND READINESS TO ASSUME A MORE INDEPENDENT ROLE IN THEIR OWN HEALTH CARE.

Medical Back-Up Plan for Emergencies

Planning for the provision of medical care and hospital facilities in the event of emergency or problems beyond the scope of the Center has been a basic consideration. (This would probably be one of the easiest problems to solve in a smaller community. With families coming from all five boroughs of New York it has taken some strategy!

From their earliest contacts families are made aware of the need and asked to arrange for "back-up" medical care. This includes general medical care in the event of an unexpected medical problem during pregnancy and obstetrical-gynecological care for both emergency and continuing care after the baby is born. Families have the option of selecting private or clinic care.

Many families have selected one of the three obstetricians on the Center's staff. This has been partly because many obstetricians in the metropolitan area, unfamiliar with the Center's program, have been skeptical. It is also due to the parents' getting to know the doctors at the Center well and having confidence in them. It has worked out well because the physicians on the staff of the Childbearing Center are aware of the philosophy of care which prevails, and can pave the way to a hospital experience more in keeping with it.

The three obstetricians are associated with three different hospitals. Families have utilized all three. One of the three hospitals is designated as the official back-up hospital. This facility and another of the three are within fifteen minutes' travel time by ambulance. A contract with a local ambulance company has facilitated transfer when labor has been more advanced or an isolate transfer was deemed necessary. All family records are in triplicate so that when transfer is necessary, the entire record can go with mother and/or baby.

Continuing care of the baby was another original area of concern. It has worked out well to have parents select and discuss plans with a pediatrician of their choice well before the 28th week of pregnancy. A letter to the pediatrician telling about the Center is provided for parents to give to the baby's doctor. Within a few hours after birth the baby is examined by the staff pediatrician. Before going home from the Center parents are encouraged to call their pediatrician to alert him to the baby's arrival so that plans can be made for continuing care of the baby. Copies of the labor record and the first newborn assessment are given to the parents to take to the pediatrician.(Second copies of these records are provided for the visiting nurse.) As soon as cord blood reports are back, the pediatrician is notified by telephone.

PARENTS CAN LEARN HOW TO TAKE A BLOOD PRESSURE, USE A STETHOSCOPE, TAKE A TEMPERATURE, EXAMINE A THROAT. IT'S NOT THAT WE EXPECT TO MAKE EXPERTS OF THEM. THE AIM IS TO REMOVE SOME OF THE MYSTIQUE AND INCREASE THEIR AWARENESS OF THEIR OWN OBSERVATIONAL CAPABILITIES.

Staffing the Birth Center

Staffing the unit was another major issue in establishing the Birth Center. Planners were asked, "Who would work in such a place?" An obstetrician, nurse-midwife team was decided upon -- obstetricians to contribute medical direction and expertise and the nurse-midwives to provide instruction and much of the care throughout pregnancy, birth, and the early postpartum period. Happily three medical "mavericks," who are also board-certified, well-established obstetricians, elected to pioneer with the unit. It has not been easy for them to weather the inevitable negative pressures instigated by such a departure from standard practice. However, their practices have begun to boom as more and more families get to know them and want to go to them for follow-up care. They may soon wish they were amoebae!

The nurse-midwife was felt to be a natural for the Center's program. Nurse-midwifery education has been directed toward the management of normal childbearing. And although not commonly known, nurse-midwives were responsible for establishing the first parent education and family centered care in this country. Nurse-midwives had staffed Maternity Center Association's successful home delivery service. The plan seemed flawless.

However, in the intervening years a metamorphosis had taken place in nurse-midwifery as programs of education and service had become established in tertiary care centers. Nurse-midwives coming to the Center were interested, enthusiastic, and dedicated, but not quite certain that the natural process could be trusted. British-trained nurse-midwives were much more comfortable, but for others a "rebirthing" was necessary to unlearn the highly technical interventionist pathology-centered approach which they had come to regard as superior maternity care. Gradually over the first year, with the help of families, vision improved. All of us have found the Childbearing Center an ideal setting in which to develop the almost lost "art" of nurse-midwifery and restore faith in the original design of the Creator. We have come to regard technology as a wonderful and life saving tool on those occasions when it is indicated, rather than an obstetric way of life.

It soon became apparent that the nurse-midwives needed help in touching all bases. A nurse-midwifery assistant role was developed with on-the-job training. Assistants took on functions of checking and restocking the labor birth and examining rooms assisting with clerical tasks, assisting with the care of families, and keeping the unit immaculate and free of pathogens. Their affectionate term for the Center is "Vesphine - Green Soap City." They have been an invaluable and enthusiastic group. There are a nurse-midwife and nurse-midwife assistant on around the clock. A second nurse-midwife is on call to assist with births or other families in labor. Two nurse-midwives and an assistant are on duty on the four days each week when office hours for antepartal care and postpartal follow-up are held.

The entire Childbearing Center Staff team meets regularly. In addition the nurse-midwives and assistants meet as a smaller group every month or more often as needed. With a continuous run of normal happenings, there is a real problem in keeping staff prepared for possible emergencies. A variety of "drills" are held at frequent intervals so that staff are kept alert to unlikely but possible situations requiring swift and skillful action.

As you may have guessed, staffing is the most costly item on the budget. This, too, relates to location. Round the clock in-house coverage might not be necessary in a smaller community. In Albuquerque, New Mexico, Eugene, Oregon, Raymondville, Texas, Englewood, New Jersey -- single pioneering nurse-midwives are taking call and caring effectively for families with much less assistance.

 PARENTS IN GENERAL, AND MOTHERS IN PARTICULAR, ARE THE PRIMARY HEALTH CARE PROVIDERS OF FAMILIES.

Many staffing patterns are possible. Centers might be staffed by physicians, experienced nurses, lay midwives and others interested in promoting truly family-centered care. Energy, flexibility, and especially wholehearted dedication are qualifications of choice for persons working in such centers.

Furnishings and Equipment

A home-like, comfortable, attractive setting where parents can come and go and whole families can gather is a must for the birth center. The family (living) room has been especially popular for much of labor. Reclining chairs for fathers to rest in have been useful, but we have learned that double beds would be better still! Both birth rooms have single labor-birth beds with oversize mattresses. On those occasions when we have had three births the couple that has had the double davenport, i.e., sofa bed in the family room, has felt especially privileged! The fully equipped kitchen is another popular family hangout before and after birth. Occasionally grandmothers move in to brew birthday feasts.

Equipment to facilitate care and obstetric management can be a large expense. It was less so for us as we were given equipment by physicians and were able to purchase some, though not all, which was "nearly new." An autoclave and washing machine have proven most useful, as has a borrowed sewing machine with which talented members of the staff have made drapes, baby blankets, wrappers, scrub dresses, etc.

The two examining rooms are equipped very much like those rooms in a doctor's office. A large mirror housed in the drawer next to the one containing speculums, enables the mother to view her own cervix during examination. One of the examining rooms is supplied with equipment for circumcision which can be done, if the parents so choose, on the seventh postpartum day.

A microscope, centrifuge for hematocrits, and "Hubie," an incubator, enable staff to perform routine laboratory work at less cost to families. All initial laboratory screening and special tests are sent to commercial or health department laboratories.

The labor-birth rooms house equipment for birth and after care of mother and baby. Supplies are labeled and tucked away in designated drawers and cabinets so that they do not predominate the home-like bedroom atmosphere. The "midwife's lamp" looks like part of the furnishings. A larger surgical lamp is kept in the hallway for those occasions when full lighting is required.

Separate packs are made for gown and towel, birth, repair of episiotomy or laceration, cervical inspection, care of the baby's eyes, baby bath and/or shampoo, etc. This separateness of sterile supplies facilitates flexibility of care. For example, after the birth, an ice cap to the perineum may suffice while priority is given to bonding of mother, father, and baby. An hour or so later, the "episiotomy pack" can be opened at leisure for repair of the perineum.

First aid equipment for mother and baby is kept in the hallway between the two labor-birth rooms. Oxygen and infant and maternal resuscitation equipment, emergency drugs, and intravenous equipment with blood expanders stand in constant readiness. Both the radiant heated bassinet and isolette transfer unit are turned on in preparation for each birth. Rarely has their use been indicated, but they are there.

Licensure

Getting licensed was an early but time-consuming problem. The Childbearing Center has operated as a "diagnosis and treatment center" after more than two years of scrutiny by the New York State Public Health Council, including its advisory bodies, the Health and Hospitals Planning Council of Southern New York, the Comprehensive Health Planning Agency of New York City, and the New York State Hospital Review Council.

There were and are now no codes which apply specifically to Childbearing Centers. We have learned that most important in setting up a Birth Center is avoidance of being drawn into conforming to hospital codes which are involved and impractical for the purpose. With legal help (a consumer volunteer if at all possible) it would be best to explore local laws and health codes to learn what is available in your locale.   In some states a center might operate under a maternity home law.   Look for codes regarding abortion clinics, surgical centers and similar services.   An interested physician could set up such a center as part of his practice. Or a hospital might set up such a unit as part of its maternity services apart from the more intensive care section.

The birth center might be incorporated by a consumer group or interested professionals. It could be operated on a profit or non-profit basis. The Childbearing Center is operated by a non-profit voluntary agency.

Various codes may dictate such items as equipment, hospital facilities, medical officers, etc., which may not always really apply. We're forced by code to have one official back-up hospital. In actual practice we use three.

The problem of keeping financially viable while preserving the highly valued features of a small service is a challenging one. Staffing, housing, housekeeping, telephone, laboratory, laundry, food, supplies, and an initial outlay for furnishings, equipment, and establishing licensure must all be considered. Fee for service must reflect all of these expenses.

Volunteer help in all forms can help to lessen costs. Innovative patterns of staffing may greatly alleviate expense. Families can be beneficiaries of considerable savings in this type alternative.

Third party payers have shown interest in out-of-hospital care. We have Blue Cross eligibility. A number of other plans have followed suit. The total care "package," which includes antepartal care, parents' classes, birth at the Center, pediatric examination, postpartal supervision, visiting nurse service and six-week examinations is costed at $750. Obstetric and hospital care are from $1500 to $2000.

Community Relations -- The "External Problems"

What happens with the birth of a childbearing center? Among the first problems confronting the planners is: Will anyone come? What will they think? These were answered when the Center opened its doors on October 1, 1975. Two types of parents came: (1) The well-informed people who definitely wanted a home or home-like birth, and (2) The more or less informed people who were reacting to traditional hospital care. Professionals and journalists came to see what a Childbearing Center was all about.

Orientation sessions were set up to describe to parents and professionals alike the philosophy and functions of the new facility. A tour was included. Close to 900 people attended orientations during the first year. The number is escalating. Referrals come from a growing number of sources.

In spite of enthusiastic public acclaim, the Center has had a large share of political problems stemming from concern about the safety of the project on the part of District II of ACOG and the New York City Department of Health. As many of you may know, early last year District II of ACOG issued a statement [1] proclaiming disapproval of out-of-hospital delivery. (See Chapter 5, pp. 33-36, for a complete reprinting of this paper.) The position paper was not adopted by the national organization.

The very thoughtful and carefully considered reply [2] by the International Childbirth Education Assn., (see Chapter 6, pp. 37-39 for ICEA reply, as well as pp. 41-42 for NAPSAC's reply) gave pause to all who would deny parents the right to make decisions regarding matters in which they have such personal investment. This statement by a prestigious consumer organization reassured the medical community and anyone concerned of parents' desires to have alternatives of care from which to choose.

IT IS NO LONGER ENOUGH TO ASSIST THE MOTHER SAFELY THRU BIRTH, THE TRUE PROFESSIONAL CHALLENGE IS TO HELP PARENTS ACHIEVE THE KIND OF BIRTH EXPERIENCE THEY DESIRE AND TO APPRECIATE EVER MORE SENSITIVELY AND OPPORTUNISTICALLY THE CRITICAL NATURE OF THE EARLY MINUTES, HOURS, AND DAYS AFTER THE BABY'S ARRIVAL,

Another political issue has been the New York City Department of Health's refusal to issue a Medicaid Number to the Center. Consequently, families with low incomes have automatically been excluded from the project. In an effort to right this situation, Maternity Center Association's Board of Directors voted to underwrite a large proportion of the cost of Medicare for eligible families until the situation can be corrected.

Harassment has taken many forms, including unsavory rumors. For example, we hear from time to time that we have been "closed."

Most recently the Center was requested to submit an application for renewal of its operating license eight months in advance. The usual time is three months. Concern has been repeatedly voiced about the 10 to 15 minute distance from a back-up hospital. The greatest concern has been focused on risks to the fetus and newborn.

In this vein, it is interesting to note that the most knowledgeable in the area of greatest concern, namely board-certified pediatricians, are among the most staunch supporters of the project. Pediatricians and their wives have been among our families. One of the babies I helped to birth recently was the Apgar 12* daughter of a pediatrician mother. Pediatricians in the community have supported our families. Many practitioners have visited the Center.

Herein, I believe, lies a clue to the dichotomy of the two related medical specialties. It is natural to be skeptical of the unknown. For example, a pediatric fellow was most specific when he came to see the Center: "Show me your resuscitation equipment!" I dutifully unveiled the radiant heat bassinet and the trays for intubation, umbilical catheterization, and the Ambubag, suction and

*For a definition of "Apgar 12" see Safe Alternatives in Childbirth, p. 25. [5]

medicine tray, the oxygen, Delee suction tubes, the sodium bicarb, and last but not least, the isolette transfer unit.

"There is one problem," I admitted, "we work so hard for babies whose responses are superior at birth, we have to practice diligently on the doll to keep up our skills."

I outlined the many elements of preventive care we consider important: nutrition during pregnancy, continued good nutrition during labor, an upright or side lying position during labor and birth, absence of stress, unmedicated births, and deep breathing with only gentle pushing to increase oxygen intake around the time of birth. The baby should cry before birth is complete and be pink to his toes as he trails over the perineum.

Gentle bulb suctioning at several levels during birth and a face down or face to side position until airways are clear, while parents' hands and warmed blankets surround the baby to prevent chilling. Then skin to skin contact with mother and/or father. Early and frequent breast feeding. I confessed, "I am a lazy midwife, and find prevention so much easier than having to deal with problems."

His reply reflected our sentiments: "I'm for prevention!" Perhaps the message is clear. We must extend hospitality to the obstetric community. It is not fair to ask to be accepted sight unseen!

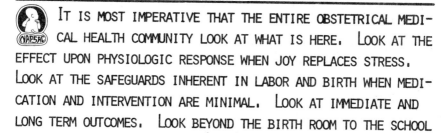

IT IS MOST IMPERATIVE THAT THE ENTIRE OBSTETRICAL MEDICAL HEALTH COMMUNITY LOOK AT WHAT IS HERE. LOOK AT THE EFFECT UPON PHYSIOLOGIC RESPONSE WHEN JOY REPLACES STRESS. LOOK AT THE SAFEGUARDS INHERENT IN LABOR AND BIRTH WHEN MEDICATION AND INTERVENTION ARE MINIMAL. LOOK AT IMMEDIATE AND LONG TERM OUTCOMES. LOOK BEYOND THE BIRTH ROOM TO THE SCHOOL ROOM, THE FAMILY, SOCIETY. LOOK!

And, we must be seen -- all the alternatives! There is more than meets the eye in a casual glance. After a year and a half in the development of an alternative, I believe it most imperative that the entire obstetrical medical health community look at what is here with all the open-minded scientific fervor of its fine tradition. Look at the effect upon physiologic response when joy replaces stress. Look at the safeguards inherent in the physiologic processes of labor and birth when medication and intervention are minimal. Look at immediate and long term outcomes. Look beyond the birth room to the school room, the family, society. Look!

Only then will our children's children and their children's children know the full heritage of care which our present knowledge, love and unwavering concern can provide.

Note: The address of the Maternity Center Association is: 48 East 92nd Street, New York, NY 10028.

CITED REFERENCES

1. American College of Obstetricians and Gynecologists, District II, Position paper on out-of-hospital maternity care, adopted, Jan. 1976. (see Ch. 5, Vol. I of these volumes)

2. Beals, P., and Beals, T., ICEA Replies to ACOG, ICEA News, 15:3-4, 1976. (see Ch. 6, Vol I of these volumes)

3. Klaus, M., and Kennell, J., Maternal-Infant Bonding, St. Louis: C.V. Mosby Co., 1976.

4. Lubic, R., Developing Maternity Services Women Will Trust, Am. J. Nurs. 75:1685-1688, 1975.

5. Lubic, R., and Hosford, M., Childbearing centers: an alternative to both hospitals and homebirth, Stewart, D., & Stewart, L., (eds), Safe Alternatives in Childbirth, 2nd ed., Chapel Hill, NC: NAPSAC, pp. 22-32, 1977.

6. Maternity Center Association, 48 East 92nd St., New York, NY 10028, Statistical Report of childbearing center, 1976, (to be published).

7. MCA Center attracts wide response, Special Delivery, Vol. VII, No. 2, Fall, 1976.

CHAPTER TWENTY TWO

SETTING UP A VIABLE HOME BIRTH SERVICE
RUN BY CNM'S, BACKED BY DOCTORS & HOSPITALS

Janet L. Epstein, C.N.M.

Health care delivery has become a topic of great interest today. Professionals and consumers alike are expressing tremendous
dissatisfaction with the medical establishment's disease orientation.
Measurement of the qualities of well being, such as productivity,
ability to cope and satisfaction is difficult, although not impossible.

Health professionals have not spent enough time studying these
issues. Perhaps Ruth Lubic, C.N.M., General Director of the Maternity Center Association in New York, is right when she speculates
that perhaps health professionals have been "seduced by the thrill of
technology and the excitement of the possibility of sharing a God
image."

Nurse-midwives everywhere are striving to move away from
that web and from that establishment and to balance the work of
health delivery and health maintenance with illness prevention and
illness treatment. After all, as nurse-midwives, we do have both
jobs.

In a very recent editorial in the Winter, 1976, issue of Journal of Nurse-Midwifery, Jean Cassidy, C.N.M., states, "Tradi-
tionally, nurse-midwives have considered themselves advocates of
the childbearing couple." Recently, a shocking accusation has challenged this position. In her book, Immaculate Deception, Suzanne
Arms stated that nurse-midwives have sold out to the "establishment." She further states that the modern nurse-midwife is far
more comfortable in the medically oriented system of maternity
care than in the family oriented system of family-centered maternity care.

The issue is not whether or not these accusations have a basis
in fact. In some cases they do and in some cases they do not. The
fact is that they have been made, and they have been given credence
by the consumer.

JANET L. EPSTEIN is President, Maternity Center Associates, Washington,
D.C.; and coauthor of "A Safe Home Birth Program That Works," and
others.

I am especially overwhelmed by misinterpretations of the American College of Nurse-Midwives' stand on out-of-hospital delivery (reproduced below):

> Where home births are a necessity, it is essential that the obstetric authorities for that area develop criteria for the practitioners to ensure the safety of the mother and infant. ACNM considers the hospital or officially approved maternity home as the site for childbirth because of the distinct advantage to the welfare of mother and child. We encourage the members of the obstetric team in hospital or maternity home settings to meet the personal needs of childbearing families by combining a family-centered atmosphere with the safety of full environmental resources and a readily available obstetric team including the physician.[1]

It is true that it is ambiguous and somewhat disparaging. The fact is, however, that many couples have opted for out-of-hospital type delivery. Suzanne Arm's accusations must make us, as nurse-midwives, try to decide what influence nurse-midwives are to have on the future direction of maternity care in this country, if any.

This is a time in our history when the population of mothers and their families is the healthiest it has ever been. The medical profession has developed the most extensive and technologically oriented methods of obstetrical care yet known. Why is it that the consumer has balked at these technological advances? Why is it that the consumer is not pleased with the medical establishment's direction?

 IT IS VITAL THAT CLIENTS BE RESPONSIBLE FOR THEIR OWN HEALTH CARE AND CONTRIBUTE AS MUCH AS THEY CAN TO THEIR OWN HEALTH MAINTENANCE.

The Founding of Our Home Birth Service

In October of 1975, Marion McCartney, a nurse-midwife, and myself established the nation's first incorporated nurse-midwifery service. Chartered under Maryland law, the Maternity Center Associates in Bethesda, as we are called, is designed to provide primary health care to childbearing women, particularly to women who desire to give birth in their own home.

THE MEDICAL PROFESSION HAS CHOSEN TO VIRTUALLY IGNORE THE PUBLIC'S DESIRE FOR HOME BIRTH AND WE FEEL NURSE-MIDWIFERY SERVICE CAN, AND SHOULD, FILL THIS VOID.

There are now three of us, all Certified Nurse-Midwives, and we practice under the general direction of two Board Certified Obstetricians whom we have employed for just that reason. Ms. McCartney and I are partners in the corporation, and jointly administer the service.

We also have an advisory committee which is composed of an obstetrician, a pediatrician, a psychiatrist, another Certified Nurse-Midwife and a consumer. Presently, this consumer is a lay midwife. This committee meets regularly to provide general advice and to participate in quality assessment activities.

We are Registered Nurses in the state of Maryland and in the other two jurisdictions over which we serve. That is, the District of Columbia and northern Virginia. For several years prior to the founding of the MCA, Inc., we served as obstetrical nurses assisting two local obstetricians who were doing home births. The day inevitably came when we "caught" a baby because a physician was unable to come to the home. The opportunity to support the couple throughout the entire childbirth experience was exhilarating for us. It occurred to us that to assist the couple throughout the entire pregnancy might be a way to humanize obstetrical care which is so cold and mechanized for the most part.

After a few such "catches," we decided to attend Georgetown University for the one-year Nurse-Midwifery course. Subsequently, we became certified by the American College of Nurse-Midwives.

Nowhere are women more aware and less patient with the "system" as in the field of their own reproductive functioning. Disenchantment is evidenced by the dramatic increase in women's gynecologic and family planning clinics, women self-help groups, and in women choosing home birth, professionally assisted or not. Some of the reasons for this disenchantment range from complaints that the service is impersonalized; that medical establishment is interventionist; that it is pathologically oriented and technologically oriented; that the medical establishment is unresponsive and inflexible; and, last but not least, that it is costly.

Some of the reasons for wanting home birth range from wanting more control; that it is more personal and friendly to have a midwife with you; that there is considerably less medical intervention, such as monitors, IV's, medications; that there is more flexibility involved; that people feel more comfortable in their own home and in their own clothing; and, of course, last but not least, it is cheaper.

The physicians with whom we worked agreed with us that the best way to satisfy the constantly increasing requests for home births was for us to attend the home births as nurse-midwives. Nurse-midwives are generally concerned with "normal women." Our experience has shown that women who want to deliver at home are quite normal.

However, what is normal? Can we screen low risk women? The medical establishment has been very good about doing research on women who are at high risk and screening these women and treating them, as they should be treated, in medical clinics with medical intervention to assist them.

However, as far as we can tell, little, if any, work has been done on what the definition is of a normal, low risk maternity patient. We reasoned that if the nurse-midwives would take care of normal women, then this would free the physicians to practice their specialties, particularly with women who are at high risk or who had complications of pregnancy.

 THE MEDICAL ESTABLISHMENT HAS BEEN VERY GOOD ABOUT SCREENING, DOING RESEARCH, AND TREATING WOMEN AT HIGH RISK. HOWEVER, LITTLE, IF ANY, WORK HAS BEEN DONE ON THE DEFINITION OF WHAT IS A "NORMAL, LOW RISK" MATERNITY PATIENT.

These physicians also agreed to act as medical directors of our service and to accept referrals. So far, our experience shows this approach to obstetrics to be practical and a satisfying of each professional skill. Furthermore, it helps to fulfill a largely unmet need among expectant mothers. That is, for home birth with continuity of care.

It fulfills the need that the consumer is demanding now, for birth alternatives. Since the medical profession has chosen to virtually ignore the public's desire for home birth, we feel nurse-midwifery service can and should fill this void. The reception of our service thus far leads us to think that similar organizations can hold promise for other areas of the country. It can be done.

Our service is medically directed and complies with the rules and regulations of the three jurisdictions in which we practice: Maryland, Virginia and the District of Columbia. This was by no means easy. It required lawyers, accountants and medical direction.

Having our own organization, however, affords us a sense of independence in caring for and assisting healthy women and their families. We believe that support and maintenance of optimum health is a unique function of nurses. This is precisely our goal within the framework of our service.

The philosophy of our service is basically very broad. We believe that childbirth should be a positive experience and that expectant parents are committed to doing what they think best for themselves and their upcoming child. In other words, we feel that parents who opt for home birth believe they are doing so because they are doing the best for themselves and their child, and not the worst, as our medical establishment would have us believe.

As professionals, we adapt our assistance to what our clients want, rather than attempt to convert them to prevailing medical philosophy. We believe that expectant parents have a right to give birth comfortably, capably and safely. We believe that a positive childbearing experience contributes to the development of a healthy family unit. Expectant parents have the right and the responsibility to be involved in their own health care.

 WE REASON THAT IF NURSE-MIDWIVES WOULD TAKE CARE OF NORMAL WOMEN, THEN THIS WOULD FREE PHYSICIANS TO PRACTICE THEIR SPECIALTIES PARTICULARLY WITH WOMEN AT HIGH RISK OR WHO HAVE COMPLICATIONS.

Finally, we believe that cultural beliefs of expectant parents should be recognized, respected and implemented if at all possible. Dr. John Knowles, President of the Rockefeller Foundation, in an essay published in Time Magazine last July stated, "The next major advances in the health of American people will result from the assumption of individual responsibility for one's own health, one that requires a change in life style for the majority of Americans."

He gives examples of such required changes, as in eating, smoking, sexual intemperance and reckless driving. Obviously, obesity, diabetes, heart disease, lung cancer, etc., can, to a more or less extent, be controlled with the quality and quantity of what he or she eats, drinks, smokes, drives, etc.

Home births is a progressive trend for the same reason. David Stewart has stated, and it is true, that home birth is a "manifestation of greater awareness and concern on the part of today's parents."[2] They are willing and able to assume this responsibility. Most of these couples are educated and knowledgeable.

Alternatives and options should always be available to all humans in all situations in life, especially in birth and even in death.

In meeting the needs of our clients, we provide comprehensive primary health care to childbearing women, including delivery at home to those who qualify as normal. Routine gynecologic services and family planning are also available. We emphasize strongly throughout emotional and physical support in health education. Clients of our home birth service are given all their primary care by nurse-midwives. And, notice I say "clients" and not "patients," because patients are not healthy; clients are healthy.

 NOTICE I SAY, "CLIENTS", AND NOT "PATIENTS", BECAUSE PATIENTS ARE NOT HEALTHY--CLIENTS ARE HEALTHY.

Consultation with and/or referral to our service's physician directors or consultants or any other medical specialists are obtained as required. Obstetrical clients are routinely seen in the office at a frequency visit of one visit a month up to 28 weeks' gestation, two visits a month up to 36 weeks' gestation, and then four visits a month up to term.

Intra-partum services are provided at home if the client meets the selection standard, or, in the hospital. In the hospital, if this is required, care is provided by the nurse-midwife and the physician working together. One prenatal home visit is also included for those clients who plan to deliver at home.

As part of our obstetrical and gynecologic care, appropriate diagnostic services are utilized at two of the large area hospitals, such as sonogram, x-ray or laboratory facilities. Presently, we are doing about 20 deliveries a month.

Teaching on an individual basis is part of our service. Every Monday three orientation sessions are given in which prospective clients come and learn how they would function within our service. We constantly stress independence and responsibility for one's own health care. When the client comes in in the morning, she reaches for her chart, checks her own urine for protein, for sugar and for nitrates, records such results on her chart and weighs herself and records that on her chart.

Clients then receive specific instruction relative to preparations specifically necessary for a home birth. She is given a list of supplies to get, how to fix her bed, the classes she should take in order to prepare herself for her childbirth experience, and when to notify the nurse-midwife -- and hopefully she does this early.

We constantly stress the fact that her body is functioning well and that she is providing for herself adequately. We try to provide a positive attitude within the service. Postpartum services include an invitation to participate in a series of three group discussions centered on new family relationships and crisis intervention which are conducted in our office. These groups are supervised by a phychiatric nurse practitioner who is employed by us. Our clients are also advised of community resources for new parents, such as Red Cross classes, parents after childbirth education sessions and a consumer group involved specifically with home birth called H.O.M.E.* These letters stand for Home Oriented Maternity Experience. I would like to note that this H.O.M.E. group particularly responds to the needs of childbearing couples who want to deliver at home. They help to prepare the couple by telling her in more detail the supplies that she needs, the risks and benefits of home birth and also parents get a chance to meet other people who have had home birth and who have had both positive and/or negative experiences.

Screening Criteria for Home Birth Couples

Home birth clients are carefully selected according to specific criteria. These have been established not only for initial acceptance, but also for the entire prenatal period and for the labor. If any criterion is not met, the client will not be accepted for home delivery. Instead, appropriate alternatives and/or interventions are suggested. In this case, one of the consulting obstetricians is available to assume direct care of her if she so chooses. In most instances, the physician and the nurse-midwife jointly manage the client's pregnancy and delivery in the hospital.

Potential home birth clients must be initially self-selected. They must expressly request home birth. They must give evidence of sufficient commitment. Alternatives to a home birth are discussed with clients, and information regarding the nature of obstetrical services in local hospitals, including "in-and-out deliveries," is provided.

---

* The address of H.O.M.E. is 511 New York Ave., Takoma Park, Washington, DC 20012. Another national organization which also offers information, classes, support and training in home birth is the Association for Childbirth at Home International (A C H I), 16705 Monte Cristo, Cerritos, CA 90701.

Clients must also meet several non-medical qualifications in order to be accepted for a home birth. These include living within certain distances of a hospital, agreeing to transfer of self and/or infant if hospital is determined necessary by the attending nurse-midwife or the consulting physician, locating a pediatrician who will agree to see the newborn within the first 24 hours, attending preparation for childbirth classes or receiving private instruction, and finally gathering together the necessary supplies and make the required preparations at home.

The history and laboratory results of a client requesting home birth must be within normal limits. "Normal limits" is defined as no evidence of any of the following: hypertension, epilepsy, active syphilis, active tuberculosis, Rh negative blood with positive antibody titers, severe anemia, diabetes, severe psychiatric disease, heart disease, multiple gestations such as twins, kidney disease, preeclampsia, abnormal vaginal bleeding, abnormal presentation or lie, and previous cesarean section.

Additionally, clients must be no younger than 15 and have a limit of 5 pregnancies. Clients accepted for home birth must appear emotionally mature and stable. Every client is evaluated clinically and by x-ray, if necessary, to rule out cephalopelvic disproportion.

Clients accepted for home birth must have a completely normal antepartum course. This means no evidence of the following: abnormal bleeding, preeclampsia, congenital abnormalities, inappropriate gestational size, multiple gestation, or unusual presentation or lie.

Labor must begin within 24 hours of ruptured membranes. The fetal head must be engaged in the primigravida after a few hours of good labor. The fetus must be in a vertex position and there must be no signs of infection or distress. Any of these abnormalities require that a client deliver in the hospital rather than in the home.

The nurse-midwife tries to make a home visit approximately two weeks before the delivery date. This is, however, getting more and more impossible since, with 20 deliveries occurring every month, a home visit is becoming impractical by the nurse-midwife.

PARENTS WHO OPT FOR HOME BIRTH BELIEVE THEY ARE DOING SO BECAUSE THEY ARE DOING THE BEST FOR THEMSELVES AND THEIR CHILD, NOT THE WORST, AS OUR MEDICAL ESTABLISHMENT WOULD HAVE US BELIEVE.

THE LAY MIDWIVES IN OUR AREA HAVE BECOME A TREMENDOUS ASSET TO US IN HELPING PROVIDE CARE FOR CLIENTS WHO WISH TO DELIVER AT HOME. THEY ARE HELPING BY MAKING THE ANTEPARTUM HOME VISIT AND BY COMING WITH US ON EACH DELIVERY TO ACT AS A BIRTH ASSISTANT.

Our Relationship with Lay Midwives

It is probably a good idea here to talk about our relationship with the lay midwives. The lay midwives in our area have become a tremendous asset to us in helping us to provide care for clients who wish to deliver at home. They are helping now by making the home visit and by coming with us on each delivery to act as a birth assistant.

We currently conduct seminars so that these lay midwives can help us when we go out on home births. The seminars include: resuscitation of newborn infants, emergency medications and how to give them, as well as just general assistance of the nurse-midwife at the time of her home birth. These midwives have become a tremendous boon to us. I must admit, I have become spoiled and that I will just not go out on a home birth without one.

The Conduct of a Home Birth

Hopefully the client calls us when she is in early labor. Since both Ms. McCartney, Ms. Vaughey and I are mothers, it is helpful to know that if a delivery is coming up what arrangements we can make for our children and car pools, if necessary. When the midwife is notified, she then goes to the mother's home. The obstetrician on call is also notified. After the baby is born, the nurse consults with the pediatrician chosen by the client.

We are guests in the client's home. We expect that she will have a place for us to sleep and some sort of small amounts of food to eat if the labor and the delivery is long.

The delivery is conducted, insofar as is safely possible, completely according to the client's wishes. If she wants a Leboyer-type of a delivery, or if she wants the father to do the delivery, this is perfectly okay with us. During the labor we encourage the client and her family to feel relaxed and in control.

The mother eats or drinks as she desires. We see no need to restrict her diet unless she, herself, elects to do so. No shaving of the perineal area is done. Rarely a small enema may be used if the mother requests it or if the lower bowel contains hard stool.

We use no drugs of any sort during labor. If analgesia or if labor stimulation is required, we feel this is best accomplished in the hospital.

The mother is encouraged to move about and use the bathroom frequently and to assume any position that is comfortable for her. The father of the baby, whenever possible, is the coach. He usually directs the rest of the family and is the major source of support to the mother. He delivers the mother approximately 50% of the time if he so desires. We do very little coaching, since the father and the mother have been prepared for childbirth in their classes. If the father is not present, we ask the mother to choose a support person whom she cares for and who cares for her.

As nurse-midwives, we feel our role is that of a specialist hired to make sure all is well. We intervene only where appropriate. We do use some medication, only if necessary, after the baby and placenta are delivered, to control hemorrhage, which very rarely occurs.

The father of the baby is encouraged to assist us during the delivery. He can choose to be as involved as he feels comfortable. We have found that an overwhelming majority of fathers are eager to help deliver their baby and express pride in doing so. Family and friends usually surround the laboring couple and offer unique support. We encourage the couple to have whomever they desire to share this exceptional experience with them.

The delivery itself proceeds with the least intervention as possible. After the head is born, we wait for the head to rotate spontaneously on its own. The mother may use vitamin E on her perineum if she desires, or hot compresses. However, we have found that a combination of vitamin E and perineal massage seem to help the mother and reduces the frequency for tears or need for episiotomies.

The cutting of the cord, once the baby has been delivered, is delayed until after the placenta has been delivered, or at least until the pulse of the cord has stopped.

We do little or no suction of the baby's nose or mouth. If we see that the baby is crying and breathing spontaneously, we feel that the baby is the best person to help get rid of the mucous, and that by suctioning the baby only interferes with this normal and natural process, which the baby is entirely capable of doing on his own. So, rarely, if ever, do we suction.

WHEN THE CLIENT COMES IN, IN THE MORNING, SHE REACHES FOR HER OWN CHART, CHECKS HER OWN URINE FOR PROTEIN, FOR SUGAR, AND FOR NITRATES, RECORDS SUCH RESULTS ON HER CHART, AND WEIGHS HERSELF.

As soon as the baby is born, the baby is placed on the mother's belly for skin-to-skin contact. Then they are both covered with warm blankets. At this point, bonding of both the mother and baby is encouraged. Usually it is quiet, and the mother and father welcome the baby together in soft low tones. Rarely do I ever hear a mother or father squeal with excitement over the sex of the baby. More often than not, I hear a soft, low voice saying, "Hello, baby; welcome, baby."

Episiotomies should be mentioned here, I guess. Episiotomies are done only if necessary, and in a very low percent of the time, approximately 5%. We repair them at home without difficulty. If we do get tears and they require repair, we try to repair those, too. We do not, however, attempt repair of third or fourth degree lacerations. In those cases, where the rectal sphincter is involved, we go to the hospital for repair by one of our consulting obstetricians. This has happened only once in approximately 250 deliveries thus far. Of course, it happened to a nurse.

Abnormal progress of labor can be treated with medical intervention and possible transfer to the hospital. The following situations require such action: elevated blood pressure, a fetus in an abnormal position, meconium stained amniotic fluid, fetal heart irregularities, prolonged labor using the criteria established by Emmanuel Friedman, excessive bleeding, unengaged vertex in the primigravida, ruptured membranes over 24 hours, or last but not least, the wishes of the client.

The nurse-midwife stays with the mother and infant until vital signs are normal, the uterus is well contracted, and the baby is nursing well and shows no signs of distress. A minimum of one hour is always desirable. If any of the following should occur, medical consultation is necessary, with possible transfer of mother and/or baby to the hospital: hemorrhage, infant weight of less than 2500 grams (or approximately 5.5 pounds), respiratory difficulty,

 THE DELIVERY, ITSELF, PROCEEDS WITH THE LEAST INTERVENTION POSSIBLE. AFTER THE HEAD IS BORN, WE WAIT FOR THE BABY TO ROTATE SPONTANEOUSLY ON ITS OWN.

such as grunting and flaring of the nostril, cardiac irregularity, congestion of the lungs, congenital abnormalities, and Apgar score of less than 7 at five minutes, prematurity, dysmaturity or post-maturity as determined by physical assessment.

In the event that the home birth proceeds abnormally, or if, in the nurse-midwife's judgment, assistance is required, the nurse-midwife has the appropriate resources available. In every home birth instance, the obstetrician on call is notified of the onset of labor and is available for telephone or on-site consultation.

The pediatrician chosen by the client is also available for consultation if a problem develops with the infant. If the mother or baby required hospitalization, the obstetrician or pediatrician admits the client to the hospital. The physicians who are consultants to the service have privileges at many of the major hospitals in the area. If the situation that requires hospitalization is of an emergency nature and does not allow time for transfer to a hospital in which the consultant is located, then the client is, of course, transferred to the nearest hospital.

Since adequate accessibility to a hospital is a prerequisite to a home birth, this situation is unlikely to occur. In an emergency the client is transferred by the rescue squad, private ambulance or car. The nurse-midwife always accompanies the client to the hospital.

 WE USE NO DRUGS OF ANY SORT DURING LABOR. IF ANALGESIA OR LABOR STIMULATION IS REQUIRED, WE FEEL THIS IS BEST ACCOMPLISHED IN THE HOSPITAL.

Statistics

At this point I think it would be appropriate to mention some of the statistics of our service, and some of our experiences that we have had. Since the inception of our service a year and a half ago, we have attempted to deliver approximately 250 women at home. Of these women, approximately 15% have ended up being transferred to the hospital for various medical reasons which have basically been non-emergency nature. Of the 20% who have been admitted to the hospital, an overwhelming majority have been primigravidas, that is, first-time mothers. Our cesarean section rate of these mothers is approximately 7%. Only one mother, who was a multipara (this was her third baby), was admitted for cephalopelvic disproportion, and had to have a cesarean section. The baby weighed over 10 pounds. Presently we are averaging about 20 deliveries a month. This really keeps us quite busy. We have very few episiotomies or tears, and we have found that our client satisfaction is extremely high. All except three out of those 250 women have breastfed. Most of them are white, middle-class and educated. We do have a low proportion of black middle-class and educated patients or clients, and a small percent of counter-culture groups. But all of our clients are extremely well-informed, particularly about nutrition, and are quite enthusiastic.

After a successful delivery at home, which occurs most of the time, the nurse-midwife completes and signs the birth certificate, fills out various forms for the information of the pediatrician, as well as for our records, and gives postpartum instructions to the client. All of these forms are included as appendices to this article.

Later, usually within 48 to 72 hours, a postpartum visit to the family is made to evaluate the condition of the mother and baby, and to provide some continuity of care. The mother is then seen in our office for a two-week checkup, and then a six-week checkup. At the six-week checkup, family planning is usually accomplished at that time. After that, we invite her back for a six-months checkup and a one-year complete gynecologic check. We also encourage the mother and the father to attend our postpartum group.

 EPISIOTOMIES ARE DONE ONLY IF NECESSARY--APPROXIMATELY 5% OF THE TIME.

Prospects for the Future

Our home birth service is extremely active -- 20 births per month. We are very happy with our results. Client satisfaction seems to be high, as reflected by the positive feedback we receive, and the results of the critique that we ask each client to fill out. We encourage these women to review their own charts and express their needs to us. This enables us to stay abreast of what kinds of birth they would like to have, and how they felt about their birth once they have had it.

We feel it is vital that clients be responsible for their own health care and contribute as much as they can to their own health maintenance. This service is proving to be a tremendous satisfaction and a joy to us as nurse-midwives. It can be a joy to other nurse-midwives also, if they would just try it.

There is a clear demand for home birth services in our area, and I am sure in all other areas in these United States. Despite some changes in obstetrical care in some of the area's hospitals, this demand is unquestionably growing. It is difficult to obtain accurate data on home birth because the majority of the medical community has chosen to turn its back on these women. They are not even interested in collecting data, because they disapprove of home births. In certain cases where women would like to go to a physician just for prenatal care, if she mentions the fact that she wants to have a home birth, these physicians will deny her this care.

Every so often a midwife will call up and express to us her desire to deliver a mother and the mother's desire to have her, the lay midwife, deliver her. We then will gladly provide prenatal care and postpartum follow-up to these clients.

According to the combined information of the two obstetricians and several nurse-midwives who currently provide home birth services in our area, approximately 300-400 women had their babies at home in 1975. This number is probably on the low side. The recent emergence of the consumer group called H. O. M. E., as I previously mentioned, which encourages and gives information about home births, attest to this growing consumer interest.

A review of the literature reveals an almost complete lack of carefully designed evaluations of home birth conducted under controlled conditions by qualified health professionals. The only exceptions to this are the studies presently being conducted by Dr. Lewis Mehl. [2] (Also see Chapters 16 and 17, Vol. 1.) The combination of a vocal and growing consumer interest in this area, along with a need for fact, prompted us to design a study as an integral part of our home birth service.

Specifically, our research will describe and evaluate home births as assisted by Certified Nurse-Midwives under medical direction and carefully selected and controlled conditions, which are similar to the ones that I have previously mentioned. We hope to characterize the women seeking home birth and to determine the effectiveness of the criteria by which we expect home birth clients. Furthermore, we want to document the pregnancy outcome of these clients, and describe the extent and nature of any complications. Lastly, we want to determine the client satisfaction with their home birth experience, whether it turned out to be what they expected, and what site they would choose for their next birth.

No where are women more aware of and less patient with the "system" as in the field of their own reproductive functions.

OUR HOME BIRTH SERVICE IS PROVING TO BE A TREMENDOUS SATISFACTION AND JOY TO US AS NURSE-MIDWIVES. IT CAN BE A JOY TO OTHER NURSE-MIDWIVES ALSO, IF THEY WOULD JUST TRY IT.

In the Washington, D.C., area, as in many other communities around the country, a significant number of expectant parents each year are seeking alternatives to hospital deliveries. Many of these parents want a childbirth experience that is safe, but also family-centered, and more important, personally meaningful. We see maternity home as another excellent alternative by providing technical facilities of the hospital with a very flexible home-like atmosphere.

Two specific examples of a maternity home setting come into mind, and those are the Booth Maternity Hospital in Philadelphia (see Chapter 8, Vol. 1) and the Maternity Center Association in New York (see Chapter 21, Vol. 2), both superior and excellent facilities.

Although changes are occurring in hospital obstetrics, they are not taking place fast enough for most of these couples. Because these couples believe they cannot achieve the experience they want in a hospital, many look to home birth as their only alternative.

We in our service feel that we are successful and safely meeting these needs. We would like to go on record as stating that:

(1) We would like to change the certified nurse-midwife image to that of the nurse-midwife as being flexible and receptive to consumer needs and demands, and

(2) That as nurse-midwives and as professionals, we will assist anyone else who wants to provide this type of care, particularly if there are no other professionals available in the area to meet these needs.

For instance, we would be willing to train other nurse-midwives or lay midwives to assist couples in providing safe home birth services.

I could go on, but perhaps it suffices to say that young parents of today are not only disenchanted with the system, but are creating alternatives for themselves, so that their personal goals of birth, whatever they may be, are achieved. They are taking the responsibilities for these decisions also. Given adequate professional assistance and support, these consumers will help to lead the way to a future in which our national health consciousness is raised to a new level of understanding and action.

CITED REFERENCES

1. J. Am. Col. Nurse-Midwives 20:15, Fall 1975.

2. Stewart, D., and Stewart, L., (eds.) Safe Alternatives in Child-birth, 2nd ed., Chapel Hill, NC: NAPSAC, 1977.

APPENDICES

The following eleven appendices present reduced reproduc-tions of most of our forms and hand-outs for clients. Most are mimeographed and so quality is not super, but it is inexpensive and quite readable. Most are mimeographed onto MCA stationary with our address, phone number, and the names of the midwives and physicians of our service. In addition to the forms shown, we also use two standard prenatal forms. One is the AMA Form (op-65)and the other is AMA-ACOG Prenatal Record Form. The following are shown:

Appendix I	The MCA Contract
Appendix II	New Gynocological Client Form
Appendix III	Prenatal Instructions
Appendix IV	Prenatal Checklist
Appendix V	Labor and Delivery Record
Appendix VI	Postpartum Record
Appendix VII	When to Call the Midwife
Appendix VIII	Our Silver Nitrate Policy
Appendix IX	Sex During Pregnancy
Appendix X	How to Use your Diaphragm Effectively
Appendix XI	Instructions for Emergency Childbirth

APPENDIX I

MATERNITY CENTER ASSOCIATES, LTD.
5415 Cedar Lane
Suite 107-B
Bethesda, Maryland 20014
(301) 530-3300

JANET L. EPSTEIN, R. N., C. N. M.   JAMES D. BREW, JR., M. D.
MARION McCARTNEY, R. N., C. N. M.   L. J. DEVOCHT, M. D.

CONTRACT

In order to ensure optimum safety to mother and infant, the preparation for home birth must be carried out jointly by the staff of the Maternity Center Associates and the home birth client.

Maternity Center Associates will provide:

1. Explanation to each client, and whomever she wishes to include, of all medical records and lab tests throughout her association with this service. (Transfer of copies of records will be available on client's request.)

2. Full explanation of all medications, treatments and tests, including possible side effects, <u>before</u> administering such services to client.

3. Complete medical history, physical screening, and evaluation of each client upon admission to the service.

4. Regular prenatal exams to ensure normal progress during pregnancy.

5. Management of labor and delivery in home if progress meets criteria accepted as normal.

6. Postpartum follow-up of mother and infant at home and in office, including family planning methods agreed upon by client and C.N.M.

Client will:

1. Request complete records from previous doctor for current pregnancy.

2. Provide name of pediatrician who will see infant within 24 hours of birth.

3. Agree to have silver nitrate used in infant's eyes.

4. Agree to transfer mother and/or infant to hospital if progress in labor is not within normal limits as defined by C.N.M.

5. Agree to consult with specialists during pregnancy for medical problems.

6. Provide maps to home.

7. Agree to purchase necessary supplies and equipment.

APPENDIX II

MATERNITY CENTER ASSOCIATES, LTD.
5415 Cedar Lane
Suite 107-B
Bethesda, Maryland 20014
(301) 530-3300

JANET L. EPSTEIN, R. N., C. N. M.
MARION McCARTNEY, R. N., C. N. M.

JAMES D. BREW, JR., M. D.
L. J. DEVOCHT, M. D.

NEW GYNECOLOGY CLIENT

Name	Age	Race	Religion	Occupation
		M	S W D S	
Home Address			Marital Status	Education
Home Telephone	Height	Weight	B/P Blood Type	Allergies
Business Address		Business Telephone		Type of Diet

FAMILY HISTORY

(Hypertension, Cancer, Diabetes, Heart Disease)

Mother: Brother(s):

Father: Sister(s):

CLIENT'S MEDICAL HISTORY

EENT: _____   G. I.: _____

Cardiac: _____   G. U.: _____

Pulmonary: _____   Endocrine: _____

Skin: _____   Neuro-Psych.: _____

Previous Surgery: _____

GYNECOLOGY HISTORY

Menarche	Length of Cycle	Number of Days	Amount	Pain
LMP		Hx Gyn Disorders and/or Sexual Problems		
Previous Pregnancies (Gravida, Para, Abortion, Primi)			Complications	
Birth Control (Type, Dates)				
Last Gyne Exam		Last Pap Smear and Result		Last G. C. Culture

(over)

Reverse Side

NEW GYNECOLOGY CLIENT

Reason for Visit:

PHYSICAL EXAM

Eyes: _____   Teeth: _____   Thyroid: _____   Throat: _____   Skin: _____

Heart and Lungs: _____

Breasts: _____

Abdomen: _____   Extremities: _____

General Body Type: _____

PELVIC EXAM

Vulva: _____

Vagina: _____

Perineum: _____

Cervix: _____

Uterus: _____

Adnexa: _____

Recto-Vaginal: _____

Impression:

Rx:

Signed: _____ Date: _____

APPENDIX III

MATERNITY CENTER ASSOCIATES, LTD.
5415 CEDAR LANE
SUITE 107-B
BETHESDA, MARYLAND 20014

(301) 530-3300

JANET L. EPSTEIN, C. N. M.
MARION McCARTNEY, C. N. M.

JAMES D. BREW, JR., M. D.
L. J. DeVOGHT, M. D.

PRENATAL INSTRUCTIONS

SUPPLIES NEEDED FOR MOTHER & DELIVERY:

* A stiff bed is best - put a piece of plywood under mattress
  if necessary.
* Cover your mattress with a plastic cover or inexpensive shower
  curtain; cover pillows also if desired.
* Small pile of newspapers.
* Plastic-lined trash receptacle.
* Glad or Giant brand plastic 18 qt. bags
* Bowl with a rounded bottom for the placenta
* Roll of paper towels
* Two dozen 4" X 4" gauze pads
* One bottle Zepherine Chloride 1:750
* One Fleet enema
* Chux bed pads (Sears or Wards underpads are less expensive,
  but must be ordered from catalog. Takes 2 weeks or so.)
* 2 oz. ear syringe
* Scissors
* White shoestrings
* Three maps with directions to place of birth. Include name &
  phone number, landmarks, etc.
* A place for the nurse-midwife to sit and/or lie down for rest
* Clean towels and washcloths
* Sanitary belt
* Hospital-size sanitary napkins
* Clean gown or pajamas

SUPPLIES NEEDED FOR THE INFANT:

* One or two old receiving blankets
* Infant's hair brush
* Diapers, pins, shirt and gown or kimono
* Clean blankets
* Rectal thermometer
* Cotton balls
* Alcohol
* Scales (Bathroom scale may be used)
* Tape measure (optional)
* Clean towels and washcloths
* Bed for baby

WHEN LABOR BEGINS: Call 530-3300 (office or answering service).

Appendix III Cont'd

MATERNITY CENTER ASSOCIATES, LTD.
5415 CEDAR LANE
SUITE 107-B
BETHESDA, MARYLAND 20014

(301) 530-3300

JANET L. EPSTEIN, C. N. M.   (Page 2)   JAMES D. BREW, JR., M. D.
MARION McCARTNEY, C. N. M.   L. J. DEVOCHT, M. D.

GENERAL PRENATAL INSTRUCTIONS

Check with the midwife a few weeks prior to your delivery date and she will give you instructions regarding prenatal home visit and when she is to be notified.

It is wise to pre-register and tour the hospital you would use as an alternative to home birth. Also, pack a bag for both mother & baby in case hospitalization is necessary.

Select a pediatrician who will agree to see your baby within 24 hours of birth either at your home or in his office. Give the pediatrician's name and telephone number to the nurse-midwife two weeks prior to delivery date.

Have all supplies ready three weeks before delivery date.

Take classes in Preparation for Childbirth (these classes are usually six weeks long and fill up early, so register by your fifth month or so).

Make up a delivery bed as follows:

    A. Cover for mattress, if desired
    B. Clean fitted sheet
    C. Plastic mattress cover or shower curtain
    D. Clean fitted sheet

After delivery, top fitted sheet and plastic mattress cover are removed and clean fitted sheet is readily available on bed.

The nurse-midwife will complete and sign your baby's birth certificate and mail it to the proper authorities. They will then send you information on obtaining copies.

ANY QUESTIONS? CALL THE OFFICE AT 530-3300. Office hours are Monday and Thursday from 9:00 a.m. to 3:00 p.m. and Tuesday from 5:00 to 10:00 p.m.

APPENDIX IV

MATERNITY CENTER ASSOCIATES

* PRENATAL CHECKLIST

ALL ITEMS must be checked off by 37 weeks for all home deliveries.

___ 1. I know my blood type, which is _____.

___ 2. Taking childbirth preparation classes
          with
          _____.

___ 3. Attending H.O.M.E. series.

___ 4. My birth assistant is _____
          _____.

___ 5. I'm pre-registered & have toured at
          _____ hospital.

___ 6. Read Emergency Childbirth by White and
          the emergency packet MCA gave us.

___ 7. Familiar with infant resuscitation
          techniques.

___ 8. Pediatrician:_____.
          Note: Home visit ___;or office visit ___.

___ 9. Midwives' 37-week double check.

___ 10. All supplies ready and set-up.

___ 11. Three maps have been distributed to my home.

___ 12. My bill is paid up, and/or insurance forms
          filled out, signed, and turned in to office.

APPENDIX V

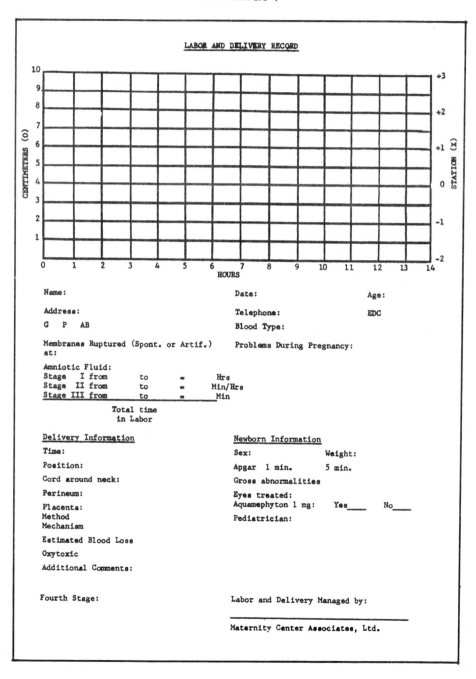

LABOR AND DELIVERY RECORD

Name: Date: Age:

Address: Telephone: EDC

G   P   AB   Blood Type:

Membranes Ruptured (Spont. or Artif.)   Problems During Pregnancy:
at:

Amniotic Fluid:
Stage I from   to   =   Hrs
Stage II from   to   =   Min/Hrs
Stage III from   to   =   Min
            Total time
            in Labor

Delivery Information   Newborn Information

Time: Sex: Weight:

Position: Apgar 1 min.   5 min.

Cord around neck: Gross abnormalities

Perineum: Eyes treated:
Placenta: Aquamephyton 1 mg: Yes____   No____
Method
Mechanism   Pediatrician:

Estimated Blood Loss

Oxytoxic

Additional Comments:

Fourth Stage: Labor and Delivery Managed by:

                                   _____

                                   Maternity Center Associates, Ltd.

APPENDIX VI

POSTPARTUM

Physical:

Weeks: _____

Wt. and B/P: _____

Bleeding: _____

Breasts and Nipples: _____

Abdomen: _____
     Muscle Tone   Fundus

Pelvic:

  Vulva: _____

  Vagina: _____

  Perineum: _____

  Cervix: _____

  Uterus: _____

  Adnexa: _____

  Recto-Vaginal: _____

Impression:

Rx:

Emotional:

Sleep: _____

Problems: _____

Infant Feeding: _____

_____

Birth Control Plan: _____
               None

Pill   IUD   Diaphragm

Foam   Condom   Rhythm

     Sterilization - Type

Signed: _____ Date:_____

POSTPARTUM

Physical:

Weeks: _____

Wt. and B/P: _____

Bleeding: _____

Breasts and Nipples: _____

Abdomen: _____
     Muscle Tone   Fundus

Pelvic:

  Vulva: _____

  Vagina: _____

  Perineum: _____

  Cervix: _____

  Uterus: _____

  Adnexa: _____

  Recto-Vaginal: _____

Impression:

Rx:

Emotional:

Sleep: _____

Problems: _____

Infant Feeding: _____

_____

Birth Control Plan: _____
               None

Pill   IUD   Diaphragm

Foam   Condom   Rhythm

     Sterilization - Type

Signed: _____ Date:_____

APPENDIX VII

MATERNITY CENTER ASSOCIATES, LTD.
5415 CEDAR LANE
SUITE 107-B
BETHESDA, MARYLAND 20014

JANET L. EPSTEIN, C. N. M.   (301) 530-3300   JAMES D. BREW, JR., M. D.
MARION McCARTNEY, C. N. M.   L. J. DeVOCHT, M. D.

WHEN TO CALL THE MIDWIFE - PREGNANCY

In general, we expect couples to use good judgment about when
to call with problems. The following is a list of guidelines
to help you decide if the situation is critical or can wait
until morning or until office hours. Naturally, all circumstances cannot be covered here, so if you're in doubt, please call.
It is better to be a little over-cautious than to always assume
it will be O.K.

1. If your membranes (bag of water) rupture prematurely
   (before 37 weeks) or if the fluid is green or yellow
   colored, call immediately. If they rupture after 37
   weeks, you may wait until morning if there are no contractions starting. If you are having contractions,
   call immediately.

2. Persistent headaches can be a sign of high blood pressure. If the headaches are not relieved by Tylenol
   or if you have been running increased blook pressure,
   call in the day time or evening.

3. Any bright red bleeding before 37 weeks should be reported immediately. Bloody show at term is sometimes
   difficult to distinguish from bleeding. Show is
   usually mucousy and less than a normal menstrual period.

4. If you have burning during urination and an increased
   frequency, it is probably a bladder infection - please
   try to call during the day time or evening; it's difficult to call in a prescription to a drug store after
   10 P.M.

5. If you have either a gastro-intestinal (or vomiting
   and diarrhea) virus or severe upper respiratory virus
   (coughing, runny nose, earache) or are running a fever,
   try to call during our day time or evening hours (see
   above reason)

6. As soon as you have regular uterine contractions and/or
   bloody show and/or ruptured membranes, call the answering
   service to notify the midwives.

APPENDIX VIII

MATERNITY CENTER ASSOCIATES, LTD.
8415 CEDAR LANE
SUITE 107-B
BETHESDA, MARYLAND 20014

JANET L. EPSTEIN, C. N. M.
MARION McCARTNEY, C. N. M.

(301) 530-3300

JAMES D. BREW, JR., M. D.
L. J. DeVOCHT, M. D.

SILVER NITRATE

Q. Why must silver nitrate be used in the baby's eyes after birth?

A. 1% solution of silver nitrate is the recommended prophylactic treatment for prevention of gonorrheal opthalmia (blindness due to gonorrheal infection contracted from the mother's birth canal) in newborns. In Maryland, Virginia and the District of Columbia, it is the law and a nurse-midwife can lose her license for failure to treat the newborn.

Q. Why not test the mother for gonorrhea and only treat those babies who need it?

A. Two reasons:

1. Although testing is available, results are unreliable. Both the method of obtaining the cultures and failure to incubate the cultures immediately (lack of facilities) result in many false negatives (the mother has gonorrhea but it does not show up on the culture).

2. Gonorrhea can be contracted at any time by the pregnant woman or her partner before delivery. The nurse-midwife cannot be responsible for deciding who may or may not have been exposed to gonorrhea. (Think about that for a moment, please.)

Q. Why not use penicillin argerol or tetracycline which appear to be less irritating?

A. The American Academy of Pediatrics' most recent statement on this subject is in support of using silver nitrate (it is supposed to be the most effective). They believe that the side effects are less of a disadvantage than missing a case of gonorrheal opthalmia by using a less potent drug. The laws here specify that silver nitrate must be used; no other substitute is acceptable.

Q. What about the damage to the infant's eyes:

A. A chemical conjunctivitis (redness, swelling, and/or discharge) can develop after using silver nitrate. These symptoms are temporary--permanent damage does not result.

Q. Does using silver nitrate interfere with bonding between the mother and infant right after birth?

A. We feel it does and in our practice we wait one hour after birth before using silver nitrate. We find that the babies do not cry if they have first had a chance to look around and to nurse before we treat their eyes.

APPENDIX IX

MATERNITY CENTER ASSOCIATES, LTD.
5415 CEDAR LANE
SUITE 107-B
BETHESDA, MARYLAND 20014
—
(301) 530-3390

JANET L. EPSTEIN, C. N. M.
MARION McCARTNEY, C. N. M.

JAMES D. BREW, JR., M. D.
L. J. DEVOCHT, M. D.

SEX DURING PREGNANCY

Enjoyment of sex during pregnancy is a healthy, satisfying part of a couple's total relationship. Intercourse is not dangerous to mother or baby and there is no medical need to restrict sex, except for a few specific instances. Female orgasm during late pregnancy will cause uterine contractions which are harmless to the baby and will not cause premature labor. (If orgasm did cause labor, induction of labor would be a simple fun procedure!) Different positions for intercourse will need to be used as the woman's abdomen enlarges. Any position which is comfortable is safe. Increased or decreased desire in women are both normal.

Under the following conditions, intercourse should be avoided:

1. After the membranes (bag of water) have ruptured - there is danger of infection then. (Also tub baths and douches are dangerous at this time.)

2. When bleeding or premature contractions occur.

3. Women who have repeated miscarriages (more than 2) should avoid intercourse during the time when they usually miscarry.

4. No intercourse before the midwife has left the room, after the baby is delivered.

The only sexual activity which has been documented as dangerous is blowing air into the vagina of a pregnant woman. This can detach the placenta from the uterine wall and cause an air embolism.

If you have questions or wish to discuss sex with the midwives, please feel free. We welcome your questions.

APPENDIX X

MATERNITY CENTER ASSOCIATES, LTD.
5415 CEDAR LANE
SUITE 107-B
BETHESDA, MARYLAND 20014
—
(301) 530-3380

JANET L. EPSTEIN, C. N. M.
MARION McCARTNEY, C. N. M.

JAMES D. BREW, Jr., M. D.
L. J. DeVOGHT, M. D.

HOW TO USE YOUR DIAPHRAGM EFFECTIVELY

1. The diaphragm and jelly or cream must be in place when you have intercourse. You may insert the diaphragm ahead of time, but if it has been in for more than two hours, use the applicator to insert extra jelly or cream.

2. Use about a teaspoonful of jelly or cream inside the dome of the diaphragm. Smear a little on the outside, and a little around the rim. Jelly and cream are equally effective, but jelly offers a little more lubrication.

3. With one hand, spread the lips of your vagina. Squat or raise one leg as you insert the diaphragm, slanting it toward the small of your back, and tuck it behind your pubic bone. Reach up and feel your cervix through the diaphragm -- make sure it's in place.

4. Practice inserting the diaphragm daily until you feel comfortable doing it, and are sure it fits well. During this "practice" period, don't depend on the diaphragm for contraception. Use something else or abstain until you are sure that you and the diaphragm are compatible!

5. The diaphragm must stay in place for 6 to 8 hours after intercourse. If you make love during that time, use the applicator to insert more jelly. This can get messy and you may switch to a condom, but

6. DO NOT REMOVE THE DIAPHRAGM FOR AT LEAST SIX HOURS AFTER LAST INTERCOURSE. If it feels uncomfortable, make an appointment to have the size re-checked. If you feel slimy, insert a tampon. Don't douche or slosh bath water into your vagina -- the sperm must be exposed to the jelly for a full six hours.

7. Remove the diaphragm by hooking your finger under the rim and pulling it out. Wash it with plain soap and water, dry, and dust it with cornstarch (NOT talcum). Keep it in the container. Do not use vaseline on the diaphragm -- the plastic will rot.

Appendix X Cont'd

MATERNITY CENTER ASSOCIATES, LTD.
5415 CEDAR LANE
SUITE 107-B
BETHESDA, MARYLAND 20014

JANET L. EPSTEIN, C. N. M.
MARION McCARTNEY, C. N. M.

(301) 530-3300

JAMES D. BREW, JR., M. D.
L. J. DeVOSHT, M. D.

(Page 2)

HOW TO USE YOUR DIAPHRAGM EFFECTIVELY

REMEMBER

The purpose of the diaphragm is to hold the spermicide close to the cervix. The diaphragm is useless without jelly or cream. Also, the fit of the diaphragm is important. If it is too small, it will slide out of place. If it is too big, it will be uncomfortable for you. HAVE YOUR SIZE RE-CHECKED EVERY YEAR. Also, every time you have a baby, whenever you have surgery in the genital area, or if you gain or lose as much as fifteen pounds.

You or your partner may develop an allergic reaction to the jelly or cream you use. Solution: Switch brands.

Either partner may insert the diaphragm . . . one couple's nuisance is another couple's foreplay.

CAUTION

Multiple intercourse may lessen the effectiveness of the diaphragm -- added jelly makes it slide around. As stated above, condoms may be prudent.

When the woman is on top, there is an increased chance that the penis may be inserted on the wrong side of the diaphragm. Watch it.

APPENDIX XI

EMERGENCY CHILDBIRTH

The information and directions included here are meant to aid anyone who needs help delivering a medically unattended home birth. It serves only as a general guide until help arrives. A fast labor can make the mother ready to deliver before the nurse-midwife or birth assistant arrive. In these cases, please summon help -- even a next door neighbor can place phone calls while the father or coach aids with the delivery. The rescue squads in the Washington Metro Area will arrive quickly with oxygen and a delivery pack to assist you. The number is 911. If you have called one nurse-midwife and she is on the way and birth seems imminent, call the other one for further advice on how to manage until help arrives.

Again, this package is not a "do it yourself" delivery guide. Its purpose is to give simple, clear instructions to follow while waiting for medical assistance. It only covers the most general course of events and cannot explain specific techniques for every type of delivery.

Read this package thoroughly and ask questions about it during your prenatal care.

Head Presentation

If the nurse-midwife has not arrived and the baby's head is visible at the vagina:

1. Call the Rescue Squad - 911.

2. Have the mother lie down and pant with each contraction.

3. Deliver the head slowly. It is preferable to have the mother push the head out gently between contractions.

4. When the head is out, check with your fingers to see if the cord is around the neck. Loosen it gently, either by pulling it over the baby's head or loosening it so the baby can deliver through it.

5. The head will then turn toward the mother's left or right. The mother should then push with the next contraction to deliver the shoulders. The top shoulder first (depress the baby's head toward the bed), then the bottom shoulder (lift the head toward the ceiling).

6. Put the baby on the mother's abdomen and cover them both.

Appendix XI Cont'd

Page 2

EMERGENCY CHILDBIRTH

Breech Presentation

If the feet or buttocks appear at the vagina first,

1. Call the Rescue Squad - 911. You must attempt to deliver in the hospital. Do not wait for the midwife.

2. Lie the mother in bed. Do not pull on the body or feet of the baby.

3. If the baby delivers spontaneously up to the shoulders, cover the body with blankets as it delivers. The mother should push with each contraction. It is imperative that she do so.

4. Gently pull down a loop of cord to prevent tension on the navel.

5. If the arms do not deliver spontaneously, reach up for the hands, one at a time and sweep them down over the face.

6. The body will turn to one side and the shoulders will deliver, the top, followed by the bottom.

7. The head is ready to deliver when the back is up (toward the ceiling). Put 2 fingers in the vagina below the head and press the vagina -- make enough room for the baby to breathe. Have the mother push until the face starts to deliver. Then she should pant and the back of the head can be delivered slowly.

Prolapsed Cord

If the membranes rupture and a loop of umbilical cord washes out with the fluid:

1. Put the mother in the knee-chest position.

2. Call the Rescue Squad - 911. The baby's oxygen supply is being cut off.

3. If the cord is still protruding in the knee-chest position, cover it with warm wet gauze pads.

4. Keep the mother in the knee-chest position even during the trip to the hospital -- it reduces the pressure on the cord.

5. Give the mother O_2 in the ambulance.

Appendix XI Cont'd

Page <u>3</u>

EMERGENCY CHILDBIRTH

Transverse Lie

If the membranes rupture and the hand presents first, <u>call the midwife
immediately</u>.

Post-Partum Hemorrhage

If a steady stream of blood (or a continuous gush) starts from the vagina,
call the Rescue Squad - 911.

1. Deliver the placenta. Have the mother bear down <u>hard</u>, and
   put gentle traction on the cord. Put the placenta up next to
   the baby. Watch that the cord does not pull on the baby's navel.

2. Massage the uterus <u>firmly</u>. Push down 2 or 3 inches below the
   mother's navel and rub firmly in a <u>deep circular motion</u>. This
   causes blood to gush out of the vagina. It helps the uterus to
   contract. <u>Keep it up</u> until help arrives. This is painful for the
   mother, but is absolutely necessary to prevent severe hemorrhage.

Care of Newborn Delivered without Medical Assistance

1. Put the baby on the mother's naked abdomen. Don't cut the cord.
   Do not let the cord pull on the baby's navel.

2. Dry the baby with blankets and cover him/her - especially dry the
   head to prevent heat loss.

3. If the baby is not crying or breathing, keep it covered with 2 or
   3 blankets and have someone call the Rescue Squad - 911.

4. Suction the nose and mouth with the bulb syringe to clear airway.

5. Tip the head back to straighten the neck and open airway.

6. Feel for a heart beat. If there is none, begin Cardio-Pulmonary
   Resuscitation.

7. Rub abdomen or soles of feet briskly to stimulate crying.

8. If the baby does not breathe in one minute, begin mouth-to-mouth
   resuscitation.

CHAPTER TWENTY THREE

THE AMERICAN COLLEGE OF HOME OBSTETRICS (ACHO):
PHILOSOPHY & PRACTICE OF PHYSICIANS IN HOMEBIRTH

Gregory White, M.D.
Mayer Eisenstein, M.D.

Dr. White

I think that all of us agree with the American College of Obstetricians and Gynecologists (ACOG) that safety is important (see Chapters 3 and 5, Vol. 1). I think most of us disagree that it can only be found in a hospital. I'm very saddened to see such a sizeable segment of our profession (i.e. ACOG), and such an important segment, progressing in a direction one hundred and eighty degrees away from the direction in which the parents are progressing. The chasm between them seems to get wider all the time.

For lack of professional attendants who will come to the home, the parents are going it alone. I don't think this is ideal. It may be because of my upbringing that I have the belief that having a skilled attendant at childbirth can make it safer for mother and baby. I think this safety is important and must never be taken for granted.

Now, there's no question but what an attendant, who is skilled but who is drunk with technology, can make it less safe. Those of us who are attending births, home or hospital, have to watch ourselves.

I'm reminded of one of the members of the American College of Home Obstetrics, who ruefully, and with a grin at his own idiocy, tells how, for his first home delivery, he carried a hospital delivery table into the home. He thought that this was one of the pieces of equipment that he couldn't very well do without. He has since learned that a bed is a very good place to deliver a baby. Some home birth physicians have, for reasons that are obscure to me, chosen to use either the kitchen or dining room table.

GREGORY WHITE is President, American College of Home Obstetrics; Founding Father, La Leche League International; and Author of book, Emergency Childbirth.

MAYER EISENSTEIN is Vice President, American College of Home Obstetrics; Author of "Home Births and the Physician;" and Co-Producer of movie, "Primum Non Nocere."

THERE IS NO QUESTION BUT WHAT A BIRTH ATTENDANT, WHO IS SKILLED, BUT DRUNK WITH TECHNOLOGY, CAN MAKE A HOMEBIRTH LESS SAFE THAN NO ATTENDANT AT ALL. FOR LACK OF QUALIFIED ATTENDANTS, SOME PARENTS ARE GOING IT ALONE; I DON'T THINK THIS IS IDEAL.

One of my old teachers told the story of a birth that he attended in Chicago Maternity Center. He was the senior man. He had been on the service three weeks. They came into the house and this woman, who was quite large, was crowning. The room was a little odd. It was behind a shop where the couple made their living, and in the long, narrow room in which they lived, they were supplementing their income by raising canaries and gold fish. They had a lot of aquariums and a lot of bird cages along the two sides of the room.

The senior man decided he had better wash his hands quickly, and he did. He instructed the junior, as was the custom at that time, to tie a couple of towels to the legs of the table. He meant, of course, the top of the legs so that the mother would have something to pull on when she was bearing down. In the middle of his scrub, he heard a loud crash, and he turned around. The new student had tied the towels to the bottom of the legs of the table, and the mother had given one tremendous heave and pulled the legs off the table. At this point, she had to grab for something, because she felt herself sliding to the floor; so she reached out her arms in both directions and tipped over a bunch of bird cages on the one hand, aquariums on the other hand. The baby was born immediately on the floor amidst flopping gold fish while canaries circled wildly overhead. Believe it or not, this is a true story.

If the American College of Obstetricians and Gynecologists should ever invite any of us to come, I won't tell them that story. It is not really typical of home births. In Chicago we've been developing along a different line.

About twenty-five years ago my wife and I, after three hospital deliveries, decided we wanted to have our baby at home. We were able to persuade our family doctor to help us out. We had our fourth baby at home. We had all the subsequent babies at home.

Some of my wife's friends who were patients of mine started asking me if I would deliver them at home. I agreed. The thing slowly built through the years. I have always delivered somewhere between 100-120 babies a year. About five years ago I was doing about 50% home deliveries. Now, it is up to about 80-90%.

I am no longer as lonesome as I used to be. Things have been expanding a little in Chicago, thank God. I dare say we are not generally accepted by our professional colleagues in doing home deliveries, but Dr. Eisenstein has been doing home deliveries for about five years now. I am proud to have had a part in training him. My son, Dr. William White, has been doing home deliveries for almost two years. I am proud to have a part in training him, too, although I have to give his mother most of the credit. But there are others. Dr. Fred Ettner is newly started in practice. Dr. Eisenstein has contributed a great deal to his training. We have also had a number of other physicians who are interested, but not yet committed. My oldest son, Joseph, has been with us on a number of home deliveries. We have had residents, mostly family practice residents (not, unfortunately, obstetric residents) go with us on home deliveries. Interns have gone with us; medical students have gone with us. Currently we have about four that are interested in going out to see home deliveries, and we are trying to accommodate them all.

We usually don't have a nurse with us, although certainly nurses and nurse-midwives have been welcomed to come with us when they have requested it. We usually go it alone, with perhaps a medical student or a fellow physician or a resident helping us.

The important thing, of course, is to try to restrain oneself from interfering in a way that would either decrease safety or decrease joy and the full participation of the couple who are "doing their thing." I have had more problem with this than the younger men, because I had some obstetric training. I think on the whole we have been pretty successful in avoiding any unnecessary interferences. But I still think that a professional attendant who knows what he or she is doing, and who is willing to sort of fade into the wallpaper and let the couple do their thing, as long as everything is going well, is still the ideal for delivery at home or anywhere else.

 I AM SADDENED TO SEE THE ACOG PROGRESSING IN A DIRECTION 180° AWAY FROM THE DIRECTION IN WHICH THE PARENTS ARE PROGRESSING.

Quite recently, in the last two years, we have been working on papers and arrangements and organization and so forth. On May 10, 1977, we had the first national meeting of the American College of Home Obstetrics. We were gratified by an attendance of a number of interested physicians. We expect our membership to grow. Below is a very brief statement of purpose of the organization, which will give you some idea of what we are trying to do.

The American College of Home Obstetrics

The American College of Home Obstetrics has been founded to gather together those physicians who wish to cooperate with families who choose to give birth in the home, the natural and traditional place for birth throughout the world and the ages. We also wish to learn from and teach each other the art of the safe supervision of home births.

Members and fellows are guided by an awareness that pregnancy, labor, and delivery are normal, physiological processes, not pathological events. We rely on these natural processes whenever feasible, reserving operative intervention of any kind or magnitude and the giving of medications for those cases where there is probability of damage to mother or baby without such intervention.

We take our ethic from the Hippocratic Oath and World Medical Society Declaration at Geneva in 1948.

We try to foster not only the welfare of our patients, mother and baby, but that of the entire family.

That explains what we are trying to do. I was going to give you what might be my view of the future of home birth in this country. The other speakers at the 1977 NAPSAC Conference, the authors of this book, have already said it.

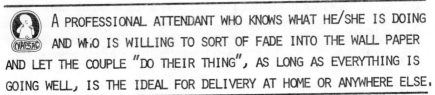

A PROFESSIONAL ATTENDANT WHO KNOWS WHAT HE/SHE IS DOING AND WHO IS WILLING TO SORT OF FADE INTO THE WALL PAPER AND LET THE COUPLE "DO THEIR THING", AS LONG AS EVERYTHING IS GOING WELL, IS THE IDEAL FOR DELIVERY AT HOME OR ANYWHERE ELSE.

Dr. Eisenstein

The first NAPSAC Conference in Washington, May, 1976, was really historical in many senses. Not only was it, in my mind, the beginning of the total rebirth of home birth in America -- it had some very interesting features.

My wife and I happened to be in New Orleans a day before the meeting. Dr. Gregory White, who was scheduled to speak at that Conference, called me up and said that a very dear friend of the family was expecting her baby any day, and he wouldn't be able to attend. Could I please come and speak in his stead?

The morning before I left for Washington I went to Cafe LeMans, which is a very famous restaurant in New Orleans. He had sent me a ten-page speech. I spent four hours writing and preparing for the speech. Then I came to Washington. I was about the fifth speaker, and everyone had said everything that I had written over those four hours. So, I figured this year I would be smarter. Since I was speaking on the second day, what I figured I would do, is not write anything until the wee morning hours before the speech.

Well, lo and behold, you see what's happened this morning. I have very, very little in a sense to add to all the excellence which I have heard this morning. So, instead of adding, I will do what I have become very famous for in the last months, and that is to be a critic. I have always tried to become an advocate, and yet everyone calls on me to become a critic.

Yesterday I received a letter from the American Sociologic Association, and they said to me, "Dr. Eisenstein, can you please attend our meeting in Chicago in September? And what we would like you to do is not present any of your work, but there are five doctors who are going to be talking before you. Can you read their papers and criticize everything that they have to say? We know you are very provocative, and the audience won't fall asleep while you are criticizing."

Well, here I go again. If you noticed me scribbling on this little yellow pad of paper, it was criticism of everything that has preceded me.

I will start first with Betty Hosford (see Chapter 21, Vol. 2). You call yourself lazy. Well, we need hundreds and hundreds of lazy people like you in this country.

We had an absolutely interesting discussion at the American College of Home Obstetrics Meeting. One doctor who came there, Dr. Brown, had been doing home births for about forty years. He trained in an institution, Rush Medical School, which closed down, he said, the year after he graduated. I understand very well, because they knew what he was about to do. Anyway, Rush Medical School was named after Benjamin Rush. Benjamin Rush was one of the signers of the Declaration of Independence. He was a physician, and his name absolutely typified the type of medicine that he practiced, and the type of medicine that has been in America for 200 years -- "rush" type of medicine. It is interesting, the physician, midwife, or medical attendant who gets the credit in our country, for birth or anything, is the one who rushes in and quickly performs some procedure. The lazy people, and I like to include myself in that, are the ones who are criticized for not wanting to do anything. But the attitude of "non-interference" is what we need to get back to and to get away from "rush medicine." This change will come about.

All right. My next criticism. Janet Epstein (see Chapter 22, Vol. 2), you said that you call your mothers "clients." Rhetoric to me doesn't make a difference, because we may use different words, but we all mean the same thing. I call them couples. Some people call them patients.

You said you give them alternatives. I listened to you for forty-five minutes. I saw no alternatives. Do you give your women drugs during pregnancy? Of course not. There is no safe alternative to that. Do you give them drugs during labor? Do you shave their perineums? Do you give them enemas? Do you give them IV fluids? Episiotomies? Stirrups? Do you encourage them to bottle feed? Of course not. You give them no alternatives.

Now that we are on alternatives, I want to criticize my good friend, Jay Hathaway, I hope you are here. You showed a movie last night that was absolutely beautiful. It lasted an hour and a half, and it was called "Alternative Childbirth" (available from Jay Hathaway Productions, 4846 Katherine Ave., Sherman Oaks, CA 91423, phone: (213) 788-6662). Thirty seconds of the film showed a horrendous medicated, spinal block, forceps delivery, and then for one hour and forty-four and a half minutes, he showed beautiful births. No alternatives, Jay!

 THERE IS ONLY ONE REASON WHY I ATTEND BIRTH AT HOME. I DON'T DO IT BECAUSE OF THE PSYCHOLOGICAL ASPECTS, ALTHOUGH THEY ARE EXTREMELY IMPORTANT & I BELIEVE THEY ARE TRUE. THE ONLY REASON I ATTEND BIRTH AT HOME IS BECAUSE IT IS MEDICALLY SAFER.

That's enough criticism. Now, we will go onto one of my functions in the American College of Home Obstetrics. As part of my training as a statistician, I have been keeping records of the births that Dr. Gregory White, Dr. William White, and myself have attended. Last year we attended approximately 300 home births. I want to, in capsule form, give you some of our findings so far.

1976 Statistics
on the White-Eisenstein Homebirth Practice
Chicago, Illinois
Total Births = 300

---

* Our cesarean section rate has been 2%.
* Our transfer to the hospital from the home, 4%.
* Our incidence of prematurity, 2.5%.
* Our incidence of episiotomy, 2%.
* And this was all accomplished with 50% first-time mothers.

Commentary on a Film Illustrating "Non-interventive" Obstetrics

I am going to show you a short film, which will last about four and a half minutes. I was very moved at NAPSAC in Washington in 1976. We showed a couple of short films, and afterwards Doris Haire came up to me and said, "Mayer, that is the first time I have ever seen a baby delivered -- a baby caught is maybe the more proper way to term it -- without the attendant pulling on the baby's head." This moved me so much, and the correspondence that I received over the year from attendants all around the country who said, "Mayer, you are right. We don't have to pull on the head when it comes normally."

There are three or four things you see in this short film segment. This is a first time mother. She will be in the pushing stage of labor. As the baby is being born, the cord will be around the neck. (Incidentally, Dr. White took very little credit. I have to criticize him also. He didn't partially train me; he completely trained me.)

I want you to observe -- the cord is around the baby's neck. One of the principles that Dr. White has taught me is that the attendant's role is never to interfere in the normal birth. The cord around the neck occurs approximately 10% of the time. If it is loose, there is no reason that you have to go cutting the cord immediately, robbing the baby of additional supply of blood.

THE CORD AROUND THE NECK OCCURS APPROXIMATELY 10% OF THE TIME. IT IT IS LOOSE, THERE IS NO REASON TO GO CUTTING THE CORD IMMEDIATELY, ROBBING THE BABY OF ADDITIONAL SUPPLY OF BLOOD.

Secondly, you will see there will be no pulling on the baby's head.

Thirdly, there will be no suctioning of the baby after it is born. Routine suction is wrong. It is absolutely wrong. Suctioning is the first means of resuscitation. And a baby that cries spontaneously does not need to be suctioned or resuscitated. Also, we have found that colostrum, the first nourishment produced by a new mother's breast, has an enzymatic effect to break down the mucous in the baby's digestive tract. When the actual milk comes in, in about two days or so, there is no mucous left, and the passageways are perfectly prepared for mother's milk. So no suctioning was needed. Furthermore, the mucous may serve an important function for the baby. It has been shown that newborns have a tendency, occasionally, to forget how to breathe. They just stop. The mucous is a little bit irritating and will cause them to cough and spit a little bit. Hence, they will start breathing again. So, in the normal birth, no suctioning, please.

Fourthly, no pulling on the placenta. We try to make this point extremely carefully. I am so pleased that I have seen so many films in the last couple of days which show births with medical attendants not pulling on the placenta.

THERE SHOULD BE NO SUCTIONING OF THE BABY AFTER IT IS BORN. ROUTINE SUCTIONING IS WRONG. IT IS ABSOLUTELY WRONG.

(Movie is shown at this point.) Editors' note: Dr. Eisenstein is available with this and other films for talks on home birth. He may be contacted directly (see addresses at end of book) or through NAPSAC.

You never get too old to learn. Last night my wife was talking to me as I was preparing some of the things I was going to say. As we viewed some films of births I attended, she said to me, "Why do you leave the babies so long before they are given to the mother?" And I said to her, "You know what happens in film. It gets out of context. It was only about thirty seconds." She says, "Well, why do you wait the thirty seconds?"

I was having a tough time answering her. Part of my training has been pediatric training, and I have always been very careful to give a complete evaluation of the newborn in the first thirty seconds of life. So, now I will have to sit and reevaluate how valuable is this really? And we are learning. We are learning a lot.

My wife also said to me, "Why do you take the baby away from the mother to cut the cord?" Well, I had to sit and think about that also. All I could say was, "That is the way I have been doing it for years. It may be wrong."

Why I Attend Birth at Home

There is only one reason why I attend birth at home. I don't do it because of the psychological aspects, although they are extremely important and I believe they are true. But the only reason why I attend birth at home is because it is medically safer. Home birth is the time-honored, safe method where birth occurs. Over and over again, on TV and radio, when someone asks me -- the first question I am always asked, "Doctor, do you think it is safe to have a baby at home?" I never answer that any more. My question to them is, "How do you know it is safe to have a baby in the hospital?" David Stewart has gone over this so eloquently (see Safe Alternatives in Childbirth, pp. 1-4). There has never been any study, ever, which has shown the hospital to be a safer place for birth to occur.

Not only has there never been a study to show that the hospital is a safer place, there has only been one major study involving tens of thousands of births comparing home versus hospital birth. It was done in the 1930's in New York, and it was done by the State Department of New York. They evaluated every birth in New York during one year of the '30's. They were having a dreadfully high maternal and infant mortality, and they were trying to blame it on the general practitioners and midwives who were delivering 50% of the babies in New York at home, as opposed to the obstetricians who were delivering the other 50% at the hospital. After one year and about four million dollars of cost, the Commission came to the conclusion that "it was almost as safe to have a baby in the hospital as at home." I want you to know that that was the last comparative study supported by hospital obstetricians. It is understandable why. After four million dollars, they couldn't even prove their point.

OVER AND OVER AGAIN, ON TV AND RADIO, THE FIRST QUESTION I AM ASKED IS "DOCTOR, DO YOU THINK IT IS SAFE TO HAVE A BABY AT HOME?" I NEVER ANSWER THAT ANY MORE. MY QUESTION TO THEM IS, "HOW DO YOU KNOW IT IS SAFE TO HAVE A BABY IN THE HOSPITAL?"

A QUALIFIED MEDICAL ATTENDANT CAN BE A MIDWIFE, GEN-
ERAL PRACTITIONER—POSSIBLY EVEN AN OBSTETRICIAN, BUT
IT IS VERY UNLIKELY THAT HE HAS RECEIVED THE SPECIAL TRAINING
IN THE ART AND SCIENCE OF HOME OBSTETRICS.

Who Should Attend a Birth

I want to speak about the attendants at a birth. And I break
them down into four groups. This is something we have been learning about more and more over the last few years. Those support
people are: (1) the husband, (2) close relatives, (3) friends, and
(4) the medical attendant. I want to speak just few words about each.

My feeling is that the husband is not the primary person at
birth. I have to be very careful when I say that, because people
may think I mean that the husband should not be present. Of course
not. The husband should always be present. But historically the
husband has never been the person who gives the major support to
the laboring woman.

Men, first of all, never have babies. And especially with the
first-time mother, the fathers can be very panicky, and this happens
very frequently. He needs support as well as the laboring woman.
When couples come to us, we encourage over and over again that
they talk either to their mother or mother-in-law and ask them to be
with them at the time of birth. Now this may or may not strike you
as a good idea at first. I can tell you what my response is. My
wife and I thought about this. "How can we ask my mother or
mother-in-law? Who are they? How could they be there?" When I
give talks like this I usually ask people in the crowd, "How many of
you would like to be present when your children have their children?"
I can tell you there won't be one person that doesn't raise their hand.

What we have to do, we have to start this family bonding right
now. (For an example of family bonding, see Chapter 18, Vol. 1.)
We have to start strengthening the family. We have been doing this
for a year and a half. The majority of women have had either their
mother or mother-in-law with them. I have never, never had a bad
experience with a mother or a mother-in-law there. They have always greatly supported the laboring woman, greatly supported their
son or son-in-law, and always made the birth experience really one
of elation. And boy, you should see what happens two years later
when the child is old enough to stay over at the grandmother's house.
That grandmother can't wait. She comes there every day. She cooks
meals.

LABOR IS HARD WORK, BUT THAT DOESN'T MEAN YOU ARE SUP-
POSED TO BE DRUGGED. WHEN MARATHON RUNNERS HIT THAT
26TH MILE, THEY ARE IN EXCRUCIATING PAIN. HAS ANYONE SAID TO
THEM, "LET US GIVE YOU A SPINAL BLOCK TO FINISH THE RACE."

One thing we have to learn is <u>not</u> to split families. We have to learn not to be independent. We have to learn to be dependent. Life is so hard, and we should try to seek as many people as we can to help us.

Equally as important at a birth is to have a close friend or relative, either a cousin, aunt or uncle, preferably a woman who has had a baby before, preferably, if you have it, a woman who has had her baby before at home. This person absolutely can relieve the husband, relieve the mother, and just strengthen the whole tie. Her job can be one of giving support. She has gone through labor, so she knows it is hard.

Labor is hard work. We have to get away from the myth that if you find the right huffing and puffing, it is going to be easy. My wife has said it has never been easy, and I believe her. That doesn't mean you are supposed to be drugged, but it is hard work. The marathon runners, when they hit that twenty-sixth mile, they are in excruciating pain. Has anyone said to them, let's give them a spinal block to finish the race?

Lastly, we come to the medical attendant. My feeling is that the medical attendant can be a midwife, general practitioner, possibly even an obstetrician, but it is very unlikely he has received the special training in the art and science of home obstetrics.

I WOULD DREAD TO SEE MEDICAL ATTENDANTS ATTEND HOME
BIRTH WHO WOULD BRING THE TECHNOLOGIC, HOSPITAL-TYPE
OF THINKING WITH THEM. SUCH THINKING WOULD NOT ONLY BE
PSYCHOLOGICALLY DAMAGING, BUT IT WOULD BE MEDICALLY DAMAGING.

I am going to have to agree very much with Betty Hosford, because I am lazy. That is the reason why I encourage all the other people to be at the birth, because I really only want to do what my job is. My job is not a labor coach. My job is not to give support during labor. My job is not a friend. That doesn't mean that I don't fill all those roles, hopefully. I talk enough when I come to someone's house. I find a hard time sitting in the corner. But I think people have to know, and this is really important, what the role of the medical attendant is.

The medical attendant is the guardian of the birth. He or she is the lifeguard. They must realize that 95% of all births are normal, and in those cases it is the role of the medical attendant not to interfere. Call it lazy. Call it standing aside. Call it sitting on your hands. But above all, they are to not interfere with the normal processes of nature. They must bring skills with them to the birth. They can't be untrained. That puts them in a category of a friend, or relative, or labor support. That is a very important role, but medical attendants have to be skilled. The untrained or poorly trained person does not help the laboring woman in the role of a medical attendant.

There are two skills the medical attendant must bring. He or she must bring the philosophical skills. These are probably the most important. These skills take care of 95% of all births. It is the philosophical attitude that "nature was very wise when she devised this system of reproduction over the thousands and thousands of years." The medical attendant must realize that nature did not intend there to be 99% of women given drugs during labor and delivery, 90% forceps in some places, and 25% cesarean section rates. Some hospitals are even up to 50% cesarean section rates. This is a philosophy that will exclude many medical attendants from attending home births. I would dread to see medical attendants attend home birth who would bring the technologic, hospital type of thinking with them. Such thinking would not only be psychologically damaging but it would be medically damaging.

Secondly, a medical attendant must bring technical skills. This is of extreme importance, because the only reason that one is hired as a medical attendant is not to catch the baby 95% of the time. My teacher, Dr. White, has mentioned in his book, Emergency Childbirth, that an eight-year-old with about three weeks of training could deliver 95% of all the babies in the world. But that does not bring what we are all interested in from a medical attendant, which is a high level of protection of health to both mother and child at the time of birth.

The medical attendant must bring skills to be able to evaluate labor. The only way you obtain this is by training with someone who is very skillful. This person must realize when labor is normal and when it is abnormal. It sounds like such a simple differentiation, but it is the major one. It is the major thing to know that there is something wrong and to decide that, "I need help," or, "I can handle it myself." The medical attendant must be skilled in the diagnoses of problems.

JUST BECAUSE SOMEONE IS AN M.D., A MIDWIFE, OR A NURSE DOES NOT, IN ITSELF, QUALIFY THEM TO BE A HOME BIRTH ATTENDANT. THE HOME BIRTH ATTENDANT'S SKILLS HAVE TO BE FAR HIGHER THAN MOST ANY OTHER SPECIALIST IN MEDICINE.

A medical attendant must also be trained in the resuscitation of the newborn. I am extremely emphatic about that. There is no place for birth attendants who cannot resuscitate newborns. These skills can be available at home. That does not mean that you have to use bulb suction on every baby. It doesn't mean you use a DeLee suction cup or tracheal catheters, but you have to have those skills.

Here again, I agree with Betty Hosford (see Chapter 21, Vol. 2), and I get nervous myself when I mention this, because the amount of times that we use resuscitation techniques are so rare that even a person who starts off very skillful, after five years, you start questioning how much you remember.

Lastly, the medical attendant must be able to use certain drugs to prevent hemorrhage after the baby is born. They must have the skill to know when they are needed, because there are drugs that are valuable. They can make the difference between a woman having a postpartum hemorrhage and just a large bleed.

All these, as I have said before, means that just because someone is an M.D., just because someone is a midwife, just because someone is a nurse, does not in itself qualify them to be a home birth attendant. We feel very strongly that the home birth attendant's skills have to be far, in a way, higher than most probably any other specialist in our medical framework. He or she takes on the ultimate responsibility of saying that, "I am going to make the evaluation. If it is normal, I am not going to interfere. If it is abnormal, I am hopefully going to help bring about a better outcome."

Change in our culture is coming about very rapidly, but it won't be instigated from within the medical profession. It should come about from consumers who will no longer go to birth attendants who do not tell them what they are going to do at the time of birth. I don't think a parent should make a decision if a cesarean section is indicated or not indicated. You hire a medical attendant for that. But I surely think it is important for every parent to ask your attendant, "What is your cesarean section rate?" If he or she says 25%, or more, I would be very leary about going back. If he or she says, "90% of all women who come to me are drugged," I would be very leary about staying there. If he or she says that, "I use forceps 50% of the time," I would be very leary about staying there.

IT IS IMPORTANT FOR EVERY PARENT TO ASK YOUR BIRTH ATTENDANT, "WHAT IS YOUR CESAREAN RATE?" IF HE/SHE SAYS, "25% OR MORE," BE VERY LEARY ABOUT GOING BACK. IF HE/SHE SAYS, "90% OF ALL WOMEN WHO COME TO ME ARE DRUGGED," OR "I USE FORCEPS 50% OF THE TIME," BE VERY LEARY ABOUT STAYING THERE.

Those aren't medical decisions. Those are consumer decisions. Those are the ones that every consumer must be aware of so they can have the highest quality input. Somebody buying a car -- it wouldn't help me at all if I ask them, "Does the carbureator work?" or does this or that work? But I would surely want to know, "How many cars came back to your shop last year? How many broke down on the road? How many tires have flats on them?" That tells me, in a sense, if it is a good car or a bad car.

A meeting like this 1977 NAPSAC Conference could not have taken place five years ago. If it would have, it would have had a handful of people instead of the more than 1000 people here. There wouldn't have been the absolute demand and enthusiasm and energy that has been generated. I think that means that change is really coming.

I just have one last thought about how this change is coming. Last year the American government decided to activate a swine flu program. How many people here had swine flu vaccine? I see about 10%. That means that about 90% of the people in this room decided that the best medical professional advice in this country was wrong.

THERE HAS NEVER BEEN ANY STUDY, EVER, WHICH HAS SHOWN THE HOSPITAL TO BE A SAFER PLACE FOR BIRTH TO OCCUR.

CHAPTER TWENTY FOUR

MATERNAL-INFANT BONDING: THE PROFOUND LONG-TERM BENEFITS OF IMMEDIATE, CONTINUOUS SKIN & EYE CONTACT AT BIRTH

Ruth D. Rice, Ph.D.

Bonding and attachment is a complex phenomenon, but it is possible to determine how affectional bonds between human mothers and their infants are established and to determine what alters or distorts this process temporarily or permanently. Because the human infant is wholly dependent upon his mother or caretaker for all his physical and emotional needs, the strength of these attachment ties may well determine whether he will survive and develop optimally. The actual cellular or chemical process by which the attachment bonds are formed between mother and child is unclear; however, there are seven time periods which are probably crucial in this process. They are: (1) planning the pregnancy, (2) confirming the pregnancy, (3) fetal movement, (4) birth, (5) seeing the baby, (6) touching the baby, and (7) caregiving (Klaus & Kennell, 1970). Since these periods are sequential in development, it may be that until each step has been fully realized, the next sequence cannot be fully developed. The first four time periods will not be discussed in this paper; however, it is felt they are equally important in the development of attachment.

A child born in the U.S. is at considerable risk, physiologically and psychologically. This great and resourceful nation, which should be able to lead the world in saving its young, ranked sixteenth in infant mortality in 1972 when compared with twenty-four other developing countries (United Nations Office of Statistics, February, 1975). The incidence of morbidity is more difficult to evaluate, but there are strong indications it is steadily increasing (Bell, 1971; James and Adamson, 1965; Perloff, 1971). An infant may survive the process of birth and even the adaptation to extrauterine life, but there is no guarantee of optimal or even reasonable health across the developmental life span (Graham, 1968).

RUTH D. RICE is a Psychologist and Family Life Specialist, National Institutes of Marriage and Family Relations; former Research Director, University of Texas; author of many publications on sensory stimulation and infant growth, learning disabilities, early maternal-infant contact, and child abuse.

A CHILD BORN IN THE U.S. IS AT CONSIDERABLE RISK—BOTH PHYSIOLOGICALLY AND PSYCHOLOGICALLY.   THIS GREAT AND RESOURCEFUL NATION, WHICH SHOULD LEAD THE WORLD IN SAVING ITS YOUNG, RANKED 16TH IN INFANT MORTALITY AMONG DEVELOPING COUNTRIES IN 1972.   MORBIDITY IS MORE DIFFICULT TO EVALUATE, BUT THERE ARE STRONG INDICATIONS IT IS STEADILY INCREASING.

There are many factors surrounding birth which may at least be partially responsible for mortality and morbidity. Some of these factors are presently undergoing considerable investigation (Balog, 1976). One such contributory factor may be the separation of mother from her newborn following birth, which hampers or even precludes bonding.

Survival in the extrauterine world necessitates the newborn making the greatest physiological adaptation of his entire life. Nearly all species of mammals maintain a continuous and very close mother-young interaction during this transitional period. But babies born in hospitals in the Western culture are more often than not separated from their mothers immediately after birth.   The result of this postpartum separation has received considerable investigation and research in the past ten years.   The evidence indicates the effects of separation to have profound and long-lasting effects of a detrimental nature on both mother and infant.

The critical or sensitive period following birth, and its effect on both maternal and infant behavior, has long been known in animal studies (Hersher, Richmond and Moore, 1963; Klopfer, Adams and Klopfer, 1964; Moore, 1968). If the animal mother is separated from her young during this period for as short a time as one to four hours, deviant mothering behavior, such as failure to care for her young, often results.   Characteristic and species-specific maternal behavior, such as nesting, retrieving, grooming, and exploring, have been observed in nonmammalian mothers immediately after delivery if the young are not removed (Rheingold, 1963).

Separation of a mother from her young during the first hour or hours after delivery in goat, sheep and cattle, generally results in rejection of the newborn animal when the two are reunited later. If the initial bonding is permitted to develop, separation at a later time does not result in rejection of the newborn animal when the two are reunited. Studies with Rhesus monkeys demonstrated that mothers who were permitted to view their infants through glass windows without having physical contact, lost interest and were unable to mother them later.

By the process of birth, the baby leaves a warm, nourishing, and familiar environment, one which has provided auditory, touch, and vestibular stimulation from the moment of conception to the moment of birth, to enter a new life which may be cold, strange, demanding, and dissatisfying. Since birth itself is an abrupt environmental change, it would appear that adjustment in the neonatal period should be facilitated by continuing the kinds and amounts of stimulation present during the fetal period (Ourth and Brown, 1961). The infant has an inborn "stimulus hunger" for such stimulation as gentle touch, body contact, body position, vestibular stimulation and sound. These stimuli are usually made available to the normal infant through the whole gamut of small acts by which an emotionally healthy mother can show her love for her child, provided she is not separated from her infant.

Tactile/kinesthetic needs or drives exist in infants which are separate from and of equal importance with the oral, anal, and phallic drives. The tactile/kinesthetic phase in utero predates the oral phase and has its own primary and specific modality of expression, which is motility. In the newborn, touch and movement are the first and dominant means of tension discharge and re-establishment of homeostasis. Touch plays a very vital role in the establishment of the mother-infant bond. Research findings indicate that attachment between mother and child is based on tactile and sensory stimulation rather than mere feeding or caregiving (Harlow, 1958; Kennell, Jerauld and Klaus, 1974; Klaus and Kennell, 1970). Harlow, Harlow, and Hansen (1963) found that monkeys who were allowed to see, but not touch, their young gradually lost interest after a period of two weeks. Viewing alone is not enough stimulus to maintain maternal interest. The human mother first uses touch to become acquainted with her baby, and later she employs it to express love. She explores his body with her fingertips, first on the infant's extremities, followed by palm encompassing contact of the trunk, and finally enfolding him in her arms, holding him close to her body (Klaus and Kennell, 1970; Rubin, 1963). Mothers who are separated from their infants after birth often have difficulty in achieving the touch progression (Klaus, Kennell, Plumb and Zuehlke, 1970).

Klaus and Kennell (1970) have studied mother-infant separation and conclude that the strength of the attachment bond and how the infant develops is dependent on how much mother and infant are together after birth. In a study where mothers were permitted to have their babies immediately after birth and were given five extra hours of contact on the first three days after delivery, it was found that these mothers spent more time fondling their babies, making eye-to-eye contact, gave more attention to their babies" development, talked to them more, and were more likely to soothe their babies if they cried. In a follow-up study two years later, these mothers were more advanced in language development and in mental and motor development than the babies whose mothers had been permitted limited contact with them in the first few days after birth. Studies have also shown that permitting nude infants to spend 45 minutes of skin-to-skin contact with their mothers, produced several interesting observations: the infants experiencing early contact with the mothers had fewer infections during the first year and gained significantly more weight. Furthermore, these infants tended to be breast fed for a longer period of time (Klaus and Kennell, 1970).

 STUDIES HAVE SHOWN THAT INFANTS EXPERIENCING EARLY CONTACT WITH THEIR MOTHERS HAVE FEWER INFECTIONS DURING THE FIRST YEAR AND GAIN SIGNIFICANTLY MORE WEIGHT.

Separation of the mother and infant may also destroy the mother's desire to breast feed her infant and produce a temporary difficulty in mother-child relationships. In a study at Duke University (1951), when compulsory rooming-in was adopted, the breast feeding rate rose more than 50% and calls from anxious mothers decreased 90% during the first week after discharge.

Touch deprivation in the infant is found to produce depression, a sense of abandonment, digestive malfunctioning, inability to maintain consistently intimate human relationships in later life, and even dwarfism (Gardner, 1972). In the past few years, a number of studies have shown that providing touch and vestibular stimulation produced quiescent behavior, increased weight gain, early development of cognitive behavior, enhancement of visual tracking and exploration, and increased the bonds of attachment (Gregg, Heffner, Korner, 1976; Ourth and Brown, 1961; Rice, 1977).

Klaus and Kennell (1970) have observed behavior common to mothers at the first postnatal contact with their nude infants as they establish affectional ties. This behavior involves an orderly, progressive transaction by the mother with the infant, such as seeking eye contact, touching, smiling, and vocalization. Such behavior is intuitively related to Bowlby's ethological theory of attachment. Bowlby (1969) theorized that in the early life of the human infant a complex array of instinctual responses are present, the function of which is to insure that the infant obtains parental care sufficient for his survival. Thus Bowlby proposed that the nature of a child's ties to his mother is a psychological attachment though this is related also to physiological satisfactions. Bowlby posed that five instinctual responses in the infant evoke maternal behavior in the mother. These responses are crying, smiling, sucking, clinging, and following. Robson (1967) and Wolff (1966) added another variable of maternal caretaking responses. The human infant's ability to attend visually, especially during the first hours, coincides with his mother's interest in his eyes.

Recent studies have shown that an infant only 3 to 27 minutes old demonstrates visual proficiency and can visually discriminate (Goren, Sarty and Wu, 1975). That is, if the infant is not sedated and does not have his vision clouded with medication. He shows a preference for face-like stimuli at a range of 6 to 13 inches, and 8 to 9 inches is known to be the fixed point of clearest vision for alert young infants (Bower, 1967; Haynes, White and Held, 1975). Within 24 hours after birth, babies have binocular vision when the visual stimulus is not more than 10 inches (Slater and Findlay, 1975).

 WHEN NOT SEDATED AND WHEN THEIR VISION IS NOT CLOUDED WITH MEDICATION, BABIES, ONLY MINUTES OLD, DEMONSTRATE VISUAL PROFICIENCY AND DISCRIMINATION AND HAVE BINOCULAR VISION WITHIN 24 HOURS AFTER BIRTH.

As the mother holds her infant to her breast, she can assume the "en face" position, and vocalize to her newborn. Her eyes are the optimal distance away, and her head, mouth, and eyes move slowly and within the circumscribed range for the infant to achieve optimum visual tracking. As the infant receives satisfaction from sucking and visual stimulation, he will also be sending stimuli, such as changes in facial expression, vocalizations and eye contact. The mother's response to such stimuli is immediate and gratifying. She responds with smiling and touching. And thus, a cyclic interaction of stimulus and response, of giving and receiving, is set up to insure the beginning of bonding and attachment.

A recently published study by Gregg, Hoffner, and Korner (1976) demonstrates that if newborns are permitted to suck and are given gentle rocking in a horizontal or semivertical direction their visual attentiveness and visual pursuit will be enhanced. The authors state that the results clearly show that it is not the upright position, as has been reported in earlier studies, which significantly influences the newborn's visual behavior, but it is the vestibular, proprioceptive stimulation and sucking which enhances this response. Thus it would appear that if the mother provided gentle rocking in a horizontal or semivertical position just prior to putting the newborn to breast, his visual processes would be stimulated and the probability of eye-to-eye contact would be enhanced.

An interesting study investigated the potential problems of maternal premedication on neonatal functioning (Conway and Brackbill, 1970). One of the conclusions reached by the authors was that since the infant's sucking behavior is one of the determinants of maternal behavior, it is not surprising to find a difference in the mother's response to the "drugged infants." Obviously of great concern is the possible detrimental role such effects may have on maternal attachment.

A study recently completed at the University of Illinois Medical Center, Chicago, (Lambesis, 1976) studied the effects on newborns when they are provided with surrogate mothering during the first four hours after birth. The surrogate mothering was an attempt to simulate the interaction which the mother and her newborn might experience if allowed to remain together after delivery. The treatment lasted 4 hours and included rocking, cuddling, and visual and verbal interaction while the baby was awake. Nonnutritive sucking to satiety was offered whenever the baby was rooting or mouthing. While asleep the baby was gently held. The babies who received this treatment had significantly less crying, which was interpreted to mean less stress, they took almost three times as much sterile water as the control group, their temperatures exhibited a more gradual rise but stabilized at two hours of life, whereas the control group was warmed by an infra-red warmer, but exhibited a continuously falling temperature following removal from the warmer. Greater fluctuations in respirations, heart rate, and systolic murmurs were heard in the control group. The study suggests that newborns can achieve physiologic adaptation with greater ease when given soothing and holding and the opportunity to suck at will. How much greater this adaptation might be if the mother supplies the infant's needs!

Dr. Gene Anderson of the University of Illinois School of Nursing (1976) has proposed a provocative hypothesis that the newborn can serve as a caregiver to its mother in a most essential and critical way. The mother and infant share a common need for generalized peristalsis during the first days following delivery, but particularly during the first few hours. If the newborn is permitted to nurse shortly after delivery, the flow of oxytocin is released, which in turn stimulates the letdown process, a form of peristalsis. Oxytocin is well known to stimulate uterine contractions (Sala, Luther, Arbello, and Cordero Funes, 1974). Peristalsis in the form of uterine contractions is a highly desirable phenomenon in the immediate postpartum mother. They are necessary to minimize the danger of postpartum hemorrhage and facilitate involution of the uterus. Sucking has also been demonstrated to promote prolactin (Shine, Williams, and Rennels, 1972). Thus the nursing activity of the human newborn not only facilitates the establishment of lactation but also serves to promote a state of equilibrium and physiological healing in the mother. From this perspective, Dr. Anderson concludes, the newborn infant would indeed seem to qualify as an effective caregiver to his mother.

It is quite possible that not only is it what the mother provides for the infant during the critical postpartum period that forms the bonds of attachment, but also the phenomenon of the newborn contributing to the restoration of physiological health and healing in the mother. Separation of the mother and infant would surely place in jeopardy this reciprocal interaction.

What about the premature infant who is not only deprived of his full share of intrauterine stimulation but is further deprived of touch and stimulation when placed in an incubator-isolette where little or insufficient stimulation may be provided? As a premature, the infant is deprived of two important factors -- the shortage of developmental time inutero and the shortened length of the period of labor. During labor, the contractions of the uterus provide massive stimulation to the fetal skin. These stimulations increase as labor advances and are extremely necessary to prepare the biological systems for postnatal functioning. But in the premature infant the period of labor is often short so that these infants not only have a disadvantage in the amount of time in utero, but also in the amount of stimulation during the labor itself.

 HOUSED IN AN INCUBATOR, THE PREMATURE INFANT IS ALMOST COMPLETELY ISOLATED FROM VESTIBULAR AND SOCIAL STIMULI AND MOST OF THE STIMULATION HE/SHE DOES RECEIVE IS OF AN INTRUSIVE AND NOXIOUS NATURE--SUCH AS INJECTIONS, GAVAGE, BLOOD TAKING, AND PHYSICAL EXAMINATIONS.

Premature nurseries have increasingly become intensive care units, housing all critically ill infants. Faced with the crisis of many sick infants, the emphasis in nursing is on biological survival. The infant is surrounded by electronic monitors, catheters, and other sorts of equipment, and keeping the life systems functioning seems to consume the total care time of hospital personnel. Little time, attention, or motivation is available to focus on emotional and social developmental needs. Housed in an incubator, the premature infant is almost completely isolated from vestibular and social stimuli and most of the stimulation he does receive is of an intrusive and noxious nature, such as injections, gavage, blood taking and physical examinations. The only time he may receive nonintrusive tactile stimulation or touch is when he self initiates it, such as moving and squirming against the bedding. Faced with the demands of keeping the biological systems functioning and often influenced by the assumption, which has yet to be researched and proved, that handling increases energy consumption, nursing personnel do not provide the cuddling, caressing and holding that the full-term and healthier infant may receive. Parents may take their cues from this model and continue to handle their premature infant less than they would a full-term baby. Consequently, it is suspected that the premature child receives less stimulation throughout his entire developmental period than the full-term child. Not only does this adversely affect his neurophysiological development, but there is a serious hazard placed on mother-infant attachment.

 IT IS POSSIBLE TO BRING PARENTS INTO THE NURSERY WITHOUT INCREASED RISK OF INFECTION. THEY CAN STROKE, CUDDLE, TALK TO, FEED, AND CARE FOR THEIR INCUBATOR BABIES. IT SHOULD BE MANDATORY FOR HOSPITAL PERSONNEL TO BE SUPPORTIVE OF AND TO ENCOURAGE THE MOTHER TO PRODUCE BREAST MILK FOR HER INCUBATOR INFANT.

There are several ways to decrease the effects of physical separation. Although it is not rational to discontinue the management of high risk infants in specialized units, it is possible to bring mothers into the nursery. Research has not indicated an increased risk in infection if parents are allowed to care for their premature babies (Klaus, et al., 1970; Korones, 1972). They can use the same sterile techniques that medical personnel use. Parents can stroke, cuddle, talk to, feed, and care for their incubator babies. They can also be taught to provide sensorimotor stimulation. It should be mandatory for hospital personnel to be supportive of and to encourage the mother to produce breast milk for her incubator infant. Nourishing her baby from her own body is one potent way the mother can facilitate her infant's growth and meet her own emotional need to be more competent in her role as a mother. In this respect, she is enhancing the probability of attachment.

In some premature nurseries today, there is a relaxation of policies so that mothers are encouraged to visit their infants and to participate in their care. This has brought about an increase in infant handling, but the handling is still affected mainly by the mother's wishes, inclinations, and confidence in herself and the severity of the infant's condition. Therefore, the infant experiences an uneven, sporadic kind of tactile stimulation, and for most premature babies, their mothers do not visit or handle them at all.

I was concerned with the lack of stimulation and holding a premature infant receives, and three years ago, conducted a research study to determine if the neurophysiological development of premature infants could be facilitated if they were provided with extra handling and holding. Since the nerve pathways from the skin are among the first to be sufficiently developed to activate and accelerate the rhythms and sequences of development, a specific technique of stroking and massaging was developed and field tested. Thirty premature infants were randomly selected to participate in the study. The mothers of 15 infants were taught to administer the stroking and rocking treatment and were instructed to provide it for 15 minutes, four times a day, for 30 days. Public Health Nurses visited the mothers daily during the 30-day treatment period to make sure the treatment was being given in a uniform way. The control group of 15 infants received the routine care prescribed by their doctors. When all infants were 4 months old, which was several weeks after the stroking and rocking treatment had ended, they were examined by a pediatrician, a psychologist, and a pediatric nurse who did not know which infants were experimental or control. The infants who had received the stroking and rocking were significantly more advanced than the control group in neurological development, weight gain, and mental functioning. (Editors' note: The instructions for this specific way to stroke and massage your baby has been placed on a cassette tape for mothers and is available from Dr. Rice. See address at end of the book.)

 TOO FREQUENTLY WE SEE PREMATURE INFANTS WHO HAVE ACHIEVED BIOLOGICAL SURVIVAL, BUT WHO ARE CRITICALLY DEFICIENT IN PSYCHOLOGICAL DEVELOPMENT DUE TO DEPRIVATION OF SENSORY, SOCIAL, AND EMOTIONAL INVOLVEMENT WITH THE MOST INFLUENCING FORCE IN THEIR LIVES--A PARENT.

Too frequently we see premature infants who have achieved biological survival but who are critically deficient in psychological development due to a deprivation of sensory, social and emotional involvement with the most influencing force in their lives -- a parent. Parents must no longer accept the "wait and see" regime which is frequently advised them by well-meaning medical personnel at the advent of a high risk infant. The infrequent and timid visitation of a mother with her incubator infant is not sufficient to change the course of events. Most premature infants probably receive some fondling in the normal course of care, but such tactile stimulation is not given consistently, is not given to all infants, is not a part of routine nursing care, and is not given frequently enough or for a long enough period of time.

A most important side effect of a mother providing sensory stimulation to her incubator infant is the measurable difference in her coping behavior, the replacement of her fear with confident responding, and the changing of her role from anxious observer to that of active participant. The cyclic interaction of mother and infant which precipitates attachment and bonding can now take place during the most critical of all time periods for the establishment of a mother-infant dyad -- the immediate post-birth period.

There is a significant correlation between prematurity and child abuse (Ambuel and Harris, 1963; Gregg and Elmer, 1969; Stern, 1973). The immediate and prolonged separation of mother and infant must surely be considered as a contributing cause. Child abuse and neglect is now one of our most severe and prevalent social problems, and this condition demands that we provide alternatives to separation of mother and premature infant.

There is sufficient research and evidence reported in the literature to validate a cause for changing the current hospital practices surrounding obstetrics and the care of our infants. As consumers of obstetric and pediatric practices, parents can, and must, begin to demand changes in the procedures that exist in most hospital settings which actually prevent, or at best hinder, not only the normal process of mother-infant attachment, but the health of the child and mother as well.

 As CONSUMERS OF OBSTETRIC AND PEDIATRIC PRACTICES, PARENTS CAN, AND MUST, DEMAND CHANGES IN MOST HOSPITAL SETTINGS WHICH ACTUALLY PREVENT, OR AT BEST HINDER, NOT ONLY THE NORMAL PROCESS OF MOTHER-INFANT ATTACHMENT, BUT THE VERY HEALTH OF THE CHILD AND MOTHER AS WELL.

CITED REFERENCES

1. Ambuel, J., and Harris, B., Failure to thrive: A study of failure to grow in height or weight, OH Med. J. 59:997, 1963.

2. Anderson, G., The mother and her newborn: Mutual caregivers, paper presented at N. Am. Soc. Psychosomatic OB/Gyn, U. of Chicago, April 10, 1976.

3. Balog, J., A new look at our infant mortality, Birth & Fam. J. 3:15-23, 1976.

4. Barnard, K., The effects of stimulation on the sleep behavior of the premature infant, Comm. Nurs. Res., (Ed.) Batey, M., 1974.

5. Bell, R., Stimulus control of parents or caretaker behavior by offspring, Dev. Psy. 4:63-72, 1971.

6. Bower, T., The development of object permanence: Some studies of existence constancy, Perception and Psychophysics, 2:411-418, 1967.

7. Bowlby, J., Attachment and loss, New York: Basic Books, Inc., Vol. 1, 1969.

8. Conway, E., and Brackbill, Y., Delivery medication and infant outcome: An empirical study, Monographs of the Soc. for Res. in Child Dev., 35: 24-34, 1970.

9. Gardner, L., Deprevation dwarfism, Sci. Am. 13:101-106, 1972.

10. Goren, C., Sarty, M., and Wu, P., Visual following and pattern discrimination of face-like stimuli by newborn infants, Ped. 56:544-549, 1975.

11. Graham, F., in lecture, 1968.

12. Gregg, C., Haffner, M., and Korner, A., The relative efficacy of vestibular-proprioceptive stimulation and the upright position in enhancing visual pursuit in neonates, Child Dev., 47:309-314, 1976.

13. Gregg, G., and Elmer, E., Infant injuries: accident or abuse, Ped. 44:434-440, 1969.

14. Harlow, H., The nature of love, Am. Psychologist, 13:673-685, 1958.

15. Harlow, H., Harlow, M., and Hansen, E., The maternal affectional system of Rhesus monkeys, in Rheingold, H., (ed.), Maternal behavior in mammals, New York: Wiley, 1963.

16. Haynes, H., White, B., and Held, R., Visual accommodation in human infants, Science, 528-530, 1965.

Cited References Cont'd

17. Hersher, L., Richmond, J., and Moore, A., Modifiability of the critical period for the development of maternal behavior in sheep and goats, Behavior, 20:311, 1963.

18. James, L., and Adamsons, K., Respiratory physiology of the fetus and new born infant, N. Eng. J. Med. 271:1352-1360, 1964.

19. Kennell, J., Jerauld, R., and Klaus, M., Maternal behavior one year after early and extended postpartum contact, Dev. Med. 10:2-10, 1974.

20. Klopfer, P., Adams, D., and Klopfer, M., Maternal "imprinting" in goats, Proc. Nat. Acad. Sci. 52:911, 1964.

21. Klaus, M, and Kennell, J., Mothers separated from their newborn infants, Ped. Clinics of N. Am. 17:1015-1037, 1970.

22. Klaus, M., Kennell, J., Plumb, N., and Zuehlke, S., Human maternal behavior at the first contact with her young, Ped. 46:187, 1970.

23. Korones, S., High-risk newborn infants, St. Louis: C.V. Mosby, 1972.

24. Lambesis, C., The effects of surrogate mothering of the transitional newborn upon physiologic stabilization, Paper presented at first annual Nat'l Found. March of Dimes Perinatal Nurs. Res. Roundtable, Chicago, Nov. 8, 1976.

25. Moore, A., Effects of modified care in the sheep and goat, in Newton, G., and Levine, S., (eds.), Early Experience and Behavior, Springfield, IL: Charles Thomas, 1968.

26. McBride, A., Compulsory rooming-in in the ward and private newborn service at Duke Hospital, JAMA 145:625, 1951.

27. Ourth, L., and Brown, K., Inadequate mothering and disturbance in the neonatal period, Child Dev. 32:287-295, 1961.

28. Perloff, J., Therapeutics of nature--the invisible sutures of sutures of "spontaneous closure", Am. Heart J. 82:581-585, 1971.

29. Rheingold, H., Maternal Behavior in mammals, New York: Wiley & Sons, 1963.

30. Rice, R., Neurophysiological development in premature infants following stimulation, Dev. Psyc. 13:69-76, 1977.

31. Robson, K., The role of eye-to-eye contact in maternal-infant attachment, J. Child Psyc. and Psychiat., 8:13-25, 1967.

Cited References Cont'd

32. Rubin, R., Maternal touch, Nursing Outlook, 11:828, 1963.

33. Sala, N., Luther, E., Arballe, J., and Cordero Funes, J., Oxytocin re-
    producing reflex milk ejection in lactating women, J. Appl. Physiology,
    36:154-158, 1974.

34. Shiino, M., Williams, G., and Rennels, E., Ultrastructural observation
    of pituitary release of prolactin in the rat by suckling stimulus, Endo-
    crinology, 90:176-187, 1972.

35. Slater, A., and Findlay, J., Binocular fixation in the newborn baby,   J.
    Exp. Child Psyc. 20:248-273, 1975.

36. Stern, L., Prematurity as a factor in child abuse, Hospital Practice, 117-
    123, May 1973.

37. Wolff, D., The causes, controls, and organization of behavior in the neo-
    nate, Psychological Issues 5:1, 1966.

38. United Nations Office of Statistics, February, 1975.

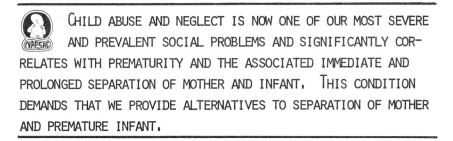

CHILD ABUSE AND NEGLECT IS NOW ONE OF OUR MOST SEVERE AND PREVALENT SOCIAL PROBLEMS AND SIGNIFICANTLY CORRELATES WITH PREMATURITY AND THE ASSOCIATED IMMEDIATE AND PROLONGED SEPARATION OF MOTHER AND INFANT. THIS CONDITION DEMANDS THAT WE PROVIDE ALTERNATIVES TO SEPARATION OF MOTHER AND PREMATURE INFANT.

CHAPTER TWENTY FIVE

WHY WOMEN MUST MEET
THE NUTRITIONAL STRESS OF PREGNANCY

Tom Brewer, M.D.
Jay Hodin

The 1977 NAPSAC Conference, as well as the one in 1976, depicts the growing concern among concerned individuals and organizations that technological approaches to childbirth obscure the basic principles of preventive obstetrical and pediatric care. The underlying consensus among those who contributed to NAPSAC's publication Safe Alternatives in Childbirth (NAPSAC, 1976), which resulted from the 1976 conference, was that until hospitals and other medical institutions begin to fulfill the needs of those they are established to serve, those dedicated to making childbirth a safe, healthy, and joyous family-oriented experience must unite and remain organized. NAPSAC has provided the forum crucial to the dissemination of information and advocacy of uncomplicated childbirth. As NAPSAC's president profoundly stated, "The outcome of birth is only in the hands of the obstetrician and the hospital staff for a short while; but the outcome of birth remains with the parents and the child for life."[1]

As hospitals and physicians become more inclined to take advantage of the recently developed (but not proven safe) medical technologies, such as elaborate laboratory testing, oxytocin challenge tests, fetal monitoring, amniocentesis, sonargrams, and other devices, principles of patient care become more oriented to the convenience of the hospital staff and that of the doctors than to the health care needs of the pregnant woman. Automated childbirth is threatening the lives and health of thousands of pregnant women and their newborns in our nation. Will obstetrics of the future be characterized by "the drama of instrumented babies under plastic bubbles

TOM BREWER is President, Society for the Protection of the Unborn Through Nutrition; Author of book, Metabolic Toxemia of Late Pregnancy, and numerous other works; he is featured in the movie, "Nutrition in Pregnancy."

JAY HODIN is Executive Director, Society for the Protection of the Unborn Through Nutrition; statistician and author of "Malnutrition and Developmental Disabilities -- A Causal Relation."

kept alive and restored to health by space-age medicine?"[2] Will "many births in the near tomorrow...take place in a setting of blinking lights, green glowing cathode-ray screens, dials and wires and tubes, "[2] or will those who recognize the inherent risks of such space-age obstetrics be able to channel medical advancements into family-centered preventive care?

Because many physicians have not learned to correctly interpret readings from the modern electronic machines, the rate of cesarean section has increased dramatically in many areas. Trained in techniques to monitor abnormal childbirth, many physicians apply them to innumerable instances of normal pregnancy, thereby converting the normal to abnormal. Premature delivery caused by over-zealous use of these modern devices can affect the newborn's health deleteriously.

The pyramiding effect of automated perinatal care, besides presenting dangers to the health of the mother and baby, camouflages some basic, physiologic processes of pregnancy and childbirth. The concept of primary prevention of complications of pregnancy and delivery and prevention of neonatal abnormalities through sound prenatal nutrition has been supplanted by secondary prevention, which consists of elaborate intensive care nurseries which electronically monitor premature babies, many of whom would have been normal size at birth. The relatively new specialty of neonatology (or perinatology), with its emphasis on treatment of abnormalities (many of which would have been unnecessary had primary prevention been applied), seems to be an appropriate addition to the medical hierarchy. The use of drugs, which are prescribed (frequently futilely) to facilitate control of weight and/or water retention during pregnancy, and restrictive dietary regimens (e.g., low-salt and/or low-calorie diets) are prime causes of prematurity, creating the need for electronic gadgetry in an attempt to prevent much of the disease, damage, and death associated with prematurity.

AS HOSPITALS AND PHYSICIANS BECOME MORE INCLINED TO TAKE ADVANTAGE OF THE RECENTLY DEVELOPED (BUT NOT PROVEN SAFE) MEDICAL TECHNOLOGIES, THE PRINCIPLES OF PATIENT CARE BECOME MORE ORIENTED TO THE CONVENIENCE OF THE HOSPITAL STAFF AND DOCTORS THAN TO THE HEALTH NEEDS OF PREGNANT WOMEN.

Why is there increased utilization of fetal monitoring when studies have shown that most cases of births of children with mental retardation, cerebral palsy, or other central nervous system impairment are not associated with complications during labor or delivery? One physician presented data to show that 70% of all such births are not complicated during labor or delivery.[3] Most of those that do have such labor and delivery abnormalities are likely to be caused by the same factor that led to the disability -- inadequate prenatal nutrition. As far back as 1897, Freud contested the prevailing medical theories that prematurity, dystocia, asphyxia, and related complications were directly related to the fetal developmental disability.[4] Instead, Freud believed the complications and disability were caused by the same developmental factor. More current studies have shown that malnutrition frequently lies at the etiology of both the pregnancy, labor, and/or delivery complication(s) and the child's disability.

Even the undue emphasis on labor and delivery on the part of childbirth education groups must be questioned and their ultimate intentions reconsidered. Not only does the gestation period encompass a greater and more comprehensive period of development than labor and delivery, but environmental (particularly nutritional) factors play a significant role in affecting the final stages of the birth process. An analysis of Social Security recipients who had a long-term disability which afflicted them before the age of 18 revealed that in 75% of the cases the disability originated during the prenatal period.[5] In 94% of the cases the disability was neurological.

 AUTOMATED CHILDBIRTH IS THREATENING THE LIVES AND HEALTH OF THOUSANDS OF PREGNANT WOMEN AND THEIR NEWBORNS IN OUR NATION.

Not only is fetal monitoring ineffective in reversing intrauterine growth retardation caused by malnutrition and other environmental factors, its use has been associated with increased complications of labor and delivery in addition to higher risks of surgery. A Department of HEW study of 483 "high risk" pregnant women who delivered at one hospital revealed the possible hazards of the utilization of fetal monitors.[6] All of the 483 women were fitted with fetal scalp electrodes and intrauterine catheters so that the fetal heart rate and uterine contractions could be monitored. With the use of a random selection procedure, in approximately half of the pregnancies, controls of the monitors were disconnected without the women's knowledge. In all of these cases, nurses monitored the fetal heartbeats without the use of electronic equipment.

The results were startling. There were two and a half more cesarean sections (40) in the electronically monitored group than in the group monitored by the nurses (16). An even more dramatic difference was observed in postpartum infections. In the monitored group 13.2% of the women experienced postpartum infections in contrast to 3.4% among the controls. In addition, pediatric evaluations showed that the health of those children born without the use of fetal monitors was, in general, superior to that of the monitored births. Five of the study group infants, in contrast to none of those whose births were monitored by nurses, needed assistance to maintain breathing two minutes after birth.

Another recent but more comprehensive study also demonstrated that greater utilization of elaborate machinery is not necessarily associated with reduced risks of complications, particularly prematurity.[7] The study analyzed nearly 300,000 births in North Carolina, where the perinatal mortality rate is much higher among nonwhites (41.0) than whites (25.7), to determine means of reducing the interracial difference in perinatal mortality. Neither the number of prenatal visits nor the level of sophistication of the obstetrical and neonatal care facilities at the hospital where the child was delivered was shown to significantly affect the perinatal mortality rate. The mortality difference was due primarily to the much higher rates of low birth weight and prematurity among nonwhites (14.0% of the nonwhite births were of less than 35 weeks' gestation and/or weighed less than 2001 grams (4 pounds 6 1/2 ounces) than whites, where 5.7% of the births were similarly premature or underweight). The authors of the study concluded:

> There is little likelihood that regionalized perinatal care will have an impact on the race differential in perinatal mortality... It appears that significant control of excess perinatal mortality among nonwhites will depend on prevention of prematurity. Since the prematurity rate for nonwhites has been increasing during the past two decades while that for whites has remained stable, the concept of preventing prematurity assumes even greater significance... If more intensive medical care is insufficient despite its great value for the newborn and the number of prenatal visits makes little difference, where are we to turn?...Few can argue against programs directed toward improving nutrition and decreasing perinatal mortality.[7]

A similar report concurred that "regionalization of perinatal services" and "sophisticated hospitals" staffed by highly trained neonatologists do not necessarily lead to an improvement in perinatal health.[8] The study showed that a marked increase in perinatal care services did not appreciably improve the outcome of pregnancy. The author wrote: "The location of the larger obstetrical services and the inclusion of the majority of medical teaching centers, as well as the existence of a large ratio of specialists per unit population in this area have not been sufficient to overcome this fault of medical care (i.e., poor maternal and infant health)."[8]

 REGIONALIZATION OF PERINATAL SERVICES AND SOPHISTICATED HOSPITALS STAFFED BY HIGHLY TRAINED NEONATOLOGISTS DO NOT NECESSARILY LEAD TO AN IMPROVEMENT IN PERINATAL HEALTH.

The prevailing nonchalance among health care professionals about the role of sound maternal nutrition in protecting the health of the pregnant woman and her newborn coupled with our preoccupation with technologically advanced medical machinery, which suppresses the concept of primary prevention, are primarily responsible for the high rates of infant and maternal mortality in the U.S. As revealed in Tables 1 and 2, the U.S. ranks 19th among all nations in infant mortality and 14th in maternal mortality.[9]

TABLE 1
NATIONS WITH A LOWER INFANT MORTALITY RATE
THAN THAT OF THE U.S. IN 1973*

	Country	Mortality Rate
1.	Sweden	9.6
2.	Finland	10.1
3.	Papua New Guinea (1971)	10.2
4.	Norway (1972)	11.3
5.	Iceland (1972)	11.6
6.	Netherlands	11.6
7.	Japan (1972)	11.7
8.	Switzerland	12.8
9.	Panama Canal Zone	14.3
10.	Luxembourg	15.5
11.	France (1972)	16.0
12.	East Germany	16.0
13.	New Zealand	16.2
14.	Liechtenstein (1969)	16.7
15.	Australia (1972)	16.7
16.	Canada	16.8
17.	Belgium	17.0
18.	Hong Kong (1972)	17.4
19.	United States	· 17.6

* Infant deaths per 1,000 live births; rates apply to 1973 unless specified otherwise.

TABLE 2
NATIONS WITH A MATERNAL MORTALITY RATE
EQUAL TO OR LOWER THAN U.S. IN 1971*

Country	Mortality Rate
1. Sweden	0.2
2. Finland	0.2
3. United Kingdom (1972)	0.3
4. Belgium (1970)	0.4
5. Netherlands	0.4
6. Czechoslovakia	0.5
7. Denmark	0.5
8. East Germany (1972)	0.5
9. Canada	0.5
10. Luxembourg (1972)	0.6
11. Austria (1972)	0.6
12. Bulgaria (1972)	0.6
13. Poland (1972)	0.6
14. United States	0.6

* Maternal deaths during pregnancy or childbirth per 100,000 females; rates apply to 1971 unless specified otherwise.

Because of our emphasis on providing elaborate intensive care nurseries equipped with modern electronic machinery and our neglect of establishing networks to prevent prematurity and low birth weight, an international comparison of low birth weight puts the U.S. in an even less favorable position than in the case of infant mortality. It is particularly startling that the incidence of low birth weight (under 5 1/2 pounds) babies in the U.S. is no lower today than it was in the early 1920's.[10, 11] As Table 3 reveals, the rate of underweight births has remained fairly stabilized in the U.S.; the rate for non-whites has increased significantly.

The U.S. incidence of low birth weight babies is 75% higher than Finland's,[12] 60% higher than Iceland's, and 25% higher than that of Japan.[13] Our rate of underweight births is even 16% higher than that of Britain [13] even though the U.S. infant mortality rate is lower.[9] In the People's Republic of China, an emphasis on preventive medicine and applied research has led to a decline in the prematurity rate to less than 3%.[14]

 TRAINED IN TECHNIQUES TO MONITOR ABNORMAL CHILDBIRTH, MANY PHYSICIANS APPLY THEM TO NORMAL PREGNANCY, THEREBY CONVERTING THE NORMAL TO ABNORMAL.

TABLE 3
U.S. LOW BIRTH WEIGHT INCIDENCE
(DATA NOT AVAILABLE FOR YEARS PRIOR TO 1950)

Year	All Births†	White	Nonwhite (1950-1967)/ Black (1968-1972)*
1950Δ	7.5%	7.1%	10.2%
1951Δ	7.6	7.1	10.8
1952	7.7	7.1	11.2
1953	7.7	7.1	11.4
1954	7.5	6.9	11.4
1955	7.6	6.8	11.7
1956	7.6	6.8	12.1
1957	7.6	6.8	12.5
1958	7.7	6.8	12.9
1959	7.7	6.8	12.9
1960	7.7	6.8	12.8
1961	7.8	6.9	13.0
1962	8.0	7.0	13.1
1963	8.2	7.1	13.6
1964	8.2	7.1	13.9
1965	8.3	7.2	13.8
1966	8.3	7.2	13.9
1967	8.2	7.1	13.6
1968	8.2	7.1	13.7
1969	8.1	7.1	13.9
1970	7.9	6.8	13.9
1971	7.7	6.6	13.4
1972	7.7	6.5	13.6

† Live births with known weight.
Δ Excludes Connecticut and Massachusetts.
* Births other than white or black are included in col. 1 (all births) but excluded from the composite of the last 2 cols. for 1968-1972.

Prenatal Nutrition and Birth Weight

Nutrition has been shown to have a more profound effect on birth weight than any other environmental factor. The relationship between prenatal nutrition and birth weight has been known for 50 years. In a study conducted in the 1920's, Acosta-Sison observed that women on poor prenatal diets were more than ten times as likely as well-fed women to give birth to a low birth weight baby.[15] (See Table 4.) As the nutritional status of the women worsened, both the maximum and average birth weights declined.

TABLE 4
RELATIONSHIP BETWEEN PRENATAL NUTRITION
AND BIRTH WEIGHT

Nutritional Status of Gravid Women	# of Women	% Low Birth Weight	Significance Level of Difference with Fairly Nourished Group
GOOD	63	3.2	p<.005
FAIR	272	11.0	---
POOR	28	33.0	p<.005

In a prospective nutrition study in 1937, low birth weight was eradicated among 750 women, approximately 82% of whom had exhibited signs of nutritional deficiencies prior to pregnancy and two-thirds of whom were clinic patients.[16] The eradication of low birth weight (in addition, no stillbirths occurred) was accomplished by increasing the women's daily nutrients well above the recommended levels, providing nutrition counseling, and administering polyvitamin therapy. To ensure proper nutritional intake throughout pregnancy, the consumption of five to six relatively small meals was encouraged. As the study progressed, the author improved the diet and vitamin supplementation regimen. Recognizing the nutritional stress of gestation (which he called the "metabolic demand in pregnancy"), he stated: "our therapeutic efforts are always directed toward improving the general nutrition of the patient, principally from natural food sources, but also with polyvitamin therapy in sufficient dosage to relieve the signs and symptoms."

The smallest child among the 750 well-fed women weighed 6 pounds 4 1/4 ounces (2482 grams). In contrast, among 750 control group women, who comprised a similar population as that of those in the study group but who received neither nutrition education nor polyvitamin supplementation, 37 (4.9%) of the infants weighed under 5 pounds (2268 grams). The probability that the difference between the two groups in the number of infants weighing under 5 pounds at birth was not caused by the nutrition regimen is less than one in 10 million.

NUTRITION HAS BEEN SHOWN TO HAVE A MORE PROFOUND EFFECT ON BIRTH WEIGHT THAN ANY OTHER ENVIRONMENTAL FACTOR AND HUNDREDS OF SCIENTIFIC STUDIES HAVE DEMONSTRATED THAT BIRTH WEIGHT IS THE MOST ACCURATE PREDICTOR OF HEALTH AND MENTAL AND PHYSICAL DEVELOPMENT.

Another notable prospective study documented the relationship between nutrition and birth weight. In this study of 216 pregnancies at Harvard University Department of Public Health, thorough dietary histories were taken of all of the pregnant women to determine their nutritional status.[17-19] Based upon the dietary information acquired through interviews with nutritionists, women were classified into five different groups according to their intake of calories and various nutrients. Unlike the aforementioned study of 1,500 pregnancies, there was no dietary intervention.

As Table 5 reveals, birth weight was shown to be directly related to prenatal diet. Infants born to women who had been on excellent or good diets weighed an average of 2 pounds 11 ounces (1219 grams) more than those born to the poorly nourished women.

TABLE 5
RELATIONSHIP OF BIRTH WEIGHT
TO PRENATAL NUTRITION

Prenatal Diet	Good or Excellent	Fair	Poor or Very Poor
Number of Infants	31	149	36
Average Birth Weight	8lb,8oz (3856 g)	7lb,7oz (3374 g)	5lb,13oz (2637 g)

The level of protein intake, which paralleled the general dietary intake, was significantly related to both birth weight and length. None of the infants born to mothers with a daily protein intake of at least 80 grams weighed under 6 pounds at birth, their median birth weight being 8 1/2 pounds (3856 grams). In contrast, 47% of the babies born to women who had an average of less than 45 grams of protein every day were of low birth weight. Among these births, the median birth weight was 5 1/2 pounds.

For every additional 10 grams of dietary protein (up to 85 to 100 grams), the birth weight increased 240 grams (8 1/2 ounces). Birth size (in terms of both weight and length) increased with every increment of dietary protein. The correlation between birth length and protein (0.80) and that of the same relationship with the effect of maternal height removed (0.78) were both significant at the 10^{-9} level of statistical significance.[18]

Not surprisingly, starvation results in a precipitious decline in birth size. During the siege of Leningrad, U.S.S.R., during World War II, amenorrhea, a decline in conception, spontaneous abortion, subnormal birth size, and infant morbidity and mortality increased dramatically as a result of inadequate food rations, severe cold, lack of heat, physical exertion, and other harsh conditions.[20] Of the 368 of 391 live births in one large clinic in Leningrad (there were 23 stillbirths) who were weighed during the first half of 1942, 49.1% were of low birth weight. Only 3.6% of the infants weighed over 3500 grams (7 pounds 11 1/2 ounces).

The general improvement in nutrition and other environmental conditions among women who delivered during the second half of 1942 was reflected in their lower incidence of low birth weight and subnormal birth length. Among births during the first half of the year, 41.2% were under 47 centimeters (18 1/2 inches) in length; only 6.5% of those born during the last six months of 1942 had a birth length of under 47 centimeters.

The mass starvation period during the winter of 1944-1945 in Holland also caused an increase in the frequency of underweight babies. Children born during the war weighed an average of 240 grams (8 1/2 ounces) less than prewar babies.[21]

 THE NEONATAL MORTALITY RATE AMONG INFANTS UNDERWEIGHT AT BIRTH IS 30 TIMES HIGHER THAN THAT OF INFANTS WHO WEIGH MORE THAN 5.5 LBS AT BIRTH.

Numerous prospective as well as retrospective studies document the direct relationship between nutrition and birth weight. In a prospective study in which a control group was selected through a random process, supplementation was shown to have a direct effect on birth weight. The low birth weight incidence among 641 pregnant women who received vitamin and/or protein supplementation was 6.4%.[22] That of 198 controls was 11.1%.

Tompkins and Wiehl observed that the birth weights of the study group women would have been much higher and the low birth weight rate lower if a larger number of women receiving protein supplementation had taken all of their allotted supplements. They declared: "Examination of the individual records of the patients taking protein supplement only shows that the poor weight status of babies of a few patients, who took less than half of the intended amount of the protein supplement, was responsible for the low average weight for the entire group."[22]

Of the women who were provided protein supplements, only 3.23% of the babies weighed less than 6 pounds (2722 grams) at birth. In comparison, 9.16% of the infants born to those who did not receive protein supplementation were under that weight at birth. In addition, the average length of gestation was lower among those who received protein and vitamin supplementation than those whose diets were not supplemented by both protein and vitamins (p<.05). Less than 8% of the women who received both supplements delivered more than one week before term.

Other studies reveal the significant effects of food supplementation on birth weight. Results from a prospective double-blind supplementation study have shown a significant effect of protein supplementation is increasing birth weight.[23-24] The average birth weight of babies born to women who received the protein supplement was 150 grams (5 1/4 ounces) greater than that of siblings who were born before their mother participated in the food supplementation program.

Another double-blind supplementation study has demonstrated similar results.[25] In this particular study the participants lived in conditions of abject poverty and were chronically malnourished, the typical prenatal diet consisting of 1500 calories and 40 grams of protein.[26] Centers provided supplements which consisted of 91 calories, 6.4 grams of protein, and vitamins and minerals in 100-milliliter containers.[24-25,27] The controls consisted of women who had approximately the same previous caloric intake and health status and were approximately of the same height as the women in the study group. These women were given a supplement which consisted of 33 calories, vitamins, and two minerals per 100 milliliters.[24] Throughout the women's pregnancies the amount of the supplement was measured and recorded. None of the women were informed as to whether they were given the nutritious supplement or the other one, which served as a placebo.

 LOW BIRTH WEIGHT BABIES ARE APPROXIMATELY TEN TIMES MORE LIKELY TO BE MENTALLY RETARDED THAN THOSE OF HIGHER BIRTH WEIGHT.

Birth weight rose as the maternal caloric intake increased.[24] This relationship was striking even when the authors adjusted birth weight for maternal height and weight, age, parity, and sex of the infant. Of the 69 women who ingested more than 31,000 supplementary calories, there was not one child who was underweight at birth. Moreover, 19% of these infants' birth weight was more than 3 1/2 kilograms (7 pounds 11 1/2 ounces). As Table 6 reveals, the incidence of underweight births was nearly four times as high among women who ingested less than 5,000 supplementary calories as those who consumed at least 20,000 supplementary calories during pregnancy.

TABLE 6
EFFECT OF SUPPLEMENTATION ON
DECREASING LOW BIRTH WEIGHT INCIDENCE

Amount of Caloric Supplementation During Pregnancy	Less Than 5,000	5,000 to 19,999	At Least 20,000 Calories
Number of Women	82	89	117
% Low Birth Weight	13.4	7.1	3.5

Unfortunately, the 288 births included in the birth weight analysis excluded cases of prematurity. The finding that supplementation increased birth weight would have probably been augmented had the premature births been included.

More than 35 years ago, Ebbs et al. documented the beneficial effects of food supplementation and birth weight.[28-29] The study consisted of 380 pregnant women who were in the second trimester, were reasonably healthy, and agreed to be confined in a hospital (for dietary administration and observation) until delivery. Thorough dietary histories for the seven-day period prior to hospital admission were taken. All of the 170 women who were found to be well-nourished were provided nutrition counseling until delivery. Ninety of the 210 poorly nourished women were selected on an alternate basis to receive food supplementation until six weeks postpartum;[29] the average duration of supplementation was 4.7 months.[28] None of the remaining poorly nourished women received supplementation or nutrition guidance.[28-29]

During the study there was little difference between the dietary intake of the 170 women who received nutrition education and the 90 whose diets were markedly improved by supplementation.

The prematurity (probably low birth weight) rate was significantly lower in the supplemented and good diet groups than in the groups of 120 poorly nourished women. In fact, the incidence of prematurity was lower among the 90 women who were provided food supplementation (2.2%) than the well-nourished group of 170 women (3.0%) even though the former women were said to have been poorly nourished through the first half of pregnancy. The prematurity incidence among the 120 poorly nourished women who received neither food supplementation nor nutrition education was 8.0%.

A food supplementation program in a low-income Mexican village where chronic malnutrition is rampant resulted in an 8% increase in birth weight.[30] In addition, during infancy, those born to women whose diets had been supplemented exhibited superior language development and were more active than other children of comparable age and socioeconomic status.

A recent individualized prenatal nutrition education program had a profound effect in increasing birth weight.[24, 31-32] Two-thirds of the 1,736 participants (less than 5% of those who enrolled in the voluntary program dropped out) had completed no more than five years of education. All participants were provided extensive nutrition education and multivitamin supplements. The 1,246 (72% of all participants) who were below the poverty level received food supplementation in the form of milk, eggs, and oranges. Even though the average length of service in the program was only 18 weeks, the program's director, Agnes Higgins, was able to enhance the women's nutritional status sufficiently (the average daily protein intake was increased from 68 to 101 grams; that for calories rose from 2,249 to 2,778) to increase birth weight and decrease infant mortality. Greater nutritional intakes were encouraged for conditions of underweight, previous undernourishment, and stress.

As caloric and protein intakes increased, birth weight rose. The average birth weight among women whose protein intake was not more than 84% of their determined requirement was 3235 grams (7 pounds 2 ounces); that of women who exceeded their protein requirements by at least 15% was 3447 grams (7 pounds 10 ounces). The overall low birth weight incidence of 6.87% was significantly lower than that of other clinic patients who received care and delivered in the same hospital as those in the program (9.04%) (p<.005). Much more impressive was the low birth weight incidence of 3.3% among women under 18 years of age. Also striking was the finding that the average birth weight of infants born to women participating in the program who had another child in the same clinic but did not, in the prior or succeeding birth(s), participate in the nutrition program was significantly higher than that of their siblings (p<.01).

TABLE 7
LOW BIRTH WEIGHT INCIDENCE
AND DURATION OF PARTICIPATION

Weeks of Nutrition Counseling	Live Births	Low Birth Weight Infants	% Low Birth Weight
1-12	519	51	9.83
13-20	499	39	7.82
At least 21	713	29	4.07
All cases	1,731	119	6.87

Even when birth weight was adjusted to eliminate the effect of other variables, it was significantly associated with length of service in the program. Birth weight was not associated with length of service among other public patients at the same hospital (i.e., the controls). The average birth weight among the 521 women who participated in the program for at least 21 weeks and who received food supplementation was 3381 grams (7 pounds 7 ounces), approximately 100 grams greater than that among women who went to private obstetricians at the same hospital. The average birth weight among other clinic patients in the same hospital (the controls) was 3127 grams (6 pounds 14 ounces), about 9 ounces less than the 521 study group women.

A case history of one of the participants unequivocally demonstrates the value of nutrition education and supplementation. The birth weights of this woman's 11 children, all of whom were delivered at the same hospital, are indicated in Figure 1. Only during her last three pregnancies was the woman a program participant. Note that the smallest of these infants weighed 1 pound 1 1/4 ounces more than the heaviest of her previous eight births, when she received no nutrition counseling. There is less than one chance in a billion that the difference between the birth weights during her first eight pregnancies and those of the last three can be attributed to chance.

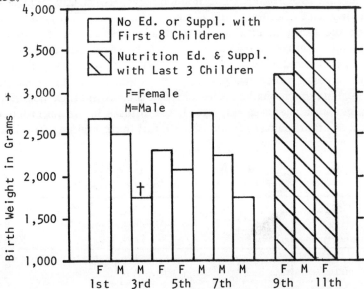

FIGURE 1. Effect of nutrition education and food supplementation on birth weight for mother of 11.

The woman's third child died at the age of one month. A physical and mental assessment of her other seven children born before she learned of the nutrition program revealed that all of them are impaired neurologically. To date, more than $300,000 of public funds have been expended for their maintenance and rehabilitation. In contrast, all three children born while the woman was enrolled in the nutrition program are in good health. The program's cost to provide her nutrition education and food supplementation was approximately $125 for each of the pregnancies.

 EVEN IN THE ABSENCE OF FOOD SUPPLEMENTATION, NUTRITION EDUCATION, WHEN PROPERLY IMPLEMENTED, CAN RESULT IN A MARKED REDUCTION IN THE INCIDENCE OF UNDERWEIGHT BABIES.

Even a briefer period of food supplementation than that provided in the aforementioned program can substantially increase birth weight. During the last four weeks of gestation, 25 low-income women were hospitalized so that protein and calorie supplementation could be administered and monitored.[33] The average daily caloric intake had been increased from 1,400 to 2,100. In addition, all of the women received iron and multivitamin tablets and protein supplementation. Slightly more than half (13) of the women were placed on a diet which provided 60 grams of protein per day (animal protein comprised 20 grams); the other 12 women received 90 grams of protein per day (which included 20 grams of animal and 30 grams of dairy protein). The average daily protein consumption had been 40 grams prior to the study. A control group of 26 women of the same economic class was utilized for comparison.

When compared with the control group, the food supplementation increased the birth weight by nearly 11 1/2 ounces, from 2704 to 3028 grams. The level of statistical significance applicable to the difference in birth weights is infinitesimal.

Iyenger theorized that the additional 30 grams of protein among the 12 women did not result in a further significant increase in birth weight because they did not receive additional calories.[33] Since a 30% deficiency can result in a 60% reduction in dietary protein being available for tissue synthesis,[34] if the additional protein supplementation had been accompanied by a somewhat proportional increase in calories, the average birth weight among the 12 women would have been much higher than that of the 13 other who received only moderate supplementation.

Even in the absence of food supplementation, nutrition education when properly implemented can result in a marked reduction in the incidence of underweight births. In one such program, the low birth weight incidence among all primigravidas (who are tradition- ally considered to be high risk) who delivered in one county during a four-and-a-half-year period was nearly five times lower than that of primigravidas of similar economic classes. The level of statis- tical significance reflecting the reduction in low birth weight is less than one billionth.

TABLE 8
INFLUENCE OF NUTRITION EDUCATION
IN LOWERING RISK OF LOW BIRTH WEIGHT

	# of Women	% Low Birth Weight
Infants born to primigravidas Receiving Nutrition Education	321	2.8
Infants born to other primigravidas Attending same County Clinic	1,237	13.7

Reviewing this dramatic decline in the low birth weight rate resulting from sound nutrition education, the scientific director of the National Institutes of Child Health and Human Development, Na- tional Institutes of Health, attributed the high rate of underweight births (13.7%) in the control group largely to the fact that many of the control group primigravidas had been placed on salt-restricted diets and had been told to restrict their weight gain,[35] both of which lead to hypovolemia and its attendant complications,[36, 38-42] and diuretics were prescribed to many.

Referring to the dramatic effects of the nutrition education program, the director declared: "These conclusions challenge the conventional wisdom, which demands constraint on weight gain by caloric restriction, a limitation of salt intake, and use of saline diuretics. None of these were used in the Brewer series . . . Why is our prematurity rate rising, a factor of life in no other advanced nation? The answer may well be in our prenatal regimens. It looks as if we can make real progress on both questions merely by feeding pregnant women."[35]

BIRTHWEIGHT HAS BEEN SHOWN TO BE DIRECTLY RELATED TO I.Q. IN THE MAMMOTH COLLABORATIVE PERINATAL STUDY BY THE U.S. DEPARTMENT OF HEW, 1972, IT WAS FOUND THAT NEARLY HALF OF ALL THE CHILDREN UNDERWEIGHT AT BIRTH HAD AN I.Q. UNDER 70.

Recognizing the protective effects of applied, scientific nutrition in the 1920's, Toverud reduced the low birth weight incidence to 2.2% by initiating a "nutrition station" at which 728 women participated.[43] Because of its success, the program was extended to several hundred additional women. It is especially noteworthy that there were no cases of clinical brain damage among the more than 1,500 liveborn infants born to women who participated in the program and who also received vitamin K. Previously, Toverud had reduced the rate of underweight births among 223 unwed mothers to 2%. The previous incidence among such women had been greater than 20%.

A well-controlled prospective study in 1944 of the effectiveness of nutrition counseling during the last trimester of pregnancy resulted in a significant decrease in the low birth weight incidence (p<.05).[45] Among the 500 women who received dietary counseling during the last three months of pregnancy, 6.2% gave birth to underweight babies. The low birth weight incidence among the 500 control group women was 10.0%.

Previous to this nutrition counseling study, the authors determined the direct relationship between prenatal nutrition and infant health by utilizing a retrospective analysis of the diets of the mothers of 300 infants.[45] While hospitalized after delivery, the mothers of 100 stillbirths, 100 low birth weight infants, and 100 normal weight babies were asked about their diets during their last trimester. To avoid inherent bias, the authors selected the 300 cases randomly from deliveries at one hospital.

TABLE 9
INFLUENCE OF NUTRITION
ON SURVIVAL AND WEIGHT AT BIRTH

Calories or Nutrient (g)	Optimum Requirements (As stated by the Authors)	Approximate Daily Intake by Group		
		Still-births	Low Birth Weight Infants	Normal-Weight Infants
Calories	2,500	1,644	1,710	1,946
Carbohydrates	350	207	217	217
Fat	80	61.4	64.9	80.4
Protein	90	52.4	54.5	72.1
High-Quality Protein	50	27.4	29.9	45.9
Calcium	1.5	0.7	0.8	1.2
Phosphorus	2.0	0.9	0.9	1.4
Iron (mg)	15.0	9.0	9.0	11.0

Mothers of the normal weight (defined as 5 1/2 pounds or more) infants, as is shown in Table 9, had been on diets which were much higher in calories, fat, protein (especially high-quality protein), calcium, phosphorus, and iron than mothers of stillbirths or low birth weight infants. Moreover, there was little difference in the nutritional intakes of women whose babies were pronounced dead at birth and those of women who gave birth to underweight infants, although the diets of the women in the latter group were somewhat superior.

Another retrospective prenatal dietary analysis also depicted the relationship between nutrition and birth weight. Discovering that protein consumption seemed to be the most accurate indicator of the quality and quantity of the entire diet, Jeans et al. formed five groups of the 404 women whose diets they analyzed based upon the women's daily protein intake.[46] The low birth weight incidence of the 177 women who had had less than 60 grams of protein daily was significantly higher than that of the 227 women who consumed at least 60 grams (4.0%) p<.02).

Among singletons, the results were even more significant (p<.01), since a set of twins in the best fed group were both underweight. Their combined weight, however, was over 10 1/2 pounds (4759 grams). More important, there were no stillbirths, neonatal deaths, or cases of congenital anomalies among the underweight infants born to the 227 best fed women. On the other hand, among the 17 low birth weight infants born to women who had less than 60 grams of protein per day, there was no stillbirth, five neonatal deaths, and four infants who had congenital anomalies.

 BIRTH WEIGHT IS MUCH MORE PREDICTIVE OF A CHILD'S SUSCEPTIBILITY TO SICKNESS AND DEATH THAN IS LENGTH OF GESTATION.

The Significance of Low Birth Weight

Why is the prevention of underweight births of such critical importance in any public health programs to safeguard infant health and child development? Hundreds of scientific studies far too voluminous to review herein have demonstrated that birth weight is the most accurate predictor of health and mental and physical development. Low birth weight infants account for two-thirds of all neonatal deaths (deaths among liveborn infants which occur within the first 28 days of life).[47] In fact, low birth weight is the eighth leading cause of death in the U.S.[10] The neonatal mortality rate among infants who were underweight at birth is 30 times higher than that of infants who weighed more than 5 1/2 pounds at birth.[48]

The authors of the aforementioned prospective nutrition education study among 500 women and those of the retrospective dietary analysis of 300 women noted:

> Neonatal mortality has shown very little improvement. By far the largest factor in these neonatal deaths is prematurity and of these premature deaths, roughly 50% occur in the first 48 hours. Most of these deaths are among the smallest and most weakly infants and it is unlikely that medical science even at the cost of more research and the spending of much time and money will save more than a few of them. A more rational method of approach to the problem would seem to be that of prevention.[45]

The birth weight is much more predictive of a child's susceptibility to morbidity and mortality than is length of gestation. Figure 2 demonstrates that birth weight is a much more accurate predictor of neonatal mortality than length of gestation.[49] Note that the mortality rate of neonates who weighed under 2000 grams (4 pounds 7 ounces) at birth is several times higher than that of those whose birth weight was over 3000 grams (6 pounds 10 ounces).

Margaret and Arthur Wynn wrote:

> One official government (Finland) estimate assumes that two children survive so severely and permanently handicapped as to become a charge to the state for every one who dies, and that reducing the causes of death does on the average reduce the numbers that are handicapped in the same proportion. Mortality rates are an indicator not only therefore of infant loss but of infant damage... The prevention of handicaps is much more economic, as well as more humane, than failure to prevent followed by care services and subsidies to the handicapped.[50]

The Collaborative Perinatal Study confirms the Wynns' estimate. The $100 million study showed that the incidence of definite neurological impairment of one-year-old children was three and a half times higher among those of low birth weight than among those of higher weight at birth.[51-52] In the mammoth study, birth weight was shown to be directly related to I.Q. at age 4.[51] More note-worthy, nearly half of all children who were underweight at birth have an I.Q. under 70.[53]

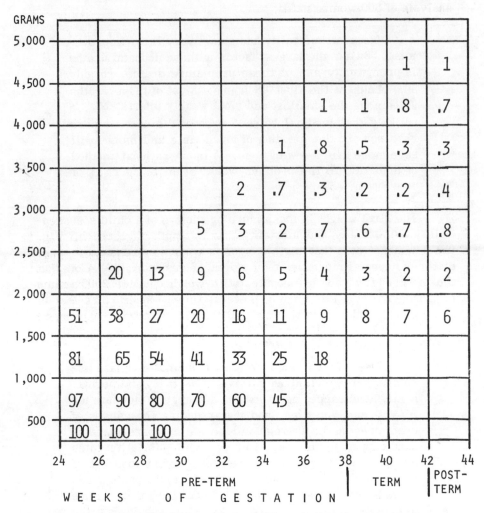

FIGURE 2. Neonatal mortality risk by birth weight & gestational age. Figures in boxes are percents of babies within the weight and age ranges of the box that die within the first 28 days after live birth. Especially note that babies born at term (38-42 weeks) but less than 2,500 grams are more likely to die than pre-term babies born at 30-36 weeks but who weigh more than 2,500 grams. (Note: 1,000 g = 2.2 lb or 2,500 g = 5.5 lb)

While developmental disabilities are more difficult to associate with low birth weight than infant death because they are less quanti- fiable, frequently under reported, and subjective analysis, the for- mer association and that between malnutrition and developmental disabilities are significant.

Low birth weight babies are approximately ten times more likely to be mentally retarded than those of higher birth weight.[54] One study of 8- to 10-year-old children showed that abstract verbal reasoning and perceptual/motor integration are more related to birth weight than they are to I.Q.[55] Approximately 35% to 40% of all low birth weight children have a diagnosable neurological abnor- mality by age 7.[56] At the age of 10, two-thirds of those who weighed no more than 1500 grams (3 pounds 5 ounces) at birth are similarly afflicted.[57]

After reviewing over 150 scientific works and analyzing data from his own studies of the effects of protein/calorie deprivation, Ben Platt stated:

> With the present state of knowledge, it must be accepted that protein-calorie deficiency, with its attend- ant ills, may lower maternal efficiency and lead to the production of underweight babies, many of whom will die before reaching two years of age, whilst among their survivors there will be some who never reach their full physical or mental potential. . . When all infants are given equal conditions both within and outside the womb, it is likely that many so-called racial characteristics will disappear.[34]

The relationship between low birth weight and neurological dysfunction becomes more meaningful when the reliability of profi- cient testing of neurologic function in predicting a child's develop- ment is considered. In one study the correlation between tests of neurological damage given during infancy and those administered more than five years later was 0.70 (p 10^{-10}).[58] In a subsequent study, neurological assessment was found to be predictive in 94% of the cases among 82 infants, which consisted of 28 controls, 30 screened normals, and 24 screened abnormals.[58]

Numerous prospective and retrospective studies reflect the high degree of association between low birth weight and subnormal development. In a study of 187 premature children who all weighed under 1500 grams (3 pounds 5 ounces) at birth, 49.7% had died with- in the first year of life.[59] Of the survivors who, at age 10 years, were given a battery of medical, neurological, psychological, EEG, and other tests, 68% were shown to be handicapped. Central nervous system disorders afflicted 49% of the children. Multiple handicaps were found among 41%. In addition, the incidence of abnormal EEG results (60%) among them was ten times higher than that usually found among normal birth weight children.

Because studies of twins (especially monozygotic twins) provide intrinsic controls of genetic and some environmental factors, they are pertinent to establishing the relationship between birth weight and development. Babson et al. examined development records of 16 sets of dissimilar-sized twins. In each case the smaller twin weighed less than 2000 grams (4 pounds 7 ounces) and at least 25% less than the larger twin at birth. I.Q., vocabulary, and language tests, and height, weight, and head circumference measurements were taken at ages ranging from 4 1/2 to 11 years. None of the examiners were aware of any child being the larger or smaller twin.

On the average, in all the tests and measurements the lower birth weight twins scored lower than the larger twins. (See Table 10.) Four of the smaller twins, in contrast to none of the larger twins, had physical defects.

TABLE 10
ASSOCIATION OF BIRTH WEIGHT
WITH VARIOUS TESTS AND MEASUREMENTS

Examination	Mean Difference Between the Higher Birth Weight Twins and the Runts	Significance Level
Vocabulary Test	2.50	ns
I.Q.	6.75	p<.05
Height	4.34 cm (1.7 in.)	p<.01
Head Circumference	1.34 cm (0.5 in.)	p<.001
Weight	3.95 kg (7 lb. 15 oz.)	p<.001

"IF ALL PROSPECTIVE HUMAN MOTHERS COULD BE FED AS EXPERTLY AS PROSPECTIVE ANIMAL MOTHERS IN THE LABORATORIES, MOST STERILITY, SPONTANEOUS ABORTIONS, STILLBIRTHS AND PREMATURE BIRTHS WOULD DISAPPEAR; THE BIRTH DEFORMED AND MENTALLY RETARDED BABIES WOULD BE LARGELY A THING OF THE PAST."

R. WILLIAMS, NUTRITIONIST

Among the nine monozygotic sets of twins, the mean differences were even greater, as revealed in the following table.

TABLE 11
ASSOCIATION OF BIRTH WEIGHT WITH I.Q.
ANS MEASUREMENTS AMONG MONOZYGOTIC TWINS

Examination	Mean Difference	Significance Level
I.Q. Head Circumference Weight Height	6.56 1.67 cm (0.7 in.) 4.81 kg (9 lb. 11 oz.) 5.89 cm (2.3 in.)	p<.05 p<.01 p<.001 p<.001

A larger study of 370 twelve-year-old children who resided at one psychiatric hospital and 370 controls showed that low birth weight is also associated with psychological disturbances.[60] The low birth weight incidence was much higher among the hospitalized, mentally ill children (14.1%) than among the controls (7.8%) (p<.005). In addition, the incidence of organic brain damage was higher among the study group children.

Many researchers have linked I.Q. and birth weight. A study involving 648 infants in which none of the examiners were aware of the children's birth weight documented the relationship between birth weight and I.Q., educational advancement, and behavior.[61] Only 1% of the children (who were tested at ages 7 or 11) who weighed over 5 1/2 pounds had moderate or severe mental, neurological, or physical handicaps. In contrast, among those whose birth weight was under 1250 grams (2 pounds 12 ounces), 64% had such abnormalities. The data in Table 12 signify that the probability that birth weight is not related to mental, physical, and/or neurological impairment is less than one in a billion.

Even when controlled by socioeconomic class, I.Q. increased as birth weight rose. Table 13 gives the distribution of I.Q. centiles by socioeconomic class based upon the I.Q. scores of the children who weighed over 5 1/2 pounds at birth. The expected distribution of I.Q. scores, assuming there was no relationship between birth weight and I.Q., would be 25% for the lowest quartile, 50% for the 25th to 75th percentile, and 25% for the highest quartile. For every socioeconomic class there were more than the expected number of children whose I.Q. was in the lowest quartile and fewer than the expected number of children whose I.Q. was in the highest quartile.

TABLE 12
ASSOCIATION BETWEEN BIRTH WEIGHT
AND RISK OF HANDICAP (514 Cases)

Birth Weight	Degree of Handicap		
	Moderate or Severe	Mild	Little Or None
1250 grams (2 lb, 12 oz) and under	64% (23)	17% (6)	19% (7)
1251-1500 grams (2 lb, 12 oz to 3 lb, 5 oz)	34% (16)	21% (10)	45% (21)
1501-1750 grams (3 lb, 5 oz to 3 lb, 13.75 oz)	19% (5)	23% (6)	58% (15)
1751-2000 grams (3 lb, 13.75 oz to 4 lb, 6.5 oz)	12% (8)	30% (20)	58% (39)
2001-2250 grams (4 lb, 6.5 oz to 4 lb, 15.5 oz)	4% (2)	23% (13)	74% (42)
2251-2500 grams (4 lb, 15.5 oz to 5 lb, 8 oz)	3% (3)	16% (19)	81% (94)
2501 grams (5 lb, 8 oz) and over	1% (2)	12% (20)	87% (143)

"THERE ARE A NUMBER OF PHENOMENA WHICH WE HAVE ACCEPTED AS 'NORMAL IN PREGNANCY' WHICH I HAVE REALIZED WERE NUTRITION-RELATED AND WHICH I DO NOT SEE IN MY PRACTICE ANY MORE...MOTHERS WHO ARE PROPERLY NOURISHED DO NOT GET STRETCH MARKS, AND THEY DO NOT SEEM TO HAVE ACCELERATION OF DENTAL CARIES OR SOFTENING OF THE GUMS. I DO NOT SEE LOSS OF HAIR, SPLITTING OF NAILS, SOFTENING OF BONES, ANEMIA, POSTPARTUM HEMORRHAGE, OR FAILURES AT NURSING. IN ADDITION, AFTER THE 4TH MONTH, MOST MOTHERS FEEL NORMAL AS FAR AS ENERGY OUTPUT."

(ONE PHYSICIAN'S OBSERVATIONS AFTER ADOPTING AN EFFECTIVE NUTRITION PROGRAM FOR HIS PREGNANT PATIENTS.)

TABLE 13
INFLUENCE OF BIRTH WEIGHT
ON DISTRIBUTION OF I.Q. SCORES
BY SOCIOECONOMIC STATUS

Socio-economic Class	I.Q. Centile	Birth Weight (g)	
		2000 and Under	2001-2500
Middle	Under 25th	55% (29)	39% (26)
	25th to 75th	36% (19)	44% (29)
	Over 75th	9% (5)	17% (11)
	Total	100% (53)	100% (66)
Working	Under 25th	64% (29)	36% (28)
	25th to 75th	25% (11)	47% (37)
	Over 75th	11% (5)	18% (14)
	Total	100% (45)	100% (79)
Lower	Under 25th	52% (14)	48% (15)
	25th to 75th	44% (12)	45% (14)
	Over 75th	4% (1)	6% (2)
	Total	100% (27)	100% (31)

Even after excluding children who had moderate or severe handicaps, a significant correlation was found between birth weight and I.Q. at ages 5 to 7. Table 14 shows the relationship between low birth weight and maladjusted behavior among 432 eleven-year-old children at all socioeconomic classes. Among children who weighed under 2001 grams at birth, 21.7% were found to be maladjusted in contrast to 8.4% of those who weighed over 2500 grams

The author concluded:

The incidence of moderate or severe handicaps increases with decreasing birthweight, particularly at weights of 2000 grams and under... Mean I.Q. scores ... fell with decreasing birthweight in all social groups ... This is not due to socio-economic factors, being equally evident when comparing children of different birthweight reared in the best (sic) homes with those reared in the worst... There is no evidence that low birthweight children 'catch up' as they become older. [61]

In a study of 50 sets of twins, whose ages ranged from 5 to 15 years, the heavier twin scored, on the average, significantly higher than the lighter twins. [62] The differences were significant at the

.1% level among the 22 sets of identical twins. For the study, the psychologist administering the I.Q. tests was not aware of any child's birth weight and tested a given set of twins on the same day to increase the reliability of the scores.

TABLE 14
RELATIONSHIP BETWEEN BIRTH WEIGHT
AND CHILDHOOD BEHAVIOR
BY SOCIAL CLASS

Socioeconomic Class	Total # of Children	% Stable	% Unsettled	% Maladjusted
Birth Weight Under 2001 grams				
Middle	42	69	24	7
Working	36	47	19	33
Lower	28	36	36	29
Birth Weight Over 2500 grams				
Middle	71	79	15	6
Working	54	70	20	9
Lower	29	45	41	14

The same author supplemented his previous findings in an analysis of the birth weights of 51 mentally retarded children, all of whom were at least six years of age at the time of the study. [63] A control group consisted of children whose I.Q.'s were over 110 and who went to the same school (in which the average I.Q. was 114) as those in the study group. The controls were matched with the retarded children for sex, age, and area of residence.

Birth weight and I.Q. were significantly associated (p<.002). In none of the cases was the birth weight of any of the 51 retarded children higher than that of his matched control. The probability that such a high correlation is due to chance (i.e., that there is no association between retardation and birth weight) is infinitesimal. Among the children of normal to high intelligence, only 3.9% were of low birth weight in contrast to 21.6% among the study group children (p<.01).

MATERNAL MALNUTRITION ALSO RETARDS THE GROWTH OF THE PLACENTA AND LOW PLACENTAL WEIGHT IS RELATED TO PERINATAL DEATH.

TABLE 15
RELATIONSHIP BETWEEN I.Q. AND BIRTH WEIGHT
AMONG 51 RETARDATES AND MATCHED CONTROLS

	Average I.Q.	Average Birth Weight	Average Birth Weight Exclusive of Low Birth Weight and/or PRemature Children
MALES Retarded Children	70	3020 grams (6 lb, 10.63 oz) (N = 25) (p<.002)	3300 grams (7 lb, 4.5 oz) (N = 20) (p<.002)
Control Group	121	3750 grams (8 lb, 4.37 oz) (N = 25)	3830 grams (8 lb, 7.25 oz) (N = 24)
FEMALES Retarded Children	67	2900 grams (6 lb, 6.37 oz) (N = 26) (p<.002	3080 grams (6 lb, 12.75 oz) (N = 20) (p<.02)
Control Group	124	3360 grams (7 lb, 6.13 oz) (N = 26)	3440 grams (7 lb, 9.37 oz) (N = 25)
N = Number of Children.			

Developmental quotient (D.Q.) has also been linked with birth weight. In one study in which 90% of the infants tested had a D.Q. between 90 and 120, 80% of those with a D.Q. under 80 were low birth weight infants.[64]

Bacola et al. studied low birth weight children to determine the rates of mental retardation, neurological dysfunction, and respiratory difficulties.[65] Of the 40 children, who were examined at an average age of 4.3 years, 12 weighed between 1000 (2 pounds 3 ounces) and 1250 (2 pounds 12 ounces) grams at birth and 28 weighed between 1250 and 1500 grams (3 pounds 5 ounces). Among the smaller birth weight children, five (42%) were mentally retarded. Half (20) of the children appeared normal, although the authors felt that many of them had minimal brain dysfunction.

Most significant, 60% of the children had had respiratory problems while infants. The incidence of respiratory distress syndrome (RDS), particularly severe RDS, was inversely proportional to birth weight. Since 80% of the deliveried were spontaneous and

cesarean sections were required in only 5% of the cases, the higher
rates of RDS, mental retardation, and other neurological impairment could not be attributed to the period of labor or the delivery
process. Among all of the mentally retarded children, severe RDS
or late apnea (breathing difficulties of at least two minutes' duration
occurring between a few hours after birth to two months of age)
and/or toxemia of late pregnancy was observed.

TABLE 16
ASSOCIATION BETWEEN BIRTH WEIGHT
AND DEVELOPMENT OF RDS

Birth Weight	Total # of Children	Incidence of RDS	Incidence of Severe RDS
1250 grams or less	12	75%	42.0%
Over 1250 grams	28	32%	3.5%

TABLE 17
RISK OF MENTAL RETARDATION
AMONG CHILDREN WITH RDS

	# of Children	Incidence of Mental Retardation Among Children with RDS
Severe RDS	6	67%
Less Severe RDS	12	8%

The relationship between RDS and low umbilical cord protein
levels has been well established. Moreover, the causal relationship
between low cord protein level and maternal malnutrition has also
been documented. In an aforementioned prospective food supplementation study, the well-fed women had cord albumin levels significantly higher than those in the malnourished group (p<.01).[33]

A study of the cord protein levels of 2,200 consecutive births
at one hospital revealed the dramatic association between low cord
protein level of 4.6 g/100 ml or less, 17.1% had RDS, whereas only
one of the 2,102 infants whose cord level was above 4.6 g/100 ml
developed RDS. The probability that the difference is due to chance
approaches one over infinity. Nineteen of the 34 infants(55.9%)were
significantly lower among those who died than the 15 who survived (p<.01). The mean protein level among the 34 infants with
RDS was 3.80 g/100 ml; that of the 2,166 who did not have the disease was 5.91 g/100 ml (p<10^{-8}).

Cord protein was also significantly associated with birth weight, length of gestation, and the occurrence of third-trimester hemorrhage. Among infants of 28 to 32 weeks' gestation who weighed between 1000 (2 pounds 3 ounces) and 1500 (3 pounds 5 ounces) grams at birth, the mean protein level was 3.8 g/100 ml. Since higher gestational age was found to be associated with a rise in colloid osmotic pressure, the author inferred that "the plasma proteins of immature infants may be not only quantitatively deficient but functionally ineffective as well."

The average birth weight among the infants who had RDS was 1570 grams (3 pounds 7 1/2 ounces). The mean length of gestation among them was 31 weeks. The author noted that the severity of RDS is also related to a decrease in cord protein.

TABLE 18

RISK OF RDS AND CONCOMITANT MORTALITY BY BIRTH WEIGHT, CORD PROTEIN LEVEL, AND LENGTH OF GESTATION

	# of Infants	% With RDS	Lvl. of Signif.	% Mortal.
Low Birth Weight	171	17.5		11.1
Birth Weight			$p < 10^{-12}$	
Over 2500 grams	2,039			*
Cord Protein of				
4.6 g/100 ml or less	98			20.4
Cord protein greater than			$p < 10^{-12}$	
4.6 g/100 ml	2,102			*
Low Birth Weight and				
Low Cord Protein				
(4.6 g/100 ml or less)	60			30.0
Normal Birth Weight				
and/or normal cord			$p < 10^{-15}$	
Protein (at least				
4.7 g/100 ml)	2,140			*
Premature (less than				
37 weeks' gestation)				
and Low Blood Protein	58			32.8
Normal Length of Gestation			$p < 10^{-15}$	
and Normal Blood Prot.	2,142			*

Many clinicians believe that low birth weight infants born at term are more prone to neurological impairment than underweight premature infants [67] and are more likely to have congenital anomalies. [10] Of 27 underweight infants born at term, 5 died, 1 was deaf, 4 had congenital heart diseases, and 6 were severely mentally retarded. [68] In addition, among the survivors, nine (41%) were mentally deficient and two (9%) had borderline intelligence. Many of the 27 mothers had nausea, developed toxemia (which will later be shown to be c a u s e d by malnutrition), and/or gained insufficient weight during pregnancy.

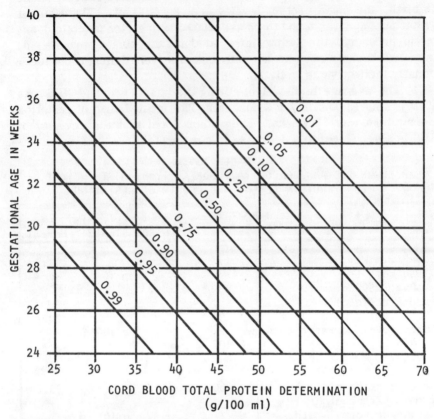

FIGURE 3. Probability that Respiratory Distress Syndrome (RDS) will develop in a given infant based on determinations of gestational age and cord blood total protein level as independent variables, with the use of the logistic function.

Effects of Prenatal Nutrition
in Reducing Infant Mortality and Improving Pediatric Health

Decades of scientific research have demonstrated the unequivocal relationship between prenatal nutrition and the condition of the newborn. This relationship, although complex, is so direct that a deficiency of even one essential nutrient can result in miscarriage, perinatal death, or the birth of a developmentally disabled child. [69]

WHILE VETERINARIANS, FARMERS, AND RANCHERS HAVE CLEARLY
DEFINED STANDARDS FOR THE MANAGEMENT OF PREGNANT ANI-
MALS, NO SUCH STANDARDS EXIST FOR HUMANS.

A noted nutritionist declared: "If all prospective human mothers could be fed as expertly as prospective animal mothers in the laboratories, most sterility, spontaneous abortions, stillbirths and premature births would disappear; the birth of deformed and mentally retarded babies would be largely a thing of the past."[69]

The pernicious effects of malnutrition are most pronounced when near-starvation is imminent. During the 17-month siege of Leningrad, amenorrhea, failure to conceive, and spontaneous abortion were common in addition to infant morbidity and mortality.[20] In one large clinic in Leningrad, the number of births declined to 79 during the second half of 1942, corresponding to the most pronounced period of starvation several months before. During the six-month period two years previous, there were 1,639 births at the same clinic. The small number of births during the entire year of 1942 (439) represented a sharp reduction from the average number of births during the previous three years of 3,869 ($p < 10^{-15}$).

Also reflecting the pronounced hunger which afflicted women who delivered during the first half of 1942 was the three and a half times higher rate of stillbirths and neonatal deaths during that period when compared to the rate during the second half of the year. Among children born in 1942, nearly 89% of them lost weight for more than three successive days after birth. Nearly 26% of all infants born during the first six months of 1942 died during that period.

The author stated:

> Hunger, vitamin deficiency, cold, excessive physical strain, lack of rest, and constant nervous tension had their effect on the health of the women, the intra-uterine development of the fetuses, and the condition of the newborn children during the siege... The cause of the unusually high proportions of premature births (defined as births under 47 centimeters in length) and of stillbirths in the first half of 1942 was hunger during pregnancy, that is, the insufficient quantity and the unsatisfactory quality of the women's food.[20]

In the previously mentioned Harvard study of 216 births, prenatal nutrition was found to be directly related to pediatric health

and r e d u c e d infant mortality. [17-19] In this double-blind study
neither the obstetricians who evaluated the health of the infants at
birth nor the pediatricians who examined them within the first two
days of life were aware of any of the mothers' nutritional status. In
addition, all of the professional examinations were performed independently.

Two-thirds of the infants born to women who had been on poor
to very poor diets were stillborn, died within the third day of life,
weighed under five pounds at birth, or had congenital defects. [17, 19]
Only 8% of the infants born to these women were determined to be in
good or superior condition. On the other hand, only 3% of the infants of mothers who had been on good or excellent diets were in
poor h e a l t h. Moreover, 94% of them were in superior or good
health.

TABLE 19
RELATIONSHIP OF PRENATAL NUTRITION
AND BIRTH WEIGHT TO NEONATAL HEALTH

	Pediatric Ratings of Infants			
	Superior	Good	Fair	Poor
Number of Infants	23	84	76	33
Average Birth Weight	8lb,2oz (3685g)	7lb,12oz (3515g)	7lb,2oz (3232g)	5lb,15oz (2693g)
Women on Good or excellent Prenatal Diet	56%	19%	1%	3%
Women on Poor or Very Poor Prenatal Diet	9%	2%	12%	79%

Numerous prospective studies p r o v i d e substantial data reflecting the critical importance of nutrition during pregnancy. Ebbs
showed that food supplementation during the second half of pregnancy
results in a marked reduction in reproductive casualty. In fact, the
90 women who were malnourished during the first half of pregnancy
and whose diets were supplemented during the latter half had lower
rates of miscarriage, stillbirths, and premature births (definition
n o t specified) t h a n the 170 women who had followed sound diets
throughout pregnancy.

Table 20, which excludes infants with gross congenital anomalies, demonstrates the relationship between maternal nutrition and
pediatric health at two weeks of age. [20] (Miscarriages and still-

births are included in the lowest pediatric rating.) Note that nutritional supplementation during the second half of pregnancy eliminated mortality and major infant morbidity, the incidence of which was 14% among the poorly nourished women.

TABLE 20
INFLUENCE OF DIET IN REDUCING RISK OF
MISCARRIAGE, STILLBIRTH, AND PREMATURE BIRTH

Type of Diet	# of Women	% Miscarriages	% Stillbirths	% Premature
Good	170	1.2	0.6	3.0
Supplemented	90	0.0	0.0	2.2
Poor	120	6.0	3.4	8.0

Among the first 250 babies examined at six months of age, there were three deaths in the poor diet group and none in either of the well-fed groups.[70] In addition, of these 250 infants, 21% of those born to women in the poor diet group, in contrast to only 5% of those born to mothers in either of the better fed groups, had had frequent colds.[28] Ebbs et al. concluded: "The application of the principles of nutrition could not be more important in any other period of life than during pregnancy."[70]

A dramatic reduction in mortality was also achieved in the prospective, controlled study of 750 pregnant women.[16] Perhaps the most revealing finding was that there were no stillbirths and only 3 infant deaths among the infants of the mothers whose diets were supplemented and who received nutrition education, in contrast to a total of 61 such deaths among the 750 controls. The author also linked inadequate nutrition, particularly vitamin A deficiency, to spontaneous abortion.

TABLE 21
PRENATAL DIET BY
CONDITION OF BABY AT AGE TWO WEEKS

Prenatal Diet Group	Condition of Baby			
	Good	Fair	Poor	Bad
Good	72.2%	23.8%	1.2%	3.0%
Supplemented	90.5%	9.5%	0.0%	0.0%
Poor	62.3%	23.7%	5.3%	8.7%

More recent prospective studies have shown similar results which are less dramatic than those in the above-mentioned study, probably because the food supplementation was of a lesser degree and nutrition education was not provided. In an aforementioned supplementation study, there were no stillbirths among the 199 women who received the largest amount of supplemented calories.[27]

TABLE 22
EFFECT OF NUTRITION ON REDUCING MODERATELY LOW BIRTH WEIGHT,
STILLBIRTH, AND INFANT MORTALITY

	Study Group		Control Group		Signif. Level of Difference
Total Number	750		750		
Births Under 5 lb (2268g)	0	(0%)	37	(4.9%)	$p<10^{-8}$
Stillbirths (rate)	0	0	20	26.7	$p<10^{-6}$
Infant Deaths (rate)	3	4.0	41	54.6	$p<10^{-7}$

Another study by the same authors documented the effects of
nutrition on child development.[27] In this study many of the 671
children (all singletons) received the same type of supplement from
6 to 15 months of age that their mothers had taken during pregnancy
and lactation. The incidence of physical growth retardation (defined
as a child's weight being under the 10th percentile) at 15 months of
age was two times higher among the 373 children whose mothers
received the smallest amount of caloric supplementation (12.3%)
than those born to the 84 women who had the greatest caloric supplementation (6.0%). In addition, the rate of low psychological test
performance was four and a half times as high in the former group
(11.0%) as in the latter (2.4%). These differences were not related
to socioeconomic or demographic variables or childhood morbidity.

The authors declared: "Intervention programs (in poor rural
populations) designed to reduce infant mortality have generally focused on the control of infectious diseases through adequate health
services and paid little attention to nutrition. These results demonstrate that nutritional interventions can help to reduce infant mortality."[27]

TABLE 23
MORTALITY BY DEGREE
OF CALORIC SUPPLEMENTATION

	# of Women	First 6 Months	More Than 6 But Less Than 9 Months	Over 9 Months But Less Than 1 Year
High Supple-mentation	199	3.0%	0.9%	0.0%
Low Supple-mentation	454	5.3%	1.2%	0.6%

More than 25 years ago, Dieckmann et al. showed that a reduction in spontaneous abortion was significantly associated with an increase in maternal protein intake (p<.002).[71] In the study, which consisted of 612 pregnant women whose diets were carefully supervised, there were also significant decreases in low birth weight and infant morbidity with improved dietary protein.

 DURING THE LAST TRIMESTER OF PREGNANCY TO THE FIRST MONTH OF LIFE, THE PERIOD OF MOST RAPID BRAIN DEVELOPMENT, MALNUTRITION CAN CAUSE IRREVERSIBLE NEUROLOGICAL DAMAGE AND PERMANENT BRAIN UNDERDEVELOPMENT.

Physiological Effects of Inadequate Maternal Nutrition

The relationship between nutrition and development as enumerated in both prospective and retrospective studies, many of which were reviewed in the previous section and prior ones, should be viewed from a more direct perspective rather than a statistical one. In fact, such studies are hardly necessary in view of the known physiological phenomena pertaining to nutrition and development. Because of our emphasis on research, which is frequently done more for research's sake than its practical applications, and our failure to apply principles of internal medicine and nutrition science, numerous pregnant women have been subjected to risks of reproductive casualty in experiments which do not ensure an adequate intake of calories and nutrients.[24]

Proper nutrition during pregnancy is a sine qua non for normal fetal development. This period of development is so rapid that an adult would be several times the size of the earth if he or she had grown at the fetal growth rate through adult life.[72] Most important, the brain develops more than any other organ during fetal development.[73] In fact, the head circumference of a newborn infant is approximately 65% of the full adult size.[47] At the age of five months, a child has approximately 80% of his or her adult capacity of brain cells.

Malnutrition directly and adversely hinders hyperplasia (cell division).[74-75] During the most rapid period of brain development, which occurs from the last trimester of pregnancy to the first month of life, malnutrition can cause irreversible neurological damage and permanent brain underdevelopment.[34,47,76] One study showed that malnutrition during pregnancy can result in a deficiency of as much as 60% of the expected number of brain cells.[75]

In the same study, the brain weight, protein, RNA, and DNA of nine infants (who were between 1/2 and 11 months of age) who had been malnourished prenatally (indicated by triangles in the figures below) were compared with the same measures of brain development of two abortuses and eight infants whose mothers had not shown signs of clinical malnutrition (indicated by circles). The number of brain cells, as measured by DNA (at the age of six months, brain DNA is nearly the adult amount [74]), was significantly lower in the malnourished group. Note that the amount of RNA and protein per brain cell were comparable in the malnourished and better nourished groups. In Figures 4-7, the lines represent the range for normal children independent of data from the study.

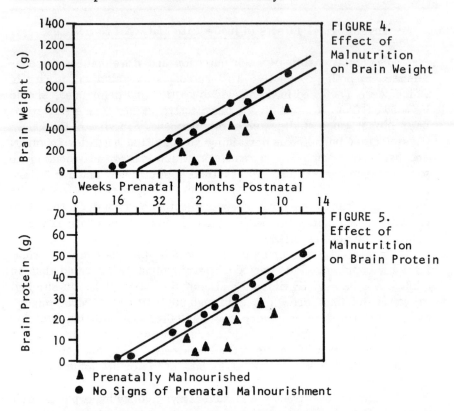

FIGURE 4.
Effect of
Malnutrition
on Brain Weight

FIGURE 5.
Effect of
Malnutrition
on Brain Protein

▲ Prenatally Malnourished
● No Signs of Prenatal Malnourishment

Malnutrition during the latter half of pregnancy leads to a reduction in the number of glial cells, [77] which are more vulnerable to malnutrition than any other form of neurological development. [30] Glial cells, which form the myelin sheath (which insulates nerve fibers) around the axons, form the foundation for the most dominant type of neurological development, myelination, which progresses from approximately age one to age four. [77]

Even more significant neurological development that glial proliferation occurs concurrently with and is dependent on glial multiplication and myelination. Impairment in the formation and development of dendrites (which conduct impulses to cells) may affect learning potential more than a reduction in the number or size of brain cells. The interneural network is adversely affected by malnutrition. [30] The size of axons, which comprise a major component of the total nerve fiber, is also stunted by intrauterine and early postnatal malnutrition.

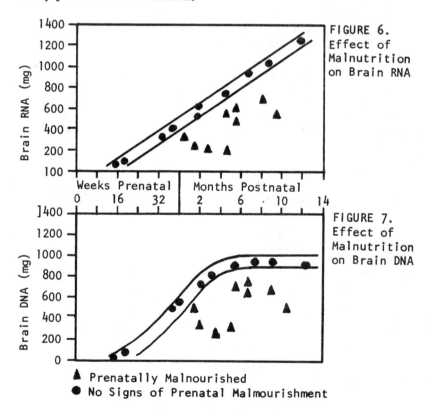

FIGURE 6. Effect of Malnutrition on Brain RNA

FIGURE 7. Effect of Malnutrition on Brain DNA

▲ Prenatally Malnourished
● No Signs of Prenatal Malnourishment

Malnutrition during the initial stages of brain development causes changes in the size, electrical activity, composition, and morphology of the central nervous system. [34] Because the cerebellum, which coordinates voluntary muscular movements, is largely developed between the 30th week of gestation and the first year of life, it is much more vulnerable to inadequate nutrition than the cerebrum,[78] which is developed over a longer period.[77]

After the age of two, poor nutrition basically retards the growth of individual brain cells.[34] Mental deficiency from malnutrition after this age, at which time brain cell proliferation has virtually ceased,[74] is much more likely to be reversible than brain underdevelopment caused by prenatal malnutrition.[34]

Maternal malnutrition also retards the growth of the placenta [26,74,79-80] and can lead to placental dysfunction and pathology.[81] Lechtig et al. discovered that malnutrition caused low birth weight primarily because of its effect on reducing the size of the placenta.[26] It is not surprising, then, that placental weight and birth weight are highly correlated.[5] The Collaborative Perinatal Study also showed that low placental weight is related to perinatal death.

TABLE 24
ASSOCIATION OF PLACENTAL WEIGHT WITH
LOW BIRTH WEIGHT AND PERINATAL MORTALITY

Weight of Placenta (g)	# Live Brths. With Known Birth Wt.	% Low Birth Wt.	Total Births	% Perinatal Mortality
0-199	122	88.5	318	86.5
200-249	311	83.6	374	33.5
250-299	1,129	51.9	1,192	9.4
300-349	3,555	26,2	3,616	2.9
350-399	6,150	12.1	6,205	1.6
400-449	7,283	5.1	7,331	1.4
450-499	5,879	2.8	5,921	1.0
500-549	3,744	1.3	3,764	1.0
550-599	2,056	0.9	2,072	1.0
> 600	1,737	0.5	1,771	2.7
TOTAL	31,966	10.13	32,564	3.03

Inadequate nutrition frequently leads to hepatic dysfunction, [36,82-83] which frequently precedes placental pathology. Hepatic storage of many nutrients, including albumin, is significantly related to birth weight.[33]

 FROM STRICTLY AN ECONOMIC STANDPOINT, PREVENTIVE OB-STETRICAL CARE IS ONE OF THE NATION'S SOUNDEST INVESTMENTS. FOR EACH CASE OF SEVERE MENTAL RETARDATION THAT IS PREVENTED, THE ECONOMIC GAIN TO SOCIETY IS MORE THAN $900,000.

Consequences of Sodium Deficiency,
A Common Cause of Toxemia

Various dramatic physiological and biochemical adjustments, particularly hormonal changes, accompany pregnancy. One major such adjustment is an increased retention of sodium, the principle electrolyte of the extracellular fluid.[85-86] Potential sodium depletion, which is frequently iatrogenic, is counteracted by a five-to tenfold increase in aldosterone, an adrenal hormone which facilitates tubular reabsorption of sodium, representing the largest pregnancy renal adjustment.[42, 86] The increase in aldosterone secretion is the last stage of the salt conservation mechanism (known as the renin-angiotensin-aldosterone homeostasis), which helps maintain a near constant concentration of sodium in the extracellular fluid. When this homeostasis is over-stressed (i.e., when the pregnant woman's sodium requirements are not met), juxtaglomerular degranulation can occur with its attendant morbidity and mortality.[87]

In an extensive study of 2,019 pregnant women, Robinson demonstrated unequivocally that sodium is an essential nutrient during pregnancy.[88] The women were divided into a high salt group (these women were told to increase their salt consumption) and a low salt group (these women were instructed to decrease their salt intake). Other than dietary sodium advice, the women in the two groups, who were of comparable age, parity, and socioeconomic status, were not placed on diverse dietary or medical regimens. The rates of miscarriage, perinatal death, toxemia, edema, and placental infarcts were much higher among the women who were told to restrict their salt consumption than among the women who were told to use additional salt.

TABLE 25
CONSEQUENCES OF SALT RESTRICTION

	# of Women	Perinatal Mortality Rate	% Toxemia	% Edema	% Placental Infarcts
Restricted Salt Intake	1,000	50.0	9.7	28.7	1.3
Increased Salt Intake	1,019	26.5	3.7	16.0	3.2

It may seem ironic that those who restricted their salt intake had the higher rate of edema, which is usually thought of as being caused by excess sodium intake. The inverted conception of the role of sodium in pregnancy edema represents one of the most misunderstood aspects of internal medicine.[36] The prevailing theory that sodium retention is a pathological condition caused by excess sodium intake has led to a vast amount of maternal and infant morbidity and mortality. Low-salt diets further deplete the woman of the essential nutrient, causing her renin-angiotensin-aldosterone mechanism to be stimulated even further to retain more sodium, the vicious cycle of which can lead to pathological edema.[84, 86]

The speculative theory that sodium should be restricted provided some justification for the drug industry to promote diuretics, which cause sodium depletion. Despite the publication of double-blind studies which conclusively demonstrated that diuretics are of no value in human pregnancy,[89-91] approximately half of all obstetricians still prescribe them.[2] Besides leading to impaired placental function [92] and fetal growth, diuretics can lead to fetal malformations,[92] neonatal thrombocytopenia,[93] hypoglycemia,[36] or electrolyte imbalance [36, 92] and maternal complications, such as toxemia [36, 41-42] or pancreatitis.[94]

The editor of a major obstetrics journal stated:

> Modern renal physiology makes it clear that the use of diuretics in pregnancy has little or no basis. In fact, they pose a significant risk of sodium depletion. The one role they might serve is in the case of heart-failure, but these instances are, of course, rare. There is a strong body of belief that diuretics may be causative of complications. The use of diuretics in pregnancy should be banned; they should be abandoned in modern prenatal care.[40]

The use of diuretics and low-salt diets can, especially in malnourished women, lead to maternal death.[38, 95] One obstetrician attributed the increase in maternal deaths from 5 to 19 during three-year periods at one hospital center largely to the indiscriminate use of low-salt diets and diuretics.[95] In reviewing the medical records of 67 maternal deaths from toxemia, he stated:

> Retrospectively, most of these deaths were unavoidable and many were the direct consequence of errors in professional judgement... Although the risk

of death from acute toxemia is higher for patients with a socioeconomic disadvantage, the majority of deaths occurred among patients receiving private care. In addition, the incidence of deaths appears to be increasing at a time when more patients are receiving private care ... Physician error contributes greatly to acute toxemic deaths. [95]

The incidence of toxemia can be sharply reduced simply by encouraging pregnant women to salt their foods to taste and refraining from prescribing diuretics. In one clinic where such management was followed, there was only one case of toxemia in 5,300 pregnancies, [41] which is far below the U.S. incidence of 7%. [96] At a nearby clinic, where the hazardous regimens are utilized, the toxemia rate was 98 times higher.

The physician supervising the former clinic explained:

> In prescribing diuretics, the physician attempts to remove fluid by reducing the tubular sodium reabsorption and thereby remove sodium from the plasma. The quantity of fluid lost in this way is then replaced by the shift of the edema fluid back to the circulation. However, if therapy is continued, or if the edema fluid does not move back into the vessels, we are removing not the fluid, but the physiological reserves of sodium. This in turn disturbs the volume homeostasis of the body fluids. As a result, all the mechanisms responsible for homeostasis are activated, and we produce all those complications that we have attempted to avoid. [41]

 DESPITE THE PUBLICATION OF DOUBLE-BLIND STUDIES WHICH CONCLUSIVELY DEMONSTRATED THAT DIURETICS (WATER PILLS) ARE OF NO VALUE IN HUMAN PREGNANCY, AS OF 1974 APPROXIMATELY HALF OF ALL OBSTETRICIANS STILL PRESCRIBED THEM. BESIDES LEADING TO IMPAIRED PLACENTAL FUNCTION AND FETAL GROWTH, DIURETICS CAN LEAD TO FETAL MALFORMATIONS, NEONATAL THROMBOCYTOPENIA, HYPOGLYCEMIA, ELECTROLYTE IMBALANCE AND MATERNAL COMPLICATIONS SUCH AS TOXEMIA OR PANCREATITIS.

Infant deaths are also associated with the administration of diuretics. In a study of more than 17,000 pregnant women, the infant mortality rate among full-term infants was 16% higher in those who had been prescribed diuretics.[97]

The FDA recently cited all of the nine drug firms which manufacture diuretics for pregnant women for promoting the drugs on no scientific basis.[98] In stating new regulations for the use of diuretics (which in essence state that the drug is contraindicated and possibly hazardous during pregnancy), the FDA noted:

> The drugs lack substantial evidence of effectiveness for all of their stated indications (i.e., hypertension of pregnancy, severe edema when due to pregnancy, prevention of the development of toxemia of pregnancy, edema of localized origin... No person requested a hearing on the indications regarded as lacking substantial evidence of effectiveness, and no comment before the Advisory Committee supported these indications... The Director of the Bureau of Drugs is unaware of any adequate and well-controlled clinical investigation... demonstrating the effectiveness of... any of the drugs for treatment of toxemia of pregnancy..."[98]

The restriction of salt during pregnancy (and the justification for the prescription of diuretics) is based upon the historically accepted, but never proven, speculation that toxemia is caused by impairment of salt excretion.[86] In reality, among toxemic women, salt retention is not a cause of toxemia but, rather, an impending sign of sodium depletion, which causes the toxemia.[99]

A major reason that the myth that sodium restriction is a prophylaxis of toxemia continues to predominate obstetrical thinking is that physiological edema is seldom differentiated from pathological edema. Physiological edema usually signifies a normal pregnancy, whereas pathological edema reflects protein/calorie, sodium, and/or related dietary deficiencies or a medical disorder unrelated to pregnancy. Differential diagnosis as well as a thorough dietary history can invariably determine the origin of the edema.[36]

Approximately 60% of all healthy pregnant women will develop edema, including generalized edema.[36, 100] A study of nonproteinuric women showed that edema was associated with a 58% reduction in perinatal mortality.[93]

TABLE 26
ASSOCIATION OF ABSENCE OF EDEMA
WITH PREMATURE DEATH

	# of Women	# of Still-Births	# of Neonatal Deaths	Perinatal Mortality Rate
No Edema of Hands or Face	2,268	33	40	32.2
Edema of Hands or Face	1,890	15	10	13.2

As has been shown above, edema, instead of being physiologic, can develop as a result of sodium deficiency. Pathological edema can also result from protein and/or calorie deficiency. This type of edema is mediated by a decrease in the plasma proteins as a result of lowered serum albumin concentration.[101-102]

By measuring the serum osmotic pressure of 65 pregnant women, all of whom were at seven months' gestation, Strauss demonstrated that the pressure was directly related to protein intake.[102] Serum osmotic pressure, serum albumin, and dietary protein were highest among the 35 nontoxemic women in the study, second highest among the 20 women who had nonconvulsive toxemia, and lowest among the 10 women who had eclampsia.

At the eighth month of gestation, 15 of the 20 nonconvulsive toxemic women were placed on a diet which consisted of 260 grams of protein and were given vitamin injections; the other 5 were placed on an isocaloric diet which provided 20 grams of protein. The osmotic pressure among the women on the high-protein diet increased by an average of 7%; that of the latter group declined 9%. Strauss noted that the average daily protein intake of the 20 women was less than 50 grams.

SODIUM (SALT) IS AN ESSENTIAL NUTRIENT DURING PREGNANCY. THE RATES OF MISCARRIAGE, PERINATAL DEATH, TOXEMIA, EDEMA, AND PLACENTAL INFARCTS WERE MUCH HIGHER AMONG WOMEN WHO WERE TOLD TO RESTRICT THEIR SALT CONSUMPTION THAN AMONG THE WOMEN WHO WERE TOLD TO USE ADDITIONAL SALT.

After three weeks on the high-protein diet, the symptoms of toxemia (including a reduction in the blood pressure of all 15 women) subsided. There was not one case of fetal mortality. The women lost an average of 6 1/2 pounds. In contrast, only two of the five toxemic women who had been placed on a low-protein diet showed a reduction in blood pressure. In addition, they gained an average of 1/2 pound.

Ross, who discovered that the incidence of eclampsia was extremely high in areas where beriberi, pellagra, and other diseases of nutritional deficiencies were found, stated: "We have been struck with the number of patients in eclampsia who are in a very poor state of nutrition... The type of patient we see in eclamptic convulsions is the patient who subsists on a 2900 calorie diet consisting of bat meat, field peas, rice, hominy, grits, cane syrup, brown gravy, lard, and cornmeal... which is deficient in Vitamins B_2, A, C, and D, iron, calcium, phosphorus, and complete proteins."[103]

Hypovolemia (and usually hypoalbuminemia) precedes the onset of metabolic toxemia of late pregnancy.[36, 104] Hypovolemia, which is frequently iatrogenic (when low-salt, low-calorie diets are recommended), is caused by a deficiency of protein, calories, sodium, and/or protein-metabolizing vitamins.[104] Also, hepatic dysfunction usually precedes the clinical symptoms of metabolic toxemia of late pregnancy. Hypoalbuminemia and hypovolemia impair the liver's ability to synthesize sufficient albumin and thereby maintain its detoxification enzymatic functions.[82-83] The fact that severe preeclampsia and eclampsia frequently result in specific hepatic ischemic or periportal lesions or infarction further indicates that maternal malnutrition leads to hepatic dysfunction.[105]

TABLE 27
ASSOCIATION OF HYPOALBUMINEMIA
WITH RISK OF TOXEMIA

	# of Women	Serum Albumin (g/100 ml)	Standard Deviation (Sic)
Toxemic	8	3.87	.03
Nontoxemic on Regular Diets	42	4.04	.04
Nontoxemic on High Protein Diets	12	4.90	.09
Nonpregnant	--	4.90	.06

In the 1930's, Dodge and Frost eradicated eclampsia by instituting a high-protein diet. Toxemic women who were placed on a
daily diet consisting of six to eight eggs, one to two quarts of milk,
meat, and legumes improved dramatically. The authors discovered
that the average serum albumin level among toxemic women was
21% lower than that of those who had been on a high-protein diet and
who didn't have toxemia. The probability that the relationship between albumin, toxemia, and protein intake (as exhibited in Table
27) is not significant is infinitesimal.

Tompkins and Wiehl also lowered the incidence of toxemia
through dietary supplementation.[156] They stated "the so-called
'toxemias of pregnancy' are in reality nutritional deficiency states."

TABLE 28
INCIDENCE OF TOXEMIA
AMONG SINGLE, VIABLE BIRTHS
BY TYPE OF SUPPLEMENTATION (IF ANY)

Group	# of Patients	% With Toxemia (Number of Cases in Parentheses)
Control	170	4.12 (7)
Vitamin Supplementation	244	3.28 (8)
Protein Supplementation	186	2.69 (5)
Protein and Vitamin Supplementation	160	0.63 (1)
TOTAL	760	2.76 (21)

In a previous prospective study of 750 pregnant women who
received nutrition education and vitamin supplementation, Tompkins
eradicated preeclampsia and eclampsia.[16] Among 750 controls
(representing women who attended the same clinic as the well-
nourished women but who did not participate in the nutrition program), there were 5 cases of eclampsia and 59 of preeclampsia,
for a total incidence of 8.6%.

TABLE 29
INFLUENCE OF PRENATAL DIET
IN REDUCING INCIDENCE OF TOXEMIA

Quality of Prenatal Diet	# of Infants	% Women Who Developed Toxemia
Excellent or Good	31	0
Fair	149	8
Poor or Very Poor	36	44

Burke a l s o demonstrated t h e relationship between prenatal diet and toxemia. [17, 19] Toxemia did not occur in any woman whose daily protein intake was at least 68 grams.

Perhaps the first physician to establish a rigorous nutrition education program for the sole purpose of reducing the incidence of toxemia, Hamlin eradicated eclampsia in 5, 000 deliveries and significantly reduced the rate of preeclampsia. [108] He observed:

> The damage (eclampsia), I believe, occurs at this stage when there is an imbalance of diet. . . The attack (to eradicate eclampsia) succeeded because it was aimed strategically at the occult basis of the disease instead of at its summit of classical late signs and symptoms.
>
> The humidcribs were often empty now. By 1949 nurses and medical students were beginning to ask why they w e r e no longer seeing enough eclamptics. . . By 1950 it was felt that one could say to the s c eptic s: 'Eclampsia will no l o n g e r afflict the patients of this hospital if the present methods o f prevention are followed meticulously.' . . . The old conception that grave pre-eclampsia with all its attendant problems and techniques of practical obstetric management, must always be with us has been disproved. [108]

Brewer, who also implemented a scientific nutrition education program, significantly reduced the incidence of metabolic toxemia of late pregnancy $(p<.01)$. [109] Retrospectively, Brewer discovered that the three women who had developed preeclampsia (none contracted eclampsia) had been inadequately nourished.

TABLE 30
EFFECT OF PRENATAL NUTRITION EDUCATION
IN DECREASING RISK OF TOXEMIA

	# of Women	Metabolic Toxemia Of Late Pregnancy
Participated in Nutrition Education Program	546	0.55%
Did Not Participate in Program	369	2.98%

For more than 20 years, Grieve, by insisting that pregnant women consume one pound of beef every day, has also nearly eradicated toxemia. [110] The differences in toxemia, abruptio placentae, and perinatal death between the 7,331 women whom he considered to be well nourished and the 4,145 whom he considered to be poorly nourished are all extraordinarily significant (p 10^{-15}).

TABLE 31
RELATIONSHIP OF ESTIMATE OF NUTRITIONAL STATUS
TO SEVERE COMPLICATIONS

	# of Women	% Toxemia (Hyper-tension, Edema, and Proteinuria)	% Abruptio Placentae	Perinatal Death Rate
Hemoglobin Level At Least 10 g/100ml and Weight Gain of Less than 39.5 lb.	7,331	.01	.03	19.2
Hemoglobin Level Under 10 g/100ml or no Greater than 12 g/100 ml and Weight Gain Greater than 39.5 lb.	4,645	.82	1.38	50.6

The fact that protein deficiency causes toxemia was verified in a recent study in which the administration of protein immediately alleviated the toxemic process.[111] Among the 37 severe toxemics who were given albumin, there was not one instance of RDS and all of their babies received high pediatric ratings.

TABLE 32
PROTECTIVE EFFECTS OF SERUM ALBUMIN
AMONG TOXEMIC WOMEN

	# of Women	Induction of Labor	Perinatal Mortality	Abruption of the Placenta
Study Group	135	5%	0.9%	0%
Control Group	297	25%	3.7%	3%

 HYPERACTIVITY IN CHILDREN IS HIGHLY ASSOCIATED WITH LOW BIRTH WEIGHT AND COMPLICATIONS DURING PREGNANCY BOTH OF WHICH ARE HIGHLY ASSOCIATED WITH INADEQUATE DIET.

Complications of Pregnancy
and Their Relationship to Child Development

Numerous complications, such as toxemia, low birth weight, abruptio placentae, and anemia, have been linked with inadequate prenatal nutrition. As will be shown herein, contrary to prevailing teachings, complications of labor and delivery are much more likely to occur among underweight births than those of higher weight. Major delivery complications, including an increase in the rate of cesarean sections, have been linked to low-weight babies born to inadequately nourished women.[17, 19]

Ebbs et al., in a prospective study of 380 pregnant women, showed the direct relationship between prenatal nutrition and lack of complications during pregnancy, labor, and delivery.[28-29] The incidence of toxemia was more than twice as high among the 120 poorly nourished women than among the 90 women whose diets had been supplemented during the latter half of pregnancy (prior to that their diets were just as deficient as those of the former group) or the 170 women who had been on good diets throughout pregnancy.[28] In addition, the duration of labor and postpartum recovery was highest among the 120 poorly nourished women.[29] Among these women, 24.2% of them had dystocia in contrast to 2.3% of the women on supplemented diets and 5.9% of those on good diets.[29] In addition, the average duration of labor was five hours shorter in the good diet group than in the poor diet group.[28] It is noteworthy that the obstetrician who diagnosed these and other complications was not aware of the group to which any of the 380 women had been placed.

TABLE 33
INFLUENCE OF PRENATAL DIET
ON COMPLICATIONS OF PREGNANCY

Quality Prenatal Diet	# of Women	% Not Having Complications	% Having Major Complications	Statistical Signif. Level Compared With Poor Diet Group
Good	170	48.5	12.2	$p<10^{-6}$
Supplemented	90	45.9	9.2	$p<10^{-5}$
Poor	120	30.3	36.2	

A similar improvement in maternal health and lowered risk of complications during delivery were achieved by Higgins, who implemented a sound prenatal nutrition program. Among the 1,736 women who participated in her program, rate of toxemia was 69% lower than that of other clinic patients and 39% less than that of private patients who received prenatal care at the same hospital.[112] Among the nutrition program's participants, who generally delivered larger babies than women who were not involved in the program, there was a much higher incidence of spontaneous deliveries and a lower rate of cesarean sections.[32]

TABLE 34
OBSTETRICAL RATING OF THE
LAST 3 to 4 MONTHS OF PREGNANCY
TO THE 6th WEEK POSTPARTUM

Quality of Prenatal Diet	Excellent	Good to Fair	Poor	Bad
Good	30.6%	54.1%	14.2%	1.1%
Supplemented	34.5%	59.6%	5.9%	0.0%
Poor	13.1%	52.9%	22.6%	11.3%

Pasamanick and Knobloch, who advanced the sophisticated concept of a "continuum of reproductive casualty"[113-114] to designate "the sequelae of harmful events during pregnancy and parturition resulting in damage to the fetal or newborn infant, and primarily localized to the central nervous system,"[113] were the first to extensively link maternal health with infant and childhood health and development. Their mammoth research disproved the prevailing theories that developmental disabilities are primarily caused by chromosomal abnormalities, genetically transmitted metabolic disturbances, and unknown causes.[115]

Their scientific research delineated an association between prenatal and perinatal complications and a gradient of reproductive casualty,[114] including, in descending order of significance, spontaneous abortion, perinatal death, cerebral palsy, mental retardation, and behavioral disorders.[116]

Knobloch and Pasamanick found toxemia, which they linked to malnutrition, to be highly associated with the birth of children who had minor degrees of cerebral palsy.[115] They also noted that among mothers of infants who had a D.Q. under 80 (90% of the infants in the study had a D.Q. between 90 and 120), the incidence of toxemia was twice that of all the mothers whose children they examined.[63]

In a prospective study they analyzed the relationship between behavior and emotional stability and birth weight.[92] In a series of examinations given at age three, the higher birth weight children received better results in the examinations which tested organization of b e h a v i o r , discrimination, judgment, emotional stability, attention span, perserverance, irritability, restlessness, and quality of integration. The authors concluded:

> The findings point to the overwhelming importance of the factors of prenatal maternal health, preschool stimulation and later educational effort which a r e the major foci in the antipoverty programs for children today. These programs should be geared to the elimination and modification of such results of poverty and deprivation as malnutrition, infection, and other forms of stress, prenatally in the mother and postnatally in the child.[93]

Table 35 summarizes the results of several well-controlled retrospective studies.[113] The data document the dramatic association between low birth weight, maternal complications, and neonatal abnormalities and various neuropsychiatric disorders.

Pasamanick et al. observed that infants who were of low birth weight and/or born to mothers who had complications during pregnancy frequently are afflicted with m i n i m a l brain damage,[113] which they felt usually originates during the prenatal period. Pasamanick also showed that hyperactivity is highly associated with low birth weight and complications.[113, 118]

In perhaps the m o s t thorough, well-controlled study of the relationship between birth weight and neurological function and intellectual potential, Knobloch et al. tested 500 singleborn, low birth weight children and compared their results with 492 higher birth weight singleton controls.[119] Developmental, neurological, and physical examinations were performed on a ll 992 infants at ages ranging from 34 to 69 weeks. The examiners were not aware of the group to which any child belonged.[119-120]

As is shown in Table 36, the rates of both neurological abnormalities and intellectual defects i n c r e a s e d as birth weight decreased.[119] Among the 57 lowest birth weight infants, 61.4% had minor neurological damage to severe intellectual deficiency; 44% of them had severe neurological or visual impairment in contrast to 2.6% among the control group infants. Moreover, none of the infants whose birth weight was u n d e r 2001 grams (4 pounds 6 1/2 ounces) h a d superior intellectual potential, whereas 6.3% of t h e normal birth weight infants were found to have such potential. The results would have been even more significant had the authors not standardized the test results of the low birth weight infants to adjust for their degree of prematurity.[119-120]

TABLE 35

ASSOCIATION OF NEUROPSYCHIATRIC DISORDERS WITH PRENATAL AND PARANATAL COMPLICATIONS

Neuro-Psychiatric Disorder	# of Children In Study Group	Low Birth Weight			Complications of Pregnancy			Neonatal Convulsions, Cyanosis or Asphyxia	
		Study Group	Control Group	Signif. Level	Study Group	Control Group	Signif. Level	Study Group	Control Group
Autism	50	21.0%	12.0%	ns	51.0%	17.0%	$p<.0005$	64.0%	28.0%
Behavioral Disorders	840	8.8%	2.8%	$p<10^{-8}$	40.9%	31.7%	$p<.0005$	4.7%	2.7%
Cerebral Palsy	561	22.0%	5.0%	$p<10^{-13}$	38.0%	21.0%	$p<10^{-10}$	--	--
Epilepsy	396	13.6%	6.4%	ns	34.8%	26.4%	$p<.05$	16.1%	5.0%
Hearing Disorders	124	16.1%	7.3%	$p<.05$	24.0%	11.5%	$p<.01$	17.1%	13.3%
Mental Deficiency	639	17.1%	8.7%	$p<.0005$	43.8%	36.2%	$p<.05$	14.2%	7.0%
Reading Disorders	205	11.5%	4.6%	$p<.05$	37.6%	21.5%	$p<.0005$	7.8%	3.9%
Strabismus	398	13.6%	7.8%	$p<.01$	22.9%	16.1%	$p<.02$	22.4%	13.8%

TABLE 36
STATUS OF DEVELOPMENT AT AGE 40 WEEKS

Birth Weight	# of Infants	Neurological Status			Intellectual Potential		
		Normal to Indeterminate Neurol. Funct.	Minimal Brain Damage Neurol.	Possible CP to Overt Neurol. Defect	Superior to High Average	Average to Dull	Borderline Defective to Defect.
1500 g or less	57	50.9%	22.8%	26.3%	5.3%	77.1%	17.6%
1501-2500g	443	76.7%	16.0%	7.2%	16.3%	81.9%	1.8%
Composite of Low Birth Wt. Group Adjusted for Birth Wt.	(500)	75.5%	16.3%	8.2%	15.7%	81.6%	2.6%
Control Group (2501 g or more)	492	88.4%	10.0%	1.6%	21.8%	76.6%	1.6%

The results of tests given at age three were highly correlated (p<.05) to the initial ones.[120] The correlation between the two test results was 0.75 among the children who, as determined by the initial tests, exhibited a neurological abnormality and/or intellectual impairment.

It is noteworthy that, in virtually all of their studies, Pasamanick et al. found no major differences in the rates of dystocia and delivery procedures,[113] thereby refuting the myth that delivery-related factors are major etiologic events in influencing infant health and the presence or extent of neurological damage. Lilienfeld and Parkhurst, in a thorough retrospective analysis of 561 consecutive singleton cerebral palsied children, determined that low birth weight and complications of pregnancy were not independenc factors influencing the development of cerebral palsy, as had been previously believed, but instead are caused by the same factor(s) that cause(s) the cerebral palsy.[121]

TABLE 37
RATIO OF OBSERVED TO EXPECTED CASES
OF CEREBRAL PALSY BY BIRTH WEIGHT
ACCORDING TO PRESENCE OR ABSENCE
OF COMPLICATIONS

Birth Weight	Cases in Which the Mother Had No Complications	All Cases
Under 1500 grams (3 lb, 5 oz or less)	22.00	15.00
1500-1999 grams (3 lb, 5 oz to 4 lb, 6.5 oz)	12.69	11.22
2000-2249 grams (4 lb, 6.5 oz to 4 lb, 15.5 oz)	3.90	3.39
2250-2499 grams (4 lb, 15.5 oz to 5 lb, 8 oz)	2.04	2.24
At least 2500 grams (5 lb, 8 oz or more)	.61	.82

In upstate New York, birth weight and complications among the 561 cerebral palsy cases were compared to like factors among infants who were born in upstate New York in 1948 and who survived the neonatal period. The low birth weight incidence among the cerebral palsied children was 22.2% in comparison to 4.8% among the neonatal survivors $(p<10^{-15})$. Nearly 38% of the former group were born to mothers who had had complications, whereas the incidence of complications among the 1948 neonatal survivors was 19% $(p<10^{-9})$. Among women who had not had complications, the low birth weight rate was six times higher among the cerebral palsy cases.

As is evident in Table 37, as birth weight increased, the incidence of cerebral palsy decreased. Note that the table, which is based on data from the group of neonatal survivors, shows that the incidence of cerebral palsy among children who weighed under 1500 grams at birth and whose mothers did not have complications during pregnancy was 22 times higher than expected from an unbiased population of neonatal survivors.

TABLE 38
INCREASED RISK OF DEVELOPING COMPLICATIONS
AMONG MOTHERS OF CEREBRAL PALSIED CHILDREN
OR STILLBIRTHS OR NEONATAL DEATHS

	Complications During Pregnancy	Abruptio Placentae	Toxemia of Pregnancy
1940-1947 Cerebral Palsy Group (517 cases)	37.8% (10^{-9})	1.0% (.01)	3.3% (.02)
Average per Year of 1942-1945 Group of neonatal Survivors (377,764 cases)	20.9%	0.3%	1.8%
Average of 1942-1945 Group of Stillbirths and Neonatal Deaths (17,820 cases)	62.4% (10^{-15})	10.8% (10^{-21})	10.3% (10^{-12})
Average of 1942-1945 Total Births (395,588 cases)	22.8%	0.8%	2.2%

Table 38 reveals the rates of complications among the cerebral palsy cases for which complete records were available and other populations. Premature separation of the placenta and toxemia, both of which have been shown herein to be caused by malnutrition, were the complications most overproportionately frequent among the mothers of the cerebral palsy population and the 1942-1945 group of mothers who gave birth to stillbirths or whose neonates died.

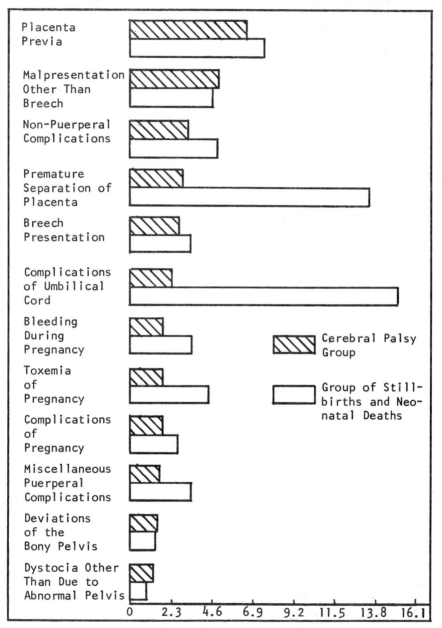

FIGURE 8. Ratio of observed to expected cerebral palsy cases and combined infant loss, by complications of pregnancy.

In Figure 8 the ratios of the actual number of instances of various complications to the expected number (as based upon a population of neonatal survivors for the cerebral palsy group and a total birth population for a group of stillbirths and neonatal deaths for the same period) are provided.

Consistent with the findings of Pasamanick et al., operative procedures used during delivery were not significantly associated with cerebral palsy births. Consequently, as evidenced by its dramatic association with low birth weight and complications of pregnancy (both of which are largely preventable by sound prenatal nutrition), cerebral palsy is primarily caused during the prenatal period.

The authors declared:

> The association of several factors of pregnancy and parturition with the development of cerebral palsy suggest the postulation and the existence of a 'continuum of reproductive wastage,' with a lethal component consisting of abortion, stillbirths, and neonatal deaths, and a sublethal component consisting of cerebral palsy and perhaps other related conditions... There appears to exist a relationship between stillbirths, neonatal deaths, and cerebral palsy. The pattern of factors, such as complications of pregnancy, prematurity, etc., which influence infant loss seems to behave in a similar manner with regard to cerebral palsy... It would appear that other congenital stigmata, such as malformations, mental deficiency, etc., should be similarly investigated in an attempt to delineate possible antecedent factors... It appears that the preventive aspect of a cerebral palsy program should be placed within the general scope of a maternal health program.[121]

Physiologically, cerebral palsy has been linked with periventricular venous infarction (death of tissue resulting from cessation of blood supply), which is a basically preventable lesion found around the cavities of the brain.[122] This lesion, which is common among premature infants, also is associated with and perhaps leads to epilepsy, mental retardation, and behavioral disorders.[123] Anoxia (oxygen deficiency), which usually results from maternal malnutrition, precedes periventricular venous infarction.

NOT ONLY IS FETAL MONITORING INEFFECTIVE IN REVERSING INTRAUTERINE GROWTH RETARDATION FROM MALNUTRITION AND OTHER ENVIRONMENTAL FACTORS, ITS USE HAS BEEN ASSOCIATED WITH INCREASED COMPLICATIONS OF LABOR AND DELIVERY IN ADDITION TO HIGH RISKS OF SURGERY.

Medical Mismanagement --
The Prevailing Obstetrical Care

The rational observer would assume that, in the light of the wealth of scientific data and implications of basic principles of internal medicine and neurology, maternal nutrition would receive top public health priority. A neurochemist and physician who extensively researched the relationship between prenatal nutrition and fetal development observed an inherent paradox in our feigned concern for infant and childhood health. He declared:

> In this country, major biomedical efforts have pinpointed a number of fatal diseases for eradication, including poliomyelitis, cancer, and cardiovascular disorders. There has been a particular emphasis on diseases that affect children, and the news media often report cases that elicit immediate and generous response from individuals and organizations. But the oldest and most persistent scourge of mankind, which most often affects children and destroys their life opportunities -- the triad of hunger, poverty, and ignorance -- is largely forgotten by the community... One would assume that medicine devoted to the care of women and children would be the most advanced part of medical research and practice. Yet nothing could be further from the truth... Why is there so much indifference to this subject of hunger, malnutrition, and starvation, when children and pregnant women, who generate instinctive sympathy and concern from almost everyone, are the most severly affected victims?[76]

Notwithstanding the reluctance of obstetricians, who seldom receive much training in nutrition, to incorporate sound prenatal nutrition as a fundamental aspect of prenatal care, it staggers the imagination to attempt to justify their insistence on drugs and restrictive diets, especially since such regimens have been linked to reproductive pathology. One survey showed that only 5% of obstetricians believe that appetite suppressants are unsafe among obese gravid women.[124] Among the obstetricians surveyed, 57% stated that they prescribe the drugs for "overweight" patients. In another survey only 57% of the obstetricians surveyed rejected the concept that the fetus behaves parasitically in extracting its nutrients regardless of the mother's nutritional intake.[125] It was not surprising that only 5% of them seemed to be aware of the protective effects of applied, scientific nutrition.

One nutritionist stated:

> Obstetricians seem to think that a low calorie diet to keep the mother's weight down is of prime importance. Many doctors even threaten to hospitalize women in the last trimester if they gain more weight than prescribed. Some patients I have seen have said their doctors have prescribed a ridiculous (weight gain) of 12-14 pounds! The doctors still prescribe a low salt diet and blindly use diuretics to hopelessly attempt to prevent swelling ... The restrictive diets these women are given daily are the most damaging regimen possible, to both mother and especially the developing fetus. Critical fetal brain development during this period can never be attained, besides the other possible damaging effects to maternal health and fetal development. It is frightening to see all these drugs the obstetricians still daily prescribe. You think they would have learned from Thalidomide that drugs and development don't mix, but it seems they want to recreate that horror in the 70's.

> The practice of weight control, salt restriction, low calorie diets, and drug use during pregnancy is still the biggest problem with the obstetrical care in the (San Francisco) Bay Area, and probably the entire U.S. These obsolete ideas are still being practiced daily, despite constant warnings from the nutritional researchers... The only answer is to inform all pregnant women of the risks they will encounter if they follow their obstetrician's philosophy, and to recommend they either find an obstetrician who has adopted the most recent methods (they are few and far between) or advise them to talk to a nutrition consultant or a university nutrition researcher in their area.[126]

A concerned supporter of good prenatal nutrition explained:

> The American medical profession appears to have
> a dragnet out during prenatal care. Or are the medical
> profession and drug industry blind regarding the nutri-
> tional needs of the expectant mother, or too ignorant or
> stiff-necked to care?

> The doctor, as one mother put it, doesn't have to
> live with the child whom he has caused to suffer brain
> damage and deformities. So a mother has to use her
> own judgment. She must discard the doctor's advice to
> restrict her weight, use drugs, and omit salt which the
> baby needs during her prenatal care. Indeed, she should
> question that doctor's whole professional outlook. Since
> the doctor's educational preparation for his profession
> does not include nutrition, the expectant mother must
> learn for herself about the nutritionally balanced diet.
> If she omits the empty calories from her diet, she will
> not put on unneeded fat. She must remember that weight
> and water gain is important for a healthy baby.[126]

While veterinarians, farmers, and ranchers have clearly defined standards for the management of pregnant animals, no such
standards exist for humans. A professor of animal husbandry stated:
"With too little salt in the diet... animals become unthrifty and in
time go to pieces. Cows deliver weak calves, or even lose their
calves. Cows may even die from salt starvation... When thinking
about salt in livestock management, keep in mind that it is: 'Profit-
able to remember, costly to forget.'"[127]

In contrast, a widely distributed booklet for pregnant women
reads: "(Your doctor) may prescribe medicines to help control your
blood pressure and/or fluid retention."[128] To toxemic women the
booklet suggests: "Do not use salt to season your food, either at the
table or in cooking."[128]

A booklet written for diabetics gives similarly pernicious
advice. It reads: "Besides insulin, your doctor may want to prescribe other medications during your pregnancy -- a diuretic, for
example, if you are retaining fluid excessively...Follow his directions carefully."[129]

 SINCE THE DOCTOR'S EDUCATIONAL PREPARATION FOR HIS/HER
PROFESSION DOES NOT INCLUDE NUTRITION, THE EXPECTANT MO-
THER MUST LEARN FOR HERSELF ABOUT A NUTRITIONALLY BALANCED DIET.

THE INSISTENCE OF WEIGHT CONTROL DURING PREGNANCY BY PHYSICIANS HAS LED TO AN INNUMERABLE NUMBER OF INSTANCES OF PREVENTABLE IATROGENIC MATERNAL AND INFANT MORBIDITY AND MORTALITY.

Another area of obstetrics which is completely misunderstood involves weight gain during pregnancy. As in the case with distorted views on salt metabolism, the use of weight control has led to an innumerable number of instances of preventable iatrogenic maternal and infant morbidity and mortality.

Weight gain has been shown to be the maternal factor which is most highly correlated with birth weight.[51] Although weight gain during pregnancy can reflect nutritional status, it is not an accurate indicator of dietary adequacy.   One reason that a dietary history and/or blood constituents analysis are more accurate means of assessing nutritional status is that, as in the nonpregnant state, a high weight gain can result from a high-calorie diet which is low in essential nutrients. Also, paradoxically, undernourished (particularly protein-deficient women) can gain a rapid amount of weight in a relatively short period of time as a result of pathological edema. As has been established herein, the edema in such women is a direct consequence of lowered colloid osmotic pressure of the plasma protein caused by hypovolemia [36, 102] and frequently leads to metabolic toxemia of late pregnancy.[36]

Since healthy, full-term children are born to women who have a normal pregnancy at a wide range of weight gain (or weight loss), subjecting a group of women to any particular weight control regimen is unscientific and potentially hazardous.[130] Hytten discovered that the distribution of weight gain during the last 20 weeks of healthy pregnancies approaches the normal statistical distribution with a mean weekly gain of one pound.[100] Because of individual differences, it is best for pregnant women to eat a diet of nourishing foods to appetite without regard for their weight gain.[36]

In a study of approximately 8,000 single live births of 37 to 44 weeks' gestation, Lowe demonstrated the direct and highly significant relationship between weight gain and birth weight.[35] The correlation between birth weight and maternal weight gain was 0.94. He showed that the relationship was not continuous, since, at and above approximately 3500 grams (7 pounds 11 ounces), birth weight does not increase as weight gain increases.

Utilizing data from the Collaborative Perinatal study, Singer et al. analyzed the association between weight gain and infant development.[131] They confirmed the findings of other researchers that age, parity, and many other factors are not related to birth weight when weight gain is one of the independent variables. The data in Table 39 show that the incidence of low birth weight is related to weight gain at the .001 significance level.

TABLE 39
CORRELATION BETWEEN
WEIGHT GAIN DURING PREGNANCY
AND INCIDENCE OF LOW BIRTH WEIGHT

Weight Gain (Pounds)	% Low Birth Weight
Loss	17.0
0-15	15.8
16-25	8.2
26-35	4.3
36 or more	3.0

They also discovered the relationship between maternal weight gain and infant size and neurological function at one year of age and that between weight gain and psychiatric, mental, and motor function at one year of age and that between weight gain and psychiatric, mental, and motor function at eight months of age. Table 40 lists infant size and the three exams in descending order of their degree of association with weight gain. All infant abnormalities except those measured by the neurological exam are significantly related to birth weight on a statistical basis. Even when the relationship between birth weight and infant abnormalities was removed from the analysis, low maternal weight gain was found to be associated with infant abnormalities.

TABLE 40
INCIDENCE OF ABNORMAL GROWTH BY WEIGHT GAIN

	0-15 Pounds (%)	16-25 Pounds (%)	26-35 Pounds (%)	Over 36 Pounds (%)
Weight	15.8	11.2	8.4	6.2
Motor Exam	11.3	8.0	6.8	5.2
Mental Exam	12.5	9.3	8.3	7.5
Height	10.1	7.5	6.5	7.3
Neurologic Test	8.8	7.5	7.9	7.1

Despite the overwhelming evidence of the potentially pernicious consequences of weight control, which is most devastating during late pregnancy (at which time fetal brain development is most rapid), obstetricians still unduly restrict weight on a routine basis. One survey showed that 95% of obstetricians restrict weight gain during pregnancy.[125] A present study showed similar results.[132] A large number of the women were reprimanded for approaching or exceeding their weight quota. One woman, who had gained 23 pounds by the ninth month of pregnancy, said: "He (the doctor) yells at me every visit. He says I eat too much. I just get so depressed. He told me my delivery is going to be harder because of my weight gain."[132]

THE ONLY ANSWER IS TO INFORM ALL PREGNANT WOMEN OF THE RISKS THEY WILL ENCOUNTER IF THEY FOLLOW THEIR OBSTETRICIAN'S PHILOSOPHY. THE DOCTOR DOESN'T HAVE TO LIVE WITH THE CHILD WHOM HE HAS CAUSED TO SUFFER BRAIN DAMAGE AND DEFORMITIES. A MOTHER HAS TO USE HER OWN JUDGEMENT. SHE MUST DISCARD THE DOCTOR'S ADVICE TO RESTRICT HER WEIGHT, USE DRUGS, AND OMIT SALT. INDEED, SHE SHOULD QUESTION THAT DOCTOR'S WHOLE PROFESSIONAL OUTLOOK.

Excerpts from Letters

The following excerpts of letters indicate that many physicians, instead of ensuring that women satisfy the nutritional stress of pregnancy, are placing them on regimens which endanger their health and the lives and health of their newborns:

I just spent the morning working with OB/GYN residents in High Risk Clinic!! One woman -- seen for Rh problem -- 34 weeks' gestation, skinny, with a total three-pound weight gain, was sent for sonar by resident for small baby. I pointed out weight gain and asked if he would like to consider the low weight gain and do some nutrition counseling. He said, "No, she looks good that way." She'll really look good with a damaged baby on her hip. Three patients today had low weight gains, small babies, and not one word about eating. Needless to say, I ran after these women and talked to them.

Excerpts from Letters Cont'd

I have a student underweight for her height who is going to a private doctor here in Miami. The doctor does not want her to gain any more than 18 pounds. One month she gained three pounds and he was very upset about it. He also told her not to salt her food. I have given her material to read and have been encouraging her to eat right.

I can't believe with all the information available that a doctor would still be prescribing this detrimental program.

I couldn't help but agree with what you said about low-calorie, no-salt diets with diuretics. My doctor is one of those that worries about weight. With my first pregnancy I had badly swollen ankles in my fourth month. He gave me water pills and took me off salf. After another month or so, when the swelling didn't get any better, he gave me a diet of 1,000 calories a day . . . None of the above three things helped. I was troubled with swollen ankles for the rest of the pregnancy.

I have been paying pretty close attention to the diet you recommended in the pamphlet "Pregnant? And Want a Healthy Child." . . . So far I have gained 20 pounds. Some of this has been as much as seven pounds a month. But I have not had the least bit of swelling in my ankles and fingers . . . The nurses and doctor are alarmed and telling me that the rapid weight gain could easily mean I will get toxemia. The doctor said any time now my ankles could swell or without any other symptoms I could start convulsing. He gave me another 1,000-calorie-a-day diet like the last one and told me to keep it to two pounds a month.

Just a few days before, he (my doctor) was called in by an associate at Stanford to assist with the worst (still living) case of metabolic toxemia of late pregnancy they'd ever seen. They treated her with diuretics because "they are the only accepted treatment in reducing the edema of toxemia -- we don't know of anything else." Well, need I tell you that she showed no improvement and gave birth to a very low birth weight baby. But then, as if that isn't enough, she went into heart failure! My God! and to think that it could've been prevented!

Excerpts from Letters Cont'd

I am a public health nurse involved in a prenatal clinic in New York City, and in spite of the convincing evidence of <u>harm</u>, the clinic physicians <u>still</u> order low-salt and weight-reduction diets. THEY GET HYSTERICAL OVER A FOUR-POUND WEIGHT GAIN IN A MONTH...P.S. I'm pregnant myself and doing my best to eat right!

I'm continually shocked that the majority of the women (I see) obtain around 1,000 calories a day, and they're usually <u>very</u> low in calcium and, of course, iron. On questioning them, I inevitably find out that their doctor has put them on a diet because he feels they're getting too heavy. I try counseling them, but few improvements are ever seen -- how can they go against their doctor, they feel.

I can't tell you how many pregnant women I've already met who've been put on diets to restrict weight gain, or who have been told to <u>lose</u> ten pounds before delivery. I myself had a low birth weight baby, due in part, I'm sure, to a diet which caused me to lose weight eacy month... Enclosed is a check for $5.00 to contribute to your cause.

I had a first child who was a low birth weight, "toxic baby" due to the severe toxemia I developed in my last trimester of pregnancy. My OB doctor restricted me to <u>liquids</u> (clear) <u>only</u> for six weeks and diuretics daily. I have never received a straight answer to my questions about toxemia and its cause... I think your works and efforts are marvelous. Please continue to help.

I am very concerned about the appalling rate of birth defects and other birth abnormalities... Also what concerns me even more is the doctors' views on nutrition (there isn't any) and drugs. Here in Philadelphia they are filling pregnant women with diuretics, appetite depressants, harmful drugs for nausea, and tranquilizers, but not anything on nutrition for their problems.

Excerpts from Letters Cont'd

I am especially pleased to learn of your organization because I obtained diet and health records of 100 welfare women and their infants while I was on the staff of the Miami Valley Project, University of Cincinnati... Of these mothers, five actually lost weight during pregnancy... Thirty-one gained less than 20 pounds... The dieticians in the clinic saw 68 women; of these they persuaded 19 to gain less than 20 pounds... Sodium restriction was imposed on 49. Diuril was prescribed for 49.

I'm still convinced that I was right to follow my judgment against my doctor's en masse methods. I see the results in friends' babies as they are born, who followed the low-calorie, low-salt diet our doctor prescribed. My little girl showed what I would consider normal and healthy development, whereas the only word that comes to mind to describe my friend's children is 'stunted.'

Enclosed is my check for $10.00 as a donation to SPUN. Please include me on your mailing list. Thank you also for sending me the materials I asked about. We need all the 'ammo' we can get to start aiming our guns at the doctors here in Columbus who are still restricting calories, salt, and essential nutrition and calmly shrugging off their patients' concerns about what these restrictions are doing to their babies. Just last night in class one "skinny" gal four and a half months pregnant stated her doctor reduced her diet to 1,000 calories because she had gained seven pounds in seven weeks (the only weight she has gained thus far in her pregnancy). I asked her what she was going to do. (We had just had the nutrition session the night before.) "I'm going to ignore him," she said proudly. "After all, he's not the one who has to live with a deformed or mentally deficient child." I couldn't have said it better.

Despite the accepted practices of weight control and salt restriction, there are, fortunately, physicians who do practice preventive obstetrical care. One physician enumerated the benefits from his emphasis on protective prenatal nutrition:

Letter from a Physician With a Nutrition Program

When I initially counsel patients with their first pregnancy visit, nutrition is strongly stressed. I do not mention limiting weight in any way but instead tell them to gain at least 25 to 30 pounds during this pregnancy and that this weight gain will be a protein weight gain. I give them a list of protein-containing foods and reassure them that much of this weight is to be gained in the first few months of pregnancy. I do not at any time, with any visit, tell the patients that they are gaining too much but instead stress only good nutrition... The patients did need constant support from me since attitudes of others around them tended to express that they were gaining too much weight or that somehow weight gain was harmful in pregnancy. I do not use diuretics in pregnancy, nor any other medications other than a good prenatal vitamin.

During the time I have been in practice here, I have managed approximately 500 obstetrical patients. I have had two patients with preeclampsia, both of whom had severe chronic diseases. One of these had systemic lupus erythematosis, the second a hereditary cholesterol problem. Both of these now have healthy babies. I have had six spontaneous premature infants. One of these was from a mother who had acute appendicitis in her sixth month of pregnancy. Three of the patients did not start prenatal care until their sixth month of pregnancy and were severely malnourished when I started with them; two of the patients had placenta praevia, and one patient was a total vegetarian whom I judged was on inadequate sources of vegetable protein.

The remainder of my patients have had normal, healthy children. One patient had a sudden infant death occur at four months of age. The mother of this baby was an epileptic requiring large doses of Dilantin to control her seizures, and this had been taken all through her pregnancy. Nearly all of my patients breastfeed their babies, and good nutrition is stressed throughout the breastfeeding time. Most of them breastfeed for six months or more. The mothers begin their first breastfeeding on the delivery table and continue to breastfeed every two to four hours throughout the hos-

Physician's Letter Cont'd

pital stay. The hospital stay in my patient group aver-
ages 24 hours. Cesarean sections taken as a group are
kept for approximately 48 hours...All cesarean section mothers nurse their babies.

In answer to the question "Do doctors in our area
limit weight gain?" I would say most still do...As an
aside, there are a number of other phenomena which we
accepted as "normal in pregnancy" which I have realized
were nutrition-related and which I do not see in my
practice any more...Mothers who are properly nourished do not get stretch marks, and they do not seem to
have acceleration of dental caries or softening of the
gums. I do not see loss of hair, splitting of nails,
softening of bones, anemia, postpartum hemorrhage, or
failures at nursing. In addition, after the fourth month
of the pregnancy, most mothers feel normal as far as
energy output. We see very quick recoveries after
pregnancy, and we do not see failures at breast-feeding
because of nutritional problems in the mother.[126]

The testimonies to the adherence of good nutrition are numerous. The following all indicate the benefits of sound prenatal nutrition:

Testimonials to Nutrition

My seven-month-old baby is a good example of optimal prenatal care. With an excellent high-protein diet and vitamin/mineral
supplements, I gained 40 pounds with no signs of toxemia or eclampsia, and needed no drugs of any kind. My son's birth weight
was 9 pounds 6 ounces, and he has been in perfect health since he
was born...

My son...now 22 months old, has the most lustrous hair,
perfect, even teeth, sparkling eyes, satiny skin, and solid body.
People marvel at him and believe it's all predestined, all genetically
controlled, and that if you have God on your side, then you'll have a
healthy baby. They just don't understand that they can take control
and insure the health of their own child.

Testimonials to Nutrition Cont'd

Having followed basically the dietary program you advocate during a pregnancy three years ago and having had a delightful pregnancy and beautiful 8 pound 14 ounce baby with an Apgar of 10, I firmly believe that you are absolutely right! . . .

I have four children and have been submitted to these drugs, thinking they are helping me, but I have found with my last two, all that was needed was to adhere to an adequate diet . . .

Why are so few obstetricians attuned to the role of maternal nutrition in protecting the health of the expectant mother and her unborn? A professor of OB/GYN reflected:

In this current flurry of interest in nutrition in pregnancy, the physician responsible for the care of pregnant women often finds himself in a difficult position. His knowledge of nutrition in general is deficient, for formal instruction in nutritional principles is notably absent from medical school curriculae and residency programs . . . This, when faced with providing nutritional advice to his patients, he all too frequently finds himself confused. [133]

Because obstetricians are not educated in the field of practical nutrition, they are susceptible to unscientific advertising claims of the drug industry. As late as 1974, diuretics and appetite suppressants were advertised in major obstetrics journals. [134] In addition, the medical profession, especially the American College of Obstetricians and Gynecologists (ACOG), have directly or indirectly sanctioned the use of medical regimens which lead to reproductive pathology. The powerful American College did not form a Committee on Nutrition until 1972. Their first position paper on maternal nutrition, which is replete with myths and unscientific speculation, was not published until December 1972. [134] A recent enumeration of the ACOG's ten-year goals did not include mention of the implementation of nutrition education for the pregnant woman or standards for the nutrition education of physicians. [135]

Because of the lack of awareness among health care professionals and the reluctance of most organizations to advocate that
pregnant women follow sound nutritional guidance and refrain from
taking drugs (unless absolutely necessary) when such advice is contrary to that given by a physician, hundreds of thousands of pregnant
women unwittingly place themselves and their unborn at risk. It is
not surprising that a major university study showed that approximately one million infants are at risk of needlessly being brain
damaged every year in the U.S.[136] Since the study was basically
confined to low-income populations, it did not consider the large
numbers of affluent women who subject themselves and their newborns to needless pathology as a result of adhering to low-salt and/
or low-calorie regimens, controlling their weight gain, and/or taking
physician-prescribed drugs.

An overt expression of the prevailing neglect to recognize the
nutritional needs of expectant mothers and their unborn is human
experimentation. Because the medical profession and others have
not advanced to the stage of instituting rigorous standards for the
management of pregnancy (as have veterinarians and ranchers),
numerous women have been subjected to cruel experimentation.

In a well-publicized study at Columbia University, pregnant
women in an area in which the low birth weight rate is 17% were
placed in 2 groups for purposes of comparing the viability of their
newborns.[137] In neither group (one group of women received a 40
gram protein supplement daily; those in the control group received
a supplement containing only 6 grams of protein) were the women
given nutrition counseling or warned of the risks of undernourishment. In another study, the women in the control group, who were
known to be consuming an average of less than 40 grams of protein
per day, were not informed of the dangers of their dietary inade-
quacies.[138] Naturally, the researchers in both studies observed
a higher incidence of reproductive casualty among the controls.

In another "scientific" study, 8 pregnant women were placed
on a diet which provided less than 25 grams of protein for a period
of five successive days.[139] It should not have surprised the researchers that their ratio of urinary urea nitrogen to total nitrogen
decreased significantly (p .01), indicating that the women were
protein deficient. The urinary urea nitrogen/total nitrogen ratio in
one woman who was placed on a diet which provided only 1500 calories and 20 grams of protein for 15 consecutive days decreased
more than 43%.

The practice of preventive medicine is probably more essential in the field of obstetrics than in any of the other medical specialties. A child born to a mother who is not exposed to proper obstetrical guidance is at risk of developing mental, physical, and/or behavioral abnormalities. Emphasizing the social and economic benefits of a practical approach to prenatal nutrition, the international publisher of perhaps the most widely circulated medically oriented publication, wrote:

"What is most baffling is that these precedents, are so important to people in terminal stages of irreversible disease, seem to have little or no bearing in regard to preventable disorders of infinitely greater incidence and of infinitely greater economic consequences. Once again, our characteristics as an activist society distort what should be the proper relationship between preventive and curative medicine. We are prepared, and we are a rich enough country, to afford $500,000,000 to $2 billion to prolong life for a few years in those with irreversibly damaged hearts and kidneys.

"Why, then, the incredible neglect annually of many thousands of pregnant women whose malnutrition causes irreversible fetal brain damage and physical anomalies in children who will for a lifetime be a burden to themselves, to their families, and to society? These are preventable conditions due to ignorance and/or lack of the most simple nutritional essentials. We seem fascinated by our mechanical facilities and technologies. It would seem that if a brain transplant were possible, our social and psychic orientation is such that we would be prepared to support a Medicare charge of $20,000 to $25,000 per "transistorized brain" transplant. Why then do we fail to make available a few hundred dollars per pregnancy to assure normal neurologic and general physical development in the unborn? Supplementation to the point of total nutritional adequacy for ALL American mothers could probably be achieved for less than the presently anticipated cost for renal dialysis of 13,000 patients. This is not to suggest that the United States need forgo either Medicare coverage for renal dialysis or for totally implantable artificial hearts but, rather, that it makes good medical sense -- indeed, common sense -- and good economics to invest in preventive

medicine for the pregnant woman and unborn child --
a venture which economically is self-liquidating and
less costly than attempts to correct, as we do now, preventable damage and its heavy economic liability.

"It seems that we still have to learn the simplest
lesson of good, preventive medicine. Why?[140]

From strictly an economic standpoint, preventive obstetrical
care is one of our nation's soundest investments. For each case of
severe mental retardation, which frequently results from inadequate
maternal nutrition, that is prevented, the economic gain to society
is more than $900,000.[141] Recognizing the extremely high rate of
preventable retardation which occurs in the U.S., a university
president declared:

"We must... prevent the occurrence of gratuitous retardation, that is, of retardation that results, not
from genetic malformation or other unavoidable causes,
but rather from social neglect. In order to do this, we
must understand the importance of nutrition, especially
the nutrition of the fetus... It is a gratuitous retardation, imposed on those children whose prenatal and early
nutrition has been defective. Only a society that has
lost its respect for human life and its concern for the
fulfillment of each individual can be indifferent to this
retardation. If we are to avoid such retardation, we
must insure that no mother, either through poverty or
ignorance, malnourishes her children in utero.

"The highest priority in American education today
should be the establishment of a national program of
nutrition and early childhood education... It is the obligation of educators at all levels -- in schools, colleges,
institutions, social agencies, and medical institutions --
to provide this education. It is the obligation of society
to see that no carrying mother or young child is undernourished because of financial need."[142]

Illustrating a case history of preventable mental retardation,
a concerned obstetrician appealed to his colleagues for the immediate implementation of primary prevention through good nutrition
as a routine, integral facet of obstetrical care. He wrote:

Patient M. was a small Mexican woman who followed her doctor's orders to the letter. A private ob/gyn specialist in California restricted her to one egg and one glass of milk a week, on the grounds that there is too much salt in milk and eggs. She was constantly advised at each prenatal visit: "Keep your weight down!" She wanted a healthy baby, so she faithfully followed her doctor's orders. Result: she gained only 14 pounds in all (from 112 to 126) and went into labor right at term. This was three months after she had been given a low-salt diet and diuretic pill to take every day; she didn't miss a day.

Her son, J.F., weighed 4 pounds, 15 ounces at birth. His blood sugar dropped to 20 mg. per cent and he had hypoglycemic convulsions repeatedly. The mother, after a normal blood loss at delivery, went into what her doctor termed "idiopathic shock" -- which we know was caused by her hypovolemia.

The boy is obviously and grossly mentally retarded and has to attend a special school for brain-damaged children. At age 15 months he was age three to four months in development and function on the Denver Grid-head drop, crossed eyes, small head. At age 18 months he still could not pull to stand or walk.

The patient had her second son after prenatal care in my clinic. During this second pregnancy she gained 50 pounds, had two eggs and a quart of milk every day, meat, vegetables, fruits, cereals, and no salt diuretics, no dietary salt restriction. She was told on each visit: "Keep eating a good diet -- salt your food to taste!" This second child, A., weighed 9 pounds at birth and is a perfect specimen.

Fellow American physicians, how long are we going to disregard the scientific evidence of the causal relationship of protein-calorie malnutrition, restriction of salt, and the dangerous use of salt diuretics to complications of pregnancy, fetal mortality, and damage to the newborn human infant?[143]

Acknowledgement

We would like to express our appreciation to Linda O'Donnell for editing and typing the manuscript.

JOIN SPUN

To counteract the lack of availability of nutrition education services for pregnant women and the prevailing nonchalance among health care professionals concerning the application of primary prevention through applied, scientific nutrition, the Society for the Protection of the Unborn through Nutrition (SPUN) was established. For five years SPUN has represented expectant mothers in their quest for services designed to make pregnancy a healthy, fulfilling, and everlasting experience. Additionally, SPUN works directly with health care agencies and providers of medical care toward establishing standards for scientific nutritional management in American obstetrics.

Membership in SPUN (17 N. Wabash, Suite 603, Chicago, IL 60602) is now available to the general public. The annual membership fee of $10.00 (which is tax-deductible) entitles members to a subscription to SPUN's newsletter and other publications pertaining to maternal and infant health care and to numerous services, such as access to audio-visual aids, referrals, and reduced or waived registration fee for special events.

A new SPUN program on the regional level is to sponsor seminars for the education and certification of community prenatal nutrition counselors. These individuals will provide SPUN services to women and medical personnel through liason with local childbirth educators and women's health facilities.

Join with other concerned individuals who are involved with the health of expectant mothers and the growth and development of their babies.

A BOOK ON NUTRITION
"What Every Pregnant Woman Should Know"
(The Truth About Diets and Drugs in Pregnancy)

A new book dealing with the mismanagement of the nutritional aspects of pregnancy by American obstetricians will be published by Random House in September 1977.   Written by Gail Sforza Brewer, with Tom Brewer, M.D., as medical consultant, it explains to mothers how they can protect themselves and their unborn from the hazards of nutritional nonchalance during pregnancy. Menus and recipes for pregnancy are included.

If not Available from your local bookstore, order from Publisher:
Random House, 201 E. 50th St., New York, NY 10022
$8.95 (plus 75¢ for postage & handling)

"IF BRAIN TRANSPLANTS WERE POSSIBLE, OUR SOCIAL AND PSYCHIC ORIENTATION IS SUCH THAT WE WOULD BE PREPARED TO SUPPORT A MEDICARE CHARGE OF $20,000 TO $25,000 PER "TRANSISTORIZED BRAIN" TRANSPLANT. WHY, THEN, DO WE FAIL TO MAKE AVAILABLE A FEW HUNDRED DOLLARS PER PREGNANCY TO ASSURE NORMAL NEUROLOGIC AND GENERAL PHYSICAL DEVELOPMENT IN THE UNBORN? SUPPLEMENTATION TO THE POINT OF TOTAL NUTRITIONAL ADEQUACY FOR ALL AMERICAN MOTHERS COULD PROBABLY BE ACHIEVED FOR LESS THAN THE PRESENTLY ANTICIPATED COST FOR RENAL DIALYSIS OF ONLY 13,000 PATIENTS."

A. SACKLER

CITED REFERENCES

1. Stewart, D., and Stewart, L., (eds.), Safe Alternatives in Childbirth, 2nd ed., Chapel Hill, NC: NAPSAC, 1977.

2. McCleary, E., New Miracles of Childbirth, New York: David McKay Co., 1974.

3. SPUN Reports, Oct 1, 1973.

4. Lilienfeld, A., and Parkhurst, E., A study of the association of factors of pregnancy and parturition with the development of cerebral palsy, Am. J. Hygiene 53:262-282, 1951. (quoting Freud, S., Die infantile cerebrallahmung, Vienna: Alfred Holder, 1897.

5. The women and their pregnancies, quoting Subcommittee on Appropriations of House of Representatives, Depts. of Labor and HEW Appropriations for 1962, U.S. Dept. HEW, p. 756, 1972.

6. ICEA News, vol 15, no 1, Jan 1976.

7. Berger, G., et al., Regionalized perinatal care: an estimate of its potential effect on racial differences in perinatal mortality in North Carolina, NC Med. J. 36:476-479, 1975.

8. Bishop, E., NC Med. J. 36:89-91, 1975.

9. Demographic Yearbook.

10. Abramowicz, M., and Kass, E., Pathogenesis and prognosis of prematurity, N.Eng. J. Med. 275:878-885, 1966.

Cited References Cont'd

11. U.S. Vital Statistics - Natality, Nat'l Cte. for Health Statistics, Vols for each of the years, 1950 through 1972.

12. Wynn, M., and Wynn, A., The protection of maternity and infancy, New York: E.H. Baker & Co., 1974.

13. Stickle, G., The health of mothers and babies: how do we stack up?, paper given at 5th Nat'l Volunteer Leadership Conf., Dec 1, 1976.

14. Observations on maternity care, and Pediatric health care in the People's Republic, Report to People's Republic of China, Nat'l Acad. of Sci., 1973.

15. Acosta-Sison, Relation between the state of nutrition of the mother and the birth weight of the fetus: a preliminary study, J. Philippine Is. Med. Assoc. 9:174-176, 1929.

16. Tompkins, W., The significance of nutritional deficiency in pregnancy: a preliminary report, J. Int'l Col. Surgeons 4:147-154, 1941.

17. Burke, B., et al., Nutrition studies during pregnancy, I. Problem, methods of study and group studied, Am. J. Ob. Gyn. 46:38-52, 1943.

18. Burke, B., et al., Nutrition studies during pregnancy, IV. Relation of protein content of mother's diet during pregnancy to birth length, birth weight, and condition of infant at birth, J. Ped. 23:506-515, 1943.

19. Burke, B., et al., The influence of nutrition during pregnancy upon the condition of the infant at birth, J. Nutrition 26:569-583, 1943.

20. Antonov, A., Children born during the siege of Leningrad in 1942, J. Ped. 30:250-259, 1947.

21. Smith, C., The effect of wartime starvation in Holland upon pregnancy and its product, Am. J. Ob. Gyn. 53:599-608, 1947.

22. Tompkins, W., and Wiehl, D., Nutritional deficiencies as a causal factor in toxemia and premature labor, Am. J. Ob. Gyn. 62:898-919, 1951.

23. Coursin, D., Maternal nutrition and the offspring's development, Nutrition Today, pp. 12-18, Mar-Apr, 1973.

24. Nutritional supplementation and the outcome of pregnancy, Nat'l Acad. of Sci. 1973.

25. Habicht, J., et al., Relation of maternal supplementary feeding during pregnancy to birth weight and other sociobiological factors, in Winick, M., (ed.), Nutrition and fetal development, New York: J. Wiley & Sons, 1974.

26. Lechtig, A., et al., Effect of moderate maternal malnutrition on the placenta, Am. J. Ob. Gyn. 123:191-201, 1975.

Cited References Cont'd

27. Lechtig, A., et al., Effect of improved nutrition during pregnancy and lactation on developmental retardation and infant mortality, in White, P., and Selvey, N., (eds.), Proceedings of Western Hemisphere Nutrition Congress 1974, Publishing Sciences Group, 1975.

28. Ebbs, J., et al., The influence of prenatal diet on the mother and child, J. Nutri. 22:515-526, 1941.

29. Ebbs, J., et al., The influence of improved prenatal nutrition upon the infant, Can. Med. Assoc. J. 46:6-8, 1942.

30. Lewin, R., Starved brains: a generation of clumsy, feeble-minded millions, Psych. Today, Sept, 1975.

31. Higgins, A., Nutrition and the outcome of pregnancy, paper presented at Can. Pub. Health annual mtg., St. John's, Newfoundland, June, 1974.

32. Higgins, A., et al., A preliminary report of a nutrition study on public maternity patients, Unpublished data.

33. Iyenger, L., Effects of dietary supplements late in pregnancy on the expectant mother and her newborn, Ind. J. Med. Research 55:85-89, 1967.

34. Platt, B., and Stewart, R., Reversible and irreversible effects of protein-calorie deficiency on the central nervous system of animals and man, World Rev. Nutri. and Dietetics 13:43-85, 1971.

35. Lowe, C., Research in infant nutrition: the untapped well, Am. J. Clin. Nutri. 25:245-254, 1972.

36. Brewer, T., Metabolic toxemia of late pregnancy: a disease of malnutrition, Springfield, IL: C.C.Thomas, 1966.

37. Brewer, T., Iatrogenic starvation in human pregnancy, Medikon, Ghent, Belgium, 4:14-15, 1974.

38. Brewer, T., Limitations of diuretic therapy in the management of severe toxemia: the significance of hypoalbuminemia, Am. J. Ob. Gyn. 83:1352-1359, 1962.

39. Lindheimer, M., and Katz, A., Sodium and diuretics in pregnancy, N. Eng. J. Med. 288:891-894, 1973.

40. Shanklin, D., Making pregnancy healthy, Med. Tribune, May 23, 1973.

41. A pregnant warning about diuretics, Med. World News, Nov 2, 1973.

42. Use of diuretics in normal pregnancies is questioned, OB/GYN News, Feb 15, 1975.

43. Toverud, G., The influence of nutrition on the course of pregnancy, Milbank Mem. Fund Quarterly 28:482-485, 1950.

Cited References Cont'd

44. Wynn, M., and Wynn, A., Nutrition counselling in the prevention of low birth-weight, Found. for Educ. and Res. in Child-bearing, London, 1975.

45. Cameron, C., and Graham, S., Antenatal diet and its influence on still-births and prematurity, Glasgow Med. J. 24:1-7, 1944.

46. Jeans, P., et al., Incidence of prematurity in relation to maternal nutrition, J. Am. Diet Assoc. 31:576-581, 1955.

47. Birch, H., and Gussow, J., Disadvantaged children: health, nutrition and school failure, New York: Grune & Stratton, 1970.

48. A study of infant mortality from linked records; comparison of neonatal mortality from two cohort studies, U.S. Dept. of HEW, 1972.

49. Lubchenco, L., et al., Neonatal mortality rate: relationship to birthweight and gestational age, J. Ped. 81:814-822, 1972.

50. Wynn, M., and Wynn, A., The protection of maternity and infancy, New York: E. H. Baker & Co., 1974.

51. Hardy, J., Birth weight and subsequent physical and intellectual developement, N. Eng. J. Med. 289:973-974, 1973.

52. The women and their pregnancies, U.S. Dept of HEW, 1972.

53. Chase, A., The great pellagra cover-up, Psych. Today pp. 83-86, Feb 1975.

54. Hurley, R., Poverty and mental retardation: a causal relationship, New York: Vintage Books, 1969, quoting Wylie, B., The challenge of infant mortality, Bull. Cleve. Acad. of Med., June, 1965.

55. Birch, H., and Gussow, J., (see 47 above), quoting Wiener, G., et al., Correlates of low birth weight: psychological status at eight to ten years of age, Ped. Res. 2:110-118, 1968.

56. Casalino, M., Intrauterine growth retardation: a neonatologist's approach, J. Reprod. Med. 14:248-250, 1975. quoting Rubin, R., et al., Psychological and educational sequelae of prematurity, Ped. 52:352-363, 1975.

57. Ob world and gynecoloty, Ross Timesaver 4:2, Jan-Feb, 1975.

58. Knoblich, H., and Pasamanick, B., Prediction from the assessment of neuromotor and intellectual status in infancy, in Zunin, J., and Jervis, G., (eds.), Psychopathology of mental development, New York: Grune & Stratton, 1967.

59. Lubchenco, L., et al., Sequelae of premature birth: evaluation of premature infants of low birth weight at ten years of age, Am. J. Dis. Child 106:101-115, 1963

Cited References Cont'd

60. Zitrin, A., et al., Pre and paranatal factors in mental disorders of children, J. Nervous and Mental Dis. 139:357-361, 1964.

61. Drillien, C., School disposal and performance for children of different birth-weight born 1953-1960, Archives of Dis. in childhood 44:562-570, 1969.

62. Churchill, J., The relationship between intelligence and birth weight in twins, neurology 15:341-347, 1965.

63. Churchill, J., et al., Birth weight and intelligence, Ob. Gyn. 28:425-429, 1966.

64. Knobloch, H., and Pasamanick, B., Mental Subnormality, N. Eng. J. Med. 266:1045-1051, 1092-1097, and 1155-1161, 1962. quoting Knobloch, H., and Pasamanick, B., Distribution of Intellectual Potential in Infant population, in The Epidemiology of Mental Disorder, Am. Assoc. for the Adv. of Sci., 1959.

65. Bacola, E., et al., Perinatal and environmental factors in late neurogenic sequelae, I. Infants having birth weights under 1,500 grams, Am. J. Dis. of Children 112:369-374, 1966.

66. Bland, R., Cord-blood total protein level as a screening aid for the idiopathic respiratory-distress syndrome, N. Eng. J. Med. 287:9-13, 1972.

67. Warkany, J., et al., Intrauterine growth retardation, Am. J. Dis. of Children 102:127-157, 1961 quoting Baird, D., Contribution of obstetrical factors to serious physical and mental handicap in children, J. Ob. Gyn. of Brit. Empire 66:743-747, 1959.

68. Knoblich, H., and Pasamanick, B., reference 64 above, 1959.

69. Williams, R., Nutrition against disease, New York: Pitman Publishing Co., 1971.

70. Ebbs, J., et al., Nutrition in pregnancy, Can. Med. A$_s$soc. J. 46:1-6, 1942.

71. Birch, H., and Gussow, J., reference 47 above, quoting Dieckmann, W., et al., Observations on protein intake and the health of the mother and baby, I. Clinical and laboratory findings, J. Am. Diet Assoc 27:1046-1052.

72. Arey, L., Developmental Anatomy, New York: W.B. Saunders, 1974.

73. Weingold, A., Intrauterine growth retardation: Obstetrical aspects, J. Reprod. Med. 14:244-247, 1975.

74. Winick, M., Changes in nucleic acid and protein content of the human brain during growth, Ped. Res. 2:352-355, 1968.

75. Winick, M., and Russo, P., The effect of severe early malnutrition on cellular growth of the human brain, Ped. Res. 3:181-184, 1969.

Cited References Cont'd

76. Shneour, E., The malnourished mind, New York: Doubleday, 1974.

77. Dobbing, J., The later growth of the brain and its vulnerability, Ped. 53:2-6, 1974.

78. Casalino, M., Intrauterine growth retardation: A neonatologist's approach, J. Reprod. Med. 14:248-250, 1975.

79. Flowers, C., Nutrition in pregnancy, Editorial, J. Reprod. Med. 7:200-204, 1971.

80. Winick, M., reference 74 above, quoting Winick, M., et al., Cellular growth in human placenta, I. Normal placental growth, Ped. 39:248-251, 1967.

81. Warkany, J., et al., Intrauterine growth retardation, Am. J. Dis. of Children 102:127-157, 1961.

82. Brewer, T., Rolf of malnutrition, hepatic dysfunction, and gastrointestinal bacteria in the pathogenesis of acute toxemia of pregnancy, An. J. Ob.Gyn. 84:1253-1256, 1962.

83. The great eclampsia mystery, or the case of the empty plaque, Med. World News, pp. 41-52, July 20, 1973.

84. Ehlich, E., Sodium metabolism in pregnancy: Current views, Contemp. Ob. Gyn. 4:17-19, 1974.

85. Pike, R., Sodium intake during pregnancy, J. Am. Diet Assoc. 44:176-181, 1964.

86. Pike, R., and Smiciklas, H., A reappraisal of sodium restriction during pregnancy, Int'l Gyn. Ob. 10:1-8, 1972.

87. Pike, R., and Gursky, D., Further evidence of deleterious effects produced by sodium restriction during pregnancy, Am. J. Clin. Nutr. 23:883-889, 1970.

88. Robinson, M., Salt in pregnancy, Lancet 1:178-181, 1958.

89. Flowers, C., et al., Chlorothiazide as a prophylaxis against toxemia of pregnancy, A double blind study, Am. J. Ob. Gyn. 84:919-929, 1962.

90. Kraus, G., et al., Prophylactic use of hydrochlorothiazide in pregnancy, JAMA 198: 128-132, 1966.

91. Weseley, A., and Douglas, G., Continuous use of chlorothiazide for prevention of toxemia of pregnancy, Ob. Gyn. 19:355-358, 1962.

92. Lindheimer, M., and Katz, A., reference 39 above, quoting Crocker, J., Renal anomalies in whole human embryonic culture, Clin Res. 20:915, 1972.

Cited References Cont'd

93. Chesley, L., Sodium, diuretic drugs, and preeclampsia, Patologia E Clin. Ostetrica E Ginecologica (Rome), 2:1-6, 1974.

94. Brewer, T., Pancreatitis in pregnancy, (letter to editor), J. Reprod. Med. 12:204, 1974.

95. Hibbard, L., Maternal mortality due to acute toxemia, Ob. Gyn. 42:263-270, 1973.

96. Williams, S., Nutrition and diet therapy, St. Louis, MO: C.V. Mosby Co., 1973.

97. Nourishing your unborn baby, Prevention, March, 1977.

98. Federal Register, 41:23989-23992, June 14, 1976.

99. Schewitz, L., Hypertension and renal disease in pregnancy, Med. Clinics of N. Am. 5:47-69, 1971, quoting Sarles, M., et al., Sodium excretion patterns during and following intravenous sodium chloride loads in normal and hypertensive pregnancies, Am. J. Ob. Gyn. 102:1-7, 1968.

100. Hytten, F., and Leitch, I., The physiology of human pregnancy, 2nd ed., New York: Blackwell Scientific Publications, 1971.

101. Shanklin, D., et al., Nutrition and pregnancy: an invitational symposium, Part One, J. Reprod. Med. 7:199-219, 1971.

102. Strauss, M., Observations on the etiology of the toxemias of pregnancy-- The relationship of nutritional deficiency, hypoproteinemia, and elevated venous pressure to water retention in pregnancy, Am. J. Med. Sci. 190: 811-824, 1935.

103. Ross, R., Relation of vitamin deficiency to the toxemia of pregnancy, S. Med. J. 120-122, 1935.

104. Bletka, M., et al., Volume of whole blood and absolute amount of serum proteins in the early stage of late toxemia of pregnancy, Am. J. Ob. Gyn. 106:10-13, 1970.

105. Toxemia--A disease of prejudice?, World Med. J. 21:70-72, 1974, quoting Sheehan, H., and Lynch, J., Pathology of toxemia of pregnancy, Edinburgh: Churchill Livingston, 1973.

106. Dodge, E., and Frost, T., Relation between blood plasma proteins and toxemias of pregnancy, JAMA 111:1898-1902, 1938.

107. Tompkins, W., and Wiehl, D., Nutritional deficiencies as a causal factor in toxemia and premature labor, Am. J. Ob. Gyn. 62:898-919, 1951.

108. Hamlin, R., The prevention of eclampsia and pre-eclampsia, Lancet 1:64-68, 1952.

Cited References Cont'd

109. Brewer, T., Metabolic toxemia of late pregnancy in a county prenatal nutrition educaion project: A preliminary report, J. Reprod. Med. 13:175-176, 1974.

110. Grieve, J., Prevention of gestational failure by high protein diet, J. Repro. Med. 13:170-174, 1974.

111. Albumin concentrate can be used for mid preeclampsia, Ob. Gyn News, Oct. 1, 1974.

112. Kitay, D., Dysfunctional antepartum nutrition, J. Reprod. Med. 7:251-256, 1971.

113. Pasamanick, B., and Knobloch, H., Retrospective studies on the epidemiology of repruductive casuality: Old and new, Merrill-Palmer Qtr. Beh. & Develop. 12:7-26, 1966.

114. Pasamanick, B., and Lilienfeld, A., Association of maternal and fetal factors with development of mental deficiency, I. Abnormalities in the prenatal and paranatal periods, JAMA 159:155-160, 1955.

115. Knobloch, H., and Pasamanick, B., Mental Subnormality, N. Eng. J. Med. 266:1045-1051, 1962.

116. Kawi, A., and Pasamanick, B., Association of factors of pregnancy with reading disorders in childhood, JAMA 166:1420-1423, 1958.

117. Knobloch, H., and Pasamanick, B., Prospective studies on the epidemiology, of repreductive casuality: Methods, finds, and some implications, Merrill-Palmer Qtr. Beh. & Devel. 12:27-43, 1966, quoting Knobloch, H. and Pasamanick, B., The developmental behavioral approach to the neurologic examination in infancy, Child Develop. 33:181-198, 1962.

118. Pasamanick, B., and Knobloch, H., reference 113 above, quoting Rogersm, M., et al., Prenatal and paranatal factors in the development of childhood behavior disorders, Copenhagen: Munksgaard, 1955.

119. Knobloch, H., et al., Neuropsychiatric sequelae of prematurity--a longitudinal study, JAMA 161:581-585, 1956.

120. Knobloch, H., and Pasamanick, B., Prematurity and development, J. Ob. Gyn. of the Brit. Commonwealth 66:729 - 731, 1959.

121. Linlienfeld, A., and Parkhurst, E., A study of the association of factors of pregnancy and parturition with the development of cerebral palsy, Am. J. Hygiene 53:262-282, 1951.

122. Taylor, E., Organic causes of minimal brain dysfunction, Cont. Med. Digest, pp. 822-823, August 1972 reviewing Tobin, A., Organic causes of minimal brain dysfunction, Perinatal origin of minimal cerebral lesions, JAMA 1207-1214, 1971.

Cited References Cont'd

123. Taylor, E., Organic causes of minimal brain dysfunction, Cont. Med. Digest, pp. 822-823, 1972.

124. Lasagne, L., Attitudes toward appetite suppressants, JAMA July 2, 1973.

125. SPUN Reports, May 15, 1975.

126. Various personal correspondences.

127. Bohstedt, G., Dairy Goat J. 46:4, 1968.

128. Toxemia of Pregnancy, Ross Laboratories.

129. Diabetes in Pregnancy, Ross Laboratories.

130. Pomerance, J., Weight gain in pregnancy: How much is enough?, Clin. Ped. 11:554-556, 1972.

131. Singer, J., et al., Relationshio of weight gain during pregnancy to birth weight and infant growth and development in the first year of life, Ob. Gyn. 31:417-423, 1968.

132. SPUN Reports, Oct. 1, 1976.

133. Kaminetsky, H., Ob. Gyn., Dec. 1972.

134. Pitkin, R., et al., Ob. Gyn. 40:773-785, 1972.

135. Russell, K., Ob. Gyn., Nov. 1973.

136. Schmeck, H., Brain harm in U.S. laid to food lack, N.Y. Times, Nov 2, 1975.

137. SPUN Reports, Jan. 15, 1973.

138. Roeder, L., Discussion: Supplementation of diets of pregnant women in Tiawan, Am. J. Clin. Nutr. 26:1143, 1973.

139. Aubry, R., et al., Maternal nutrition, I. The urinary urea nitrogen/total nitrogen ratio as an index of protein nutrition, Am. J. Ob.Gyn. 114:198-203, 1972.

140. Sackler, A., Who shall live and who shall die?, Medical Tribune, Dec. 19, 1973.

141. Conley, R., The economics of mental retardation, Baltimore: Johns Hopkins Univ. Press, 1973.

142. Silber, J., Nutrition's role in learning, NY Times, Nov. 16, 1975.

143. Brewer, T., Doctors' Debate, letter to editor, Med. Tribune, Feb-Mar, 1973.

CHAPTER TWENTY SIX

PREGNANT? AND WANT A HEALTHY CHILD: SPECIFICS OF A WELL-BALANCED DIET

Tom Brewer, M.D.

You are one of over three million women who are having a baby in the United States each year.

In recent years, pregnant women in our country have been less healthy than pregnant women in many other countries. An increasing number of premature and "low birth weight" babies are being born. This is primarily caused by the failure of our doctors to recognize the role of nutrition in pregnancy.

Instead of emphasizing good diet many American doctors who care for pregnant women prescribe low calorie, low salt diets for "weight control." Many doctors also still depend on drugs such as diuretics (water pills) and amphetamines (diet pills) to try to prevent diseases during pregnancy.

This routine type of treatment is dangerous to both mother and baby. But you can avoid danger by good nutrition throughout your pregnancy. We now know that most pregnancy diseases and complications are caused by poor diets -- by lack of enough good foods during pregnancy.

The methods of good diet described here have been used with success in my practice in over 7,000 pregnancies over a twelve-year period in the prenatal clinics of Contra Costa County, California.

When you understand what a good pregnancy diet is and how important good foods really are, you will be able to protect yourself and your baby from many complications.

The Importance of Diet

If you are an expectant mother, you must eat a good, nutritious, balanced diet every day during your pregnancy. A good diet is the best insurance that your baby will be healthy and strong, with a normal weight at birth!

TOM BREWER is President, Society for the Protection of the Unborn Through Nutrition; Author of book, Metabolic Toxemia of Late Pregnancy, and numerous other works; he is featured in the movie, "Nutrition in Pregnancy."

The Dangers of Bad Diet

Forty years of medical research has proved that bad diets during pregnancy cause:
1. Stillborn babies.
2. Low birth weight or premature babies.
3. Brain-damaged babies with less intelligence.
4. Hyperactive babies with more irritability.
5. Infection-prone babies with more illness.

A good diet will protect your baby from these troubles.

Bad diets cause diseases in mothers, too:
1. Metabolic Toxemia of Late Pregnancy (MTLP) -- a disease caused by too little high quality proteins and vitamins in the diet. Women with MTLP suffer convulsions or "fits," coma, heart failure, fat in their livers, bleeding into their livers and often death for both mother and baby. It is estimated that in the United States 30,000 babies die each year of MTLP -- and thousands more live with damage to their brains. They suffer cerebral palsy, epilepsy and other nervous system disorders.

A good diet will protect you and your baby from MTLP.
2. Anemias ("low blood") -- caused by not enough iron, vitamins and/or protein in the diet.

A good diet will protect you from anemias.
3. Abruption of the Placenta or "Afterbirth" -- a disease in which the afterbirth tears loose inside the mother's womb, often before labor begins; the mother bleeds and the baby dies in 50% of the cases.

A good diet will protect you and your baby from Abruption.
4. Severe infections of the lungs, kidneys and liver.

A good diet will protect you and your baby from severe infections.
5. Miscarriage -- if the mother does not have a good diet, the placenta grows imperfectly and cannot meet the needs of the developing baby, so a miscarriage results.

A good diet will protect you and your baby from miscarriages.

What is a Good Nutritious, Balanced Diet?

When you are pregnant, you need more of good quality foods than when you are not pregnant. To meet your own needs and those of your developing baby, you must have, every day, at least:

1. One quart (four glasses) of milk -- any kind: whole milk, low fat, skim, powdered skim or buttermilk. If you do not like milk, you can substitute one cup of yoghurt for each cup of milk.

2. Two eggs.

3. Two servings of fish, shellfish, chicken or turkey, lean beef, veal, lamb, pork, liver or kidney.

   Alternative combinations include:
   Rice with: beans, cheese, sesame, milk
   Cornmeal with: beans, cheese, tofu, milk
   Beans with: rice, bulgar, cornmeal, wheat noodles, sesame seeds, milk
   Peanuts with: sunflower seeds, milk
   Whole wheat bread or noodles with: beans, cheese, peanut butter, milk, tofu

   For each serving of meat, you can substitute these quantities of cheese:

Brick - 4 oz.	Longhorn - 3 oz.
Camembert - 6 oz.	Meunster - 4 oz.
Cheddar - 3 oz.	Monterey Jack - 4 oz.
Cottage - 6 oz.	Swiss - 3 oz.

4. Two servings of fresh, green leafy vegetables: mustard, beet, collard, dandelion or turnip greens, spinach, lettuce, cabbage, broccoli, kale, Swiss chard.

5. Five servings of whole grain breads, rolls, cereals or pancakes: wheatena, 100% bran flakes, granola, shredded wheat, wheat germ, oatmeal, buckwheat or whole wheat pancakes, corn bread, corn tortillas, corn or bran or whole wheat muffins, waffles, brown rice.

6. Two choices from: a whole potato (any style), large green pepper, grapefruit, lemon, lime papaya, tomato (one piece of fruit or one large glass juice).

7. Three pats of margarine, Vitamin A enriched, or butter.

Also include in your diet:

8. A yellow or orange-colored vegetable or fruit five times a week.

9. Liver once a week.

10. Table salt: SALT YOUR FOOD TO TASTE.

11. Water: DRINK TO THIRST.

It is not healthy for you and your unborn baby to go even 24 hours without good food!

Certain Things May Prevent You From Having a Good Diet

A good diet sounds simple, doesn't it? But it isn't so simple in our society. Many things may happen to prevent you from eating and digesting a good diet each day throughout pregnancy.

You may believe that the foods you see widely advertized on TV and in magazines give you and your baby the proteins, vitamins and minerals you need. Foods such as: boxed cereals, white bread, potato chips, soft drinks, candy, french fries, commercial cakes and cookies provide expensive, useless "empty" calories. When you spend money on these foods, you are not getting your money's worth of good nutrition. The first items to put in your shopping cart are the foods on the good diet list!

Another situation which may interfere with your good diet is the nausea and vomiting, or heartburn, indigestion and loss of appetite which many women experience in pregnancy. This problem must be corrected quickly, with the help of your doctor, so that you can resume your good eating habits.

If you are overweight at the beginning of your pregnancy, you may think that now is a good time to try to lose some of that extra weight. Pregnancy is not the time to go on a low-calorie diet. There is recent evidence that your baby's brain is growing at its most rapid rate during the last two months of pregnancy. Mothers who follow low-calorie diets risk stunting the growth of their babies' brains.

The Doctor May Stand Between You and Good Nutrition

Misinformation about diet:

You will often meet a doctor, in a private office or in a clinic, who doesn't really understand the life-and-death importance of a good diet for you and your baby.

You may not be told anything about the need for a good diet for you and your baby.

You may be told that diet "isn't too important" for your health or for the health of your unborn child. Don't believe it!

You may be told that salt, ordinary table salt, is harmful to you and your baby. Don't believe it! Continue to salt your food to taste.

Misinformation about weight gain:

You may be told to go on a starvation-type diet if you "gain too much weight." Don't go on a starvation diet! The food you eat every day while you are pregnant builds the bones, muscle and brain of your baby. Pounds gained while you are on a good diet protect and prepare you for labor and breast feeding.

If you gain a few extra pounds during this pregnancy from eating a nutritious, balanced diet, it won't hurt you or the baby -- even if you gain 50 or 60 pounds. Worry if you don't gain enough.

Misinformation about dangerous drugs:

You may be given "diet pills" to take away your appetite, drugs like Dexidrene or "speed" (amphetamines). Don't take them!

These drugs are not healthy for you. They are not healthy for your unborn baby. Who would give a baby "speed?" Every drug you take passes quickly into the placenta or afterbirth, then into the baby's bloodstream and body.

The amphetamines are given to kill the hungry mother's appetite. They also give her an unnatural boost. They relieve depression, make her feel she is working smoother and living a healthful life -- even though she is not getting enough to eat. In this way, amphetamines cover up her problem of poor nutrition.

You may be given diuretics or "water pills" during your pregnancy. The immediate effect of these pills is to cause your body to eliminate water excessively. They dry you up. They dry up your baby. Don't take them!

These drugs are <u>not</u> needed to have a healthy pregnancy and a healthy baby; however, the private drug industry has widely promoted diuretics and amphetamines for use in mothers. These "hard sell" promotions, along with the low calorie, low salt diet and indifference of many doctors toward pregnancy nutrition, have created a grave health hazard for American women and their unborn children.

Water pills have damaged many pregnant w o m e n and their babies. Reported bad effects listed by the d r u g companies who, nevertheless, continued to advertise them, include:

loss of appetite, stomach irritation, nausea and vomiting, diarrhea, constipation, cramping, muscle spasm, jaundice, pancreatitis, hyperglycemia, high blood pressure, dizziness, headache, thrombocytopenia, glycosuria, aplastic anemia, skin rash, weakness, restlessness, photosensitivity.

The doctor often prescribes these drugs to "treat" the <u>normal</u> swelling that occurs during pregnancy" If you have been eating a good, well-balanced, nutritious diet, you will probably have swelling of your feet, hands and face -- normally.

If the swelling bothers you, lie down a few minutes with your feet elevated. You can repeat this simple remedy several times a day if needed.

Remember: It is not healthy for you and your unborn baby to go even 24 hours without good food!

Reprints of this article available from Nutrition Action Group, 14 Truesdale Drive, Croton-On-Hudson, NY 10520; or SPUN, Suite 603, 17 N. Wabash, Chicago, IL 60602. 50-200 copies, 10¢ each. 250 or more, 5¢ each. Rates are post paid. For a complimentary copy, send self-addressed stamped envelope.

CHAPTER TWENTY SEVEN

BREASTFEEDING, "NATURAL MOTHERING,"
AND WORKING OUTSIDE THE HOME

Merilyn Salomon, M.A.
Victoria Schauf, M.D.
Anne Seiden, M.D.

"In a well-ordered society, there should be no difficulty in arranging work and mothering so that every woman who wants can do both. In fact, it could be easily arranged, and at a fraction of the expenditure we now place on defense, for both father and mother to work and yet be together with their children throughout a substantial portion of their early lives."

-Ashley Montagu

The theme of this book is "Twenty-First Century Obstetrics Now." We view this to be a workable synthesis of the best in traditional obstetrics and child-rearing, backed up by twentieth century medical technology where it is needed. The question has been how to retain the advantages which the technological revolution has brought us in obstetric care, without allowing technology to damage the relationship between mother and infant.

This question in obstetrics is one which appears in many other arenas of life in 1977; it is a basic ecological question that also confronts industry and agriculture. To what extent is it possible to have the industrial productivity of which this society is capable without, for example, impairing clean air, clean water, and human dimensions of the quality of life?[1]

MERILYN SALOMON is a Ph.D. Doctoral candidate, School of Social Service Administration, University of Chicago.

VICTORIA SCHAUF is an Associate Professor, Department of Pediatrics, College of Medicine, University of Illinois.

ANNE SEIDEN is Director of Research, Institute for Juvenile Research, State of Illinois; and author of numerous papers, book reviews, book chapters on the psychiatric aspects of pregnancy, birth, sex, and women.

THE QUESTION WHETHER MOTHERS CAN HUMANLY REAR INFANTS AND STILL BE ECONOMICALLY PRODUCTIVE HAS ONLY BEEN ASKED SINCE THE INDUSTRIAL REVOLUTION. IN PREVIOUS AGRICULTURAL, HUNTING OR GATHERING SOCIETIES WOMEN WERE ALWAYS ECONOMICALLY PRODUCTIVE; THEIR LABOR WAS NEEDED FOR THE SURVIVAL OF THE TRIBE OR COMMUNITY.

The same ecological question that we ask about obstetrics presents itself in the fourth trimester and beyond -- the beginning of lactation and the other dimensions of child nurturance. That question is: "How can mothers and infants and the rest of their families live in an industrial society and be part of it, without impairing the natural bonding mechanisms that are essential to the quality of infant life?"[2]

The question whether mothers can humanly rear infants and still be economically productive has only been asked since the Industrial Revolution. Previously, in agricultural and horticultural and hunting and gathering societies, women were always economically productive; their labor was needed for the survival of the tribe or the community.[3] By and large, they went about their business with their infants attached to their bodies. Since the Industrial Revolution we have seen the creation of special workplaces, such as factories, often radically unsuited to the needs of infants. This has produced a conflict between the needs of infants and the conditions of work, which has not been easy to solve. Our society has been experimenting with methods of solving that conflict ever since, and many of the compromises made in solving it have not been very successful.

One particular compromise arose and was epitomized in Victorian England among the middle class (a relatively small part of the population, but the one which produced the most writing), and has come to be seen as "traditional." The world of productive work was normatively assigned to men, and was viewed as crass, dirty, and dangerous, while the world of human values, including esthetic and religious values as well as childrearing, was largely assigned to women, and viewed as finer, higher, and nobler.[4]

This preserved a space in which it was possible to rear children humanly, but at a considerable cost. For women, that cost was ghettoization, isolation from the economic base of society and from the power that goes with it; for men, isolation from those things in life which for many of us really give life its value. For children, the cost was extreme vulnerability: only those children whose mothers obtained a protective ghetto had any chance at a good human life. Dickens chronicled the terrible fate of orphans and children of single mothers, who might as well have been orphans, when their mothers went to work in the sweatshop and left the children to the factory or the streets. The alternative was the workhouse, where parents and children were separated. [5]

In present-day America, most children are still born to a married couple, though that percentage is decreasing [6], and the percentage of marriages which rupture during the children's childhood is increasing. When marriages break, the overwhelming majority of children remain with the mother. Typically she seeks employment, since in the vast majority of cases the father fails to meet his child support obligations. [7] At present, one quarter of our children (and close to one half of our black children) do not live with both natural parents [8]; by age 18 some 35-45% of all children will spend five years or more in a single-parent home. [9] While there remains a sizeable proportion of families in which the mother can count on a protective space in which to do her childrearing, many are unable to do so, because the costs of isolation in the protected space are too great. But the persistence of the Victorian ideal has impeded women's entrance into the economic life of industrial society. [10] Proper childcare is seen as something which must be private, like sexual intercourse. [11] Powerful taboos against nursing the child in public remain in some quarters. Childish behavior itself is seen as taboo. Children, like mental patients, must be hidden from the public view. All of these factors have profound effects on children, and on the psychology of mothering. [12]

Therefore, the mother who enters the public arena of work today faces special problems. She is expected almost to pretend that her children do not exist. They should be kept away from her, in some private space, cared for by someone else during most of their waking hours. The mother has two options, neither of them very satisfactory for most women: to join the ghetto with the children, or to join the adult public arena and leave her children behind. The first option may work if the marriage endures and the husband commands a sufficient income to buy support for the children and recreational escape opportunities for the mother. Since both the stability of the husband's income and the durability of the marriage are often fragile, even the woman who does not plan employment is in a vulnerable position for childrearing. At the same time, the mother who is employed may suffer guilt about the effects of her employment on her children, though reviews of literature in this area do not support that guilt. [13, 14, 15]

THE MOTHER WHO ENTERS THE PUBLIC ARENA OF WORK FACES SPECIAL PROBLEMS. AT WORK SHE IS EXPECTED ALMOST TO PRETEND THAT HER CHILDREN DO NOT EXIST. SHE FACES DANGER OF CRITICISM FROM BOTH SIDES: FROM THOSE WHO MIGHT CRITICIZE HER BECAUSE OF HER WORKING AND FROM THOSE WHO MIGHT CRITICIZE HER BECAUSE OF HER COMMITMENT TO HER CHILD. FOR THE NURSING MOTHER THIS CRITICISM IS NOT TRIVIAL BECAUSE IT IS A STRESS THAT CAN INHIBIT LET-DOWN AND LACTATION.

All of this conflict is as unnatural as many of the birth customs which have been addressed elsewhere in these volumes. Humans are social animals; very few people are such loners as to deal well with isolation from the public arenas of our society. In fact, one study showed that if women become clinically depressed, their recovery is more rapid if they are employed outside the home.[16] Two major studies showed, disturbingly, a sharp drop in self-reported happiness among married women with small children, compared with childless married women.[17, 18]

Hence, in present American culture, several patterns have contributed to a radical detachment of mothers from childrearing. More and more mothers are employed [19]; those who do not work tend to rely on recreational pastimes to rejoin the tribe. Women often do not nurse their children, either because of their "work," or because they "do not want to be tied down." For example, one busy physician told us his wife did not nurse their baby because she valued remaining free to take skiing vacations with her husband and their friends, a rare opportunity for closeness with him and them.

In sharp contrast, a mothering pattern called "natural mothering" has been described in a number of recent publications.[20, 21] It is usually seen as including more or less constant mother-child contact during the first year or two of life, and breastfeeding the child when the child wishes to be fed. It is generally seen as incompatible with paid employment outside the home. This mothering pattern is offered as a corrective to the above described pattern of detachment from childrearing. But we feel that it needs to be expanded; otherwise the mother who must be employed may feel that the "natural mothering" approach is not available to her, which would then contribute unwittingly to a further polarization of mothering styles.

In summary, two important contemporary trends related to women's changing roles pose contradictions for the working mother: the trend toward increasing employment of women and the trend towards returning to breastfeeding and "natural mothering." Thus far in this country there has been little commitment to consolidating these trends, although other countries have done so.[22] Many working women in America have believed it impossible to have both a satisfying nursing relationship and a career or job outside the home. Most literature on breastfeeding is designed for the woman who is a full-time mother and housewife. Even the few exceptions, such as Cahill's Breastfeeding and Working? [23] may induce guilt about working by offering nursing advice to the working mother only as a second best solution. The unfortunate result for many working women has been to deny themselves both the real advantages of breastfeeding and the real emotional and practical assistance of a nursing support group in doing so.

Many working women have not tried to breastfeed, because they thought it would be impossible. Others have breastfed for the weeks they were home with the baby before returning to work, then given it up, feeling it would be impossible to manage breastfeeding and working at the same time. Other women have made irreversible plans to leave a job in order to devote full time to mothering, only to find that they were lonely, cranky, unsatisfied, and unable to be the kind of mother they had hoped to be.

It is, however, possible to both breastfeed and work. The two-fold purpose of this paper is (1) to present medical, psychological, and practical reasons why it is best for a working mother (or any mother) to breastfeed and (2) to present some practical measures for merging the two commitments of working and mothering.

Before going on, we should note an oddity of language which has some real significance. The word "work" is conventionally used to refer to paid employment, however light; the very heavy work often done by housewives is often correspondingly neglected. Thus a housewife with twelve children and no washing machine is not referred to as a "working mother." A woman whose job as a receptionist poses few demands might find it strange that her eight hours of paid employment are referred to as "work," but her other heavier labor at childcare, shopping, laundry, cleaning, and cooking are not. For convenience in this paper we have followed the conventional usage, and by "working mother" we refer to a woman employed outside the home. However, we are not happy with that usage.

THERE ARE MANY MEDICAL ADVANTAGES FOR BREASTFEEDING ON THE SIDE OF THE BABY. HOWEVER, FAR FROM BEING AN ALTRUISTIC ENDEAVOR ON THE PART OF THE MOTHER, BREASTFEEDING HAS DISTINCT MEDICAL ADVANTAGES FOR HER AS WELL.

Medical Advantages of Breastfeeding: For All Mothers; For Working Mothers

Breastfeeding provides medical benefits that are not available to the bottle fed baby. These may be summarized as follows: Human milk contains antibodies, cells, enzymes, and other factors for nonspecific resistance to infections that affect human infants. Breastfed babies are less likely to develop allergies. Human milk contains iron which the human infant can use more readily than the iron in cow's milk. Breastfed babies appear to develop a better appetite control mechanism.

Newborn babies are especially vulnerable to infection in the first six weeks of life. During this time of life, the human baby does not manufacture many antibodies [24], thus the antibodies from human milk become especially important. Other factors in human milk which may protect the baby against infection include: enzymes (lactoperoxidase, lysozyme) which promote chemical reactions which kill bacteria; leucocytes, which are cells that may limit or prevent the spread of infection; a milk protein which binds the iron which bacteria need for growth (lactoferrin); L. bifidus growth factor; anti-staphylococcal factor; and complement components. [25] The immunity conferred by human milk during this period may last longer than the actual nursing period. Therefore even a short period of nursing has advantages. The working mother should make every effort to nurse at least during her maternity leave. For some, this will lead to more extended nursing. In any case, even a limited period of nursing is beneficial.

In the past, physicians have thought that the antibodies in human milk were digested by the infant, thus losing their antimicrobial activity. Upon further investigation, it has been found that the particular molecular structure of the secretory antibody in human milk and colostrum is relatively resistant to both stomach acid and to digestive enzymes. It has also been found that an infant's stomach has very little acid in comparison with an adult human. Secretory antibodies in mother's milk protect the respiratory and gastrointestinal tract [26], the major portals of infection in a baby.

Human milk favors the growth of non-pathogenic bacteria in the bowels. Bottle fed babies are more likely to be colonized by potentially pathogenic bacteria, which could make the baby sick at a later time. Antibodies to those pathogens are not present in the baby at birth, but gradually develop during the first year of life. [24] Breastfed infants who do develop diarrhea, do not get hypertonic dehydration, a severe salt imbalance that occurs in bottle fed babies. [27]

All babies get colds, but bottle fed babies may get more seriously ill. A study of common respiratory pathogen, respiratory syncytial virus, showed that pneumonis and wheezing as complications of this infection were more common in bottle fed babies than in breastfed babies of high socio-economic class. Antibodies to this virus are uniformly present in human colostrum and milk. [28] Even affluent parents need to be concerned about respiratory infections in babies since these are common even with good living conditions. (The average child gets six to eight respiratory infections a year.)

Ear infections have been said to be more common in bottle fed infants. [29] This may partly be due to the fact that they are given the bottle while lying on their backs, thus allowing the milk to flow into the middle ear. [30] The eustachean tube in the infant is straighter than in the adult, so the milk has an easy route into the ear. Bottle fed babies seem to be more prone to tooth decay, possibly the result of prolonged exposure of teeth to milk.

Cow's milk alone or as part of a formula may be harmful to human infants. [31] Cow's milk proteins are foreign to humans and quite allergenic to babies [32], particularly to babies who are not receiving secretory antibodies from their mother's milk. The intestine is rather permeable during the first six weeks of life and may allow the absorption of foreign proteins such as those present in cow's milk. These absorbed foreign proteins may sensitize the infant and lay the foundations for food allergies. After about six weeks, the local immune response of the baby helps prevent absorption of foreign proteins. [26]

Bottle fed babies are often fed supplements and so may be exposed early to a variety of potential allergens, such as eggs and cow's milk. In recent years pediatricians have recognized the increased occurrence of intestinal symptoms (colic, vomiting and diarrhea), eczema and allergy in bottle fed babies. These considerations in the decision to breastfeed are especially important in families which have a tendency to allergy (up to one quarter of us all).

Allergens in the mother's diet can possibly be transferred to a nursing infant, but this is much less likely than the potential allergies for a bottle fed infant. If a breastfed baby develops an allergy, the mother's diet can be changed to eliminate the source of allergy. It is also important to consider what medications a potential nursing mother will be taking. If anti-convulsant drugs, such as phenobarbital and dilantin, are required for epilepsy, nursing is contraindicated. Most drugs, including antibiotics, may be safely used. Even if the antibiotic is passed from the mother to the milk, an insignificant amount is absorbed by the infant. [33]

Although both cow's milk and human milk contain little iron, iron deficiency anemia is uncommon in breastfed babies during the first six months of life. A healthy, term baby will have received enough iron during pregnancy that no iron supplement will be needed initially. Iron is needed after about six months of life, the time when solid foods containing iron should be introduced. [34] Vitamin D is required by all babies, who are not exposed to sunlight, for the prevention of rickits. For this reason it has been customary to add it to formulas and to provide supplementation for breastfed infants.

There seems to be better development of appetite control in breastfed babies. [35] The reason is unknown, but it may be that the thick, rich hind milk may act as a signal to the breastfed baby that the feeding is over. Many bottle fed babies are overweight. The reason again is unknown, but it may be that with a bottle one cannot tell when the baby is full. The risk of obesity for babies is that once fat has developed, the fat cells remain for life. Obesity with all its attendant physical and psychological problems can then remain a lifelong problem even with no organic, genetic, or other predisposition.

Thus far, the medical advantages for breastfeeding seem to lie on the baby's side. However, far from being an altruistic endeavor on the part of the mother, breastfeeding has distinct medical advantages for her. The suckling of the infant immediately after birth promotes uterine contraction and reduces the risk of postpartum bleeding. Further suckling helps the uterus return quickly to the pre-pregnancy condition. Lactation gives a woman the sense of physical well-being. The delayed return of menstrual periods is enjoyed by some. Lactation infertility has been used as a form of contraception. It does result in decreased population growth, but is unreliable on an individual basis, especially if supplementary feedings are given. It is relatively easier for the lactating mother to control her weight, as extra calories are used for milk production. Some authorities feel that there is a decreased incidence of breast cancer in women who breastfeed.

A possible hazard of human breastfeeding may be environmentally introduced pollutants. The extent of this hazard is unknown. However, pollutants may also occur in cow's milk or in other foods. Fruits and vegetables eaten by the mother should be carefully washed to prevent DDT contamination of the milk. A woman should not give up the known benefits of breastfeeding for the potential hazards of pollutants. (However, political action should be taken to control introduction of toxic substances into the environment.)

Of concern are the highly toxic chemical contaminants, the polychlorinated biphenyls (PCB) and poly-brominated biphenyls (PBB). These are industrial products which have been introduced into farm areas of Michigan and which have contaminated game fish. PCB's and PBB's are fat soluble, non-biodegradable toxins and are excreted from the body primarily in milk. The level of toxicity is not known; food contaminated with these and other industrial and agricultural pollutants should be avoided. [36]

In a few situations, nursing should be discontinued for medical reasons. In most cases, the mother can express milk from her breast to maintain lactation and resume breastfeeding later. Most infections in mother or infant do not have to end nursing. However, if the mother has active tuberculosis, she should be separated from the infant. Rarely, a newborn will become severely jaundiced as a result of an unusual effect of some maternal hormones present in the milk. In this case, the pediatrician may decide it is necessary to stop nursing temporarily. Illness in the infant does not require interruption of nursing unless the baby is so sick that it must be fed intravenously. If possible, a mother of a sick infant should accompany the baby to the hospital and continue nursing there.

ANY AMOUNT OF BREASTFEEDING IS IMPORTANT. EVEN A LITTLE BIT HELPS. A MOTHER CAN KNOW SHE HAS PROVIDED HER INFANT WITH THE BEST NUTRITION IT COULD HAVE.

While these medical advantages of breastfeeding apply to all mothers, they apply more strongly, not less so, to working mothers. After all, the love of a mother for her children does not diminish if the mother has interests outside the home. All mothers want to protect their babies from illness. In some ways, working mothers have even greater needs to provide this protection. Infants whose mothers work away from home, like infants in families with school children, may be exposed to infections carried home from others. Most parents feel guilty when their children get sick. Working mothers often feel guiltier when their babies become ill; they may feel that the child's illness would not have occurred if they had re-

mained at home.   With breastfeeding, many infant illnesses occur
less often.   In the event of illness, the nursing mother knows that
she has done her best to prevent this for her baby.

Providing proper care for a sick child is a greater problem
for a working mother than for a mother who is staying at home with
her infant.   The working mother may have to take time off from her
job to stay home with the child or to take the child to the doctor. She
may lose income and may have to pay for a doctor. Employers often
look with disfavor upon women who take time off to care for sick
children, and absenteeism among women then becomes an often
spurious argument against professional advancement and salaries
commensurate with those paid to men. [37] The prevention of disease
in the infants of working women is especially important, both in
terms of the mother's psychological well-being and in terms of the
convenience for her in managing both job and mothering.

Psychological Advantages of Nursing for the Working Mother

Once nursing is established, it is an easy approach to infant
feeding.   This is particularly important to the mother with multiple
commitments. With full breastfeeding, there is no formula preparation, sterilization, refrigeration and heating.   Babies swallow less
air and need less burping; they need fewer baths, because they smell
better; they have fewer illnesses.   If the baby sleeps in the same
bed, the mother does not need to get up out of bed or fully awake to
feed the baby at night.

The mutuality established between mother and baby is the
most important psychological advantage of nursing and is particularly important to the working mother who is likely to be separated
from her infant due to her job.   The closeness and sensuality of
breastfeeding are basic animal interactions, as breastfeeding was
intended to be.   The sensuality adds strength and earthiness to the
bond with the baby, much as the parents' sexual relationship ties
them together.   The baby is not a passive recipient of milk; it is an
active participation in a vigorous, mutual, reciprocal relationship
between mother and child.   The mother needs the baby to empty her
breasts. The baby needs the milk and the sucking obtained from the
mother's breasts.   These needs are very concrete, and the nursing
pair participates together as physiology creates the natural situation
to meet the psychological needs of both.

An increased possibility for emotional contact between mother
and infant comes with physical contact. [38, 39] The closeness of
breastfeeding is not fully duplicated by the fully clothed mother

holding a bottle. Holding, cuddling, soothing, eye to eye contact, movement, rocking, and skin to skin contact are all likely to occur in breastfeeding and to lead to a better relationship between the nursing pair.

Because working women are often encouraged to feel a destructive kind of guilt about both working and having children, breastfeeding provides an important source of confidence in her mothering which the working mother needs. She knows that by producing and giving nourishment through her own body she is giving her child all the nutritional, medical, and psychological advantages of human milk. Many women experience a specific surge of maternal feeling at the time of suckling itself [40], strengthening the bond between mother and infant, which are so important for the working mother to develop. All of these advantages help the working mother to deal with time spent away from her child at work.

Beyond the mother-infant dyad, breastfeeding has the potential for favorable psychological impact on the rest of the family. The baby's need for feeding from the mother is intuitively obvious to even very young siblings. When allowed to they are often eager to cuddle up close to the nursing pair (a large bed, or a quilt on the floor facilitates this). This is a more natural form of participation for the very young sibling than are interactions around the bottle which poses conflict between the two possibilities of taking the bottle oneself versus imitating mother by feeding the baby (which the young child cannot do safely). The father's role of helping out in other ways is also more clearly delineated than when he tries to be just like mother in holding the bottle. Pride in his own distinctive contribution is probably facilitated when his role is as a father in his own right and not as a second-best "mother." These issues may be especially important in families where the fact that both work may tend to blur role differentiations, and in some cases arouse rather basic anxieties about gender identification.

Practical Aspects of Nursing Management for the Working Mother

One theme emerges from conversations with mothers who nurse and work: continued breastfeeding success upon return to work seems to be associated with how well breastfeeding is initially established. Conversely, mothers are more often frustrated and disappointed in their attempts to coordinate nursing and work, when the attempt to do so is made on what is not yet stabilized breastfeeding.

While it is important for all mothers to insure every condition for a good beginning mothering and breastfeeding relationship the early post-partum period is an especially critical time for the mother who plans to resume outside commitments. All mothers who juggle their priorities to provide an optimal early nursing environment. That investment will be more than repaid in a thriving nursing relationship later.

A WOMAN WHO DECIDES TO BREASTFEED IS PREPARING TO DO SOMETHING WHICH, IN OUR CULTURE, IS DIFFERENT. A WOMAN WHO DECIDES TO BOTH WORK AND BREASTFEED IS PREPARING TO DO SOMETHING EVEN MORE UNUSUAL. WHAT SHE IS ABOUT TO DO MAY BE DIFFICULT.

Preparation for Nursing

A woman who decides to breastfeed is preparing to do something which in our culture is different. A woman who decides to both work and breastfeed is preparing to do something even more unusual. What she is about to do may be difficult. She must know what she wants; and she needs support from other people, other working women, her friends and family, in order to accomplish her goals. A working mother must consider what kinds of support are available to her in her decision to both breastfeed and to work, and she must be able to adapt and create the supportive systems which she need to back up choices. She and her family should educate themselves about the physiological and emotional requirements for nursing before hand. The family should become informed and be prepared to give the mother whatever assistance she needs to both nurse and work; and the working mother herself ought to become aware of her own probably resistance to seeking help, asking for advice, and allowing herself to be cared for.

The prospective mother should begin preparing for the early nursing environment as well as for her eventual return to work. The general preparation for the optimal early nursing environment will help smooth the later return to work. If one phase goes well, it paves the way for success in the next phase. The preparations include making arrangements for a leave of absence from work, assistance with the housework and other children, and future substitute caretakers (babysitters or daycare).

All plans should be made with an "open-door" policy, that is, with a flexibility that allows for change once the mother has some idea of her baby's temperament and rhythms, a sense of her own recovery from childbirth, and a chance to deal with unforeseen complications or problems post-partum. Prior flexible planning is strongly advised, however, because removing concerns about the future makes it possible for the nursing relationship to begin in a stress-free environment, which affects the greatest chance of success.

A mother, especially the first time mother, ideally should plan to take a minimum of four weeks away from full-time work, and preferably six weeks. The nursing relationship is rarely fully established (that is, with a well-conditioned let-down reflex and adequate milk supply) before one month, and it can take as long as two and one half months for the mother to fully "learn" to nurse. Nevertheless, the mother who cannot make these arrangements should not abandon the idea of breastfeeding. If she is strongly motivated and has immediate access to good breastfeeding advice - and good luck - there is still a very high probability of success. In some work situations a very early return to work may be necessary, but it may not need to be full-time. In other situations, some of the work can be done at home, or the baby taken to work. These modifications are not always essential, but the mother will find things easier if she uses as many supportive options as possible.

In traditional cultures no special preparations for breastfeeding are made. Nursing mothers typically walk around with their breasts exposed to the air and sun or wear loose-fitting garments, and young girls learn nursing and techniques of breast care from the time they are able to see. In our culture, however, prospective mothers must consciously educate themselves in the mechanics and physiology of breastfeeding, as well as inform themselves concerning the management of breast engorgement, breast infection, and the prevention of nipple soreness. Women may also need to identify any problems in breast construction which will require special preparations -- such as a breast shield or special exercises for inverted nipples.

The same "natural" approach to nipple care found in traditional society is recommended in our industrial society. Soap should be avoided so that natural skin oils will be kept at a maximum. The breast should be exposed to air, and, if possible, to sun. Very judicious use of a sun-lamp (no more than 30 seconds on each breast twice a week) may be substituted for natural sunlight. The breasts may be toughened by removing the bra or cutting holes in tips of the cups and exposing them to friction with clothing. The most effective and enjoyable technique for toughening the nipples (following the natural approach) is through use. The baby toughens the nipples post-partum by sucking. Prenatally, an obvious aid to toughening the nipples is to have someone suck them. These forms of preparation may be especially important to the woman with fair or tender skin. But in any case, lack of preparation should not discourage the mother who makes a last minute decision to breastfeed.

A working woman who expects to be separated from her infant will need some means of manually expressing milk to maintain milk supply, to feed the baby while she is absent, and to take care of breast engorgement when she is away from the baby for an extended period of time. Knowledge of manual expression also makes it possible to deal with interruptions of nursing caused by maternal illness, or other emergency situations, making it possible for the baby to continue to receive the mother's milk.

The woman should begin to practice hand expression of colostrum prenatally. Hand expression is the most economical, most portable, and generally comfortable means of manual expression. However, if the mother is not at ease with hand expression during the early post-partum period, she may want to consider the use of a breast pump.

FOR THE WOMAN WHO CHOOSES A HOME BIRTH, INSURING EARLY MOTHER-INFANT CONTACT AND PROPER INITIATION OF BREAST-FEEDING WILL NOT BE A PROBLEM. A WOMAN WHO HAS A HOSPITAL DELIVERY MUST CAREFULLY CHOOSE A HOSPITAL AND MAY HAVE TO BE ASSERTIVE IN HER DEMANDS TO INSURE A GOOD BEGINNING.

Optimal Early Nursing Environment

Good beginnings are the key to the initiation and success of the nursing relationship. Good nursing beginnings require an alert infant who is available to the mother for suckling. For the woman who chooses a home birth, insuring early mother-infant contact will not be a problem. A woman who has a hospital delivery must carefully choose a hospital to guarantee that:

(1) The nursing relationship will begin early. Preferably the baby will be given to her immediately after birth; in all cases nursing should begin within one hour of birth, as an early beginning is most likely to promote nursing success.

(2) She will be allowed unrestricted nursing with her infant. A hospital with a rooming-in policy is desirable; otherwise the baby must be brought to the mother when it is hungry. This will stimulate milk production and allow the infant to regulate its own food intake.

(3) Minimal anesthesia and analgesia -- preferably none -- will be used. If the mother has received too many drugs during delivery, they may be transferred to the baby who may then be sleepy or uninterested in nursing.[41,42] A sleepy baby may have difficulty swallowing.

(4) The baby will be given no food supplements. Sometimes there is a delay between birth and the initiation of nursing for observation of the infant; or observation may be required later for medical reasons. The mother should insist that the infant be given no supplement during this time so that it will be ready for the breast when brought to her.

One way to obtain these or other conditions for a hospital delivery is for the mother to ask about them in advance. She may interview the obstetrician in detail (and choose another if he or she refuses to cooperate). If the mother is using a clinic service, she has the same right to information -- either from the resident or nurse in charge. Again, the refusal of the staff to cooperate is an indication that the woman should seek other sources of obstetric care.[43] The mother should remember, however, that even in hospitals which have a policy of promoting early and extended mother-infant contact, she may have to insist on these policies being enforced. She must be assertive in her demands to insure herself and her infant a good beginning in early nursing.

THE MOTHER SHOULD BE CAUTIONED AGAINST EXPECTING COMPETENT NURSING ASSISTANCE AT THE HOSPITAL, EVEN IF THAT HOSPITAL HAS ROOMING-IN AND A PRO-BREASTFEEDING ATTITUDE. THE MOST REALISTIC APPROACH IS TO EXPECT LITTLE OR NO HELP.

Facilitating the Let-Down Reflex

The body takes care of most of the physiological preparation for breastfeeding. Milk production almost always occurs without difficulty, mediated by prolactin secreted by the anterior pituitary in response to sucking. The crying and sucking of the baby also stimulate the mother's "let-down" reflex, mediated by release of oxytocin from the mother's posterior pituitary.[44] This results in the release of milk into the milk ducts and thence into the sucking baby's mouth. The more the baby sucks, the more milk is produced for release.

Although the body has physiologically prepared for breastfeeding, the milk does not always appear. As many experts on breastfeeding have pointed out, the body produces milk, but milk production is not the same as milk giving.[45-49] Giving milk depends on the adequate function of the "let-down" response. Niles Newton, in particular, documented the fact that the let-down response that is affected by fatigue, anxiety, insensitive remarks, and other stressful situations.[46] In fact, stress is the primary factor which interferes with the let-down response. Every woman has a different stress tolerance, a different level at which stress begins to interfere with the let-down response. If nursing fails, it is almost never a failure of milk production, but rather the failure of the let-down response.

It is essential therefore to insure rest and relaxation in the first post-partum week, in order to permit the let-down response to operate. The woman who has a home birth should make it a point to obtain the necessary household assistance from family and others to relax and indulge herself in the post-partum period. The woman who has a hospital delivery must be very careful not to immediately return to her normal schedule when she returns home from the hospital. The care which she received at the hospital must be reinforced by additional care when she returns home.

It is widely believed that the most critical day for lactation failure is the day the woman comes home from the hospital. E. Robinson Kimball, a supportive pediatrician who encourages breastfeeding in the Illinois area, advises a woman who wants to nurse to literally go to bed with her infant for three days after they return home from the hospital. She should be removed from routine responsibilities and surrounded by items that make her feel good, and have her favorite food and drinks served to her in bed. (Wine and beer, in moderate quantities, are traditional aids to relaxation.) Tranquilizers should not be casually used since there are animal data showing damaging effects on the newborn nervous system.[50-52] This does not mean they should never be used; comparable human data are simply not available.

For working mothers, rest and relaxation pose particular important issues. The early weeks of nursing are a time when a mother has a legitimate right to think of nothing but her own and her baby's pleasure. She owes it to herself and her family to rest as much as she needs, so that she will regain the strength she needs to carry out her several roles. In our somewhat Puritan culture, self-indulgence is often frowned upon, and the working mother is especially prone to demanding a great deal of herself. Care that leads to successful nursing is a well-deserved indulgence.

The working mother should therefore be aware of the fact that the character traits which most help her on the job -- her independence and motivation to achieve, for instance -- may not be the ones which help most with nursing. The working mother should understand that she may get different kinds of rewards from nursing than she will get from her job. Breastfeeding is not a rational, predictable process which can be organized and controlled as some jobs are. It is emotional, intuitive, sensual, and enjoyable, and responsive to the baby's needs, which are not necessarily scheduled, especially not right after birth.

What the working, nursing mother can expect is a well-nourished healthy infant who is getting the best nutrition. However, this may be a different kind of achievement than she may expect from her job or from housework.

The working mother's expectations of accomplishing too much during early nursing, and her pride in her independence may prevent her from asking for help. Any woman needs help when she is beginning the nursing relationship, especially a first-time mother. She must overcome the anti-dependency sentiments of this society, which she has probably internalized, in order to obtain the help she needs. The working mother, like any other mother, may not know what she needs for beginning nursing, however experienced she is in other areas. She should consider the support of a doula, a nursing instructor, and of other working mothers in a working, nursing mother's support group.

Arranging for a Doula

Only in advanced industrial societies are women expected to assume individual responsibility through the entire reproductive cycle, because we no longer have the rituals and institutions which provide care for a new mother in more "primitive" societies. By contrast, in a study of over 300 cultures and several animal species, Dana Raphael found that all contained some form of institutionalized emotional and physical support for new mothers. She referred to individual(s) who "mothered the mother" as the doula:

> We have adopted to describe the person who performs this function -- the doula -- the word comes from the Greek, and in Aristotle's time meant 'slave.' Later it came to describe a woman who goes into the home and assists a newly delivered mother by cooking for her, helping with the other children, holding the

baby, and so forth. She might be a neighbor, a relative, or a friend, and she performs her task voluntar-
ily and on a temporary basis.

It is in the latter context that we use the term
"doula" as a title for those individuals who surround,
interact with and aid the mother at any time within the
perinatal period, which includes pregnancy, birth, and
lactation.

The function of the doula varies in different cultures from a little help here and there to complete
succoring, including bathing, cooking, carrying and
feeding. Whatever the doula does, however, is less
important than the fact that she is there. [49]

The doula may do household or domestic chores, care for other
children, instruct the mother in nursing and infant care, or simply
provide psychological support and comfort. Her primary task is to
shield the mother from pressures and stress which could interfere
with the establishment of lactation. Dana Raphael goes as far as to
state, "I doubt that breastfeeding can proceed in our bottle feeding
culture without a doula. It would be the rare woman, indeed, who
manage such a feat, particularly with her first child."

The doula may be a friend or relative, or she might be a
hired assistant. It does not necessarily take money to arrange a
doula. Some women's mothers are happy to act as the doula and
thus assist in the care of a new grandchild. Other women may be
reciprocal doulas for each other. Most importantly, the doula must
be committed to breastfeeding and to being helpful and supportive to
the new mother in all ways.

Obtaining a Nursing Instructor

"How often should I nurse?" "How do I know when the milk
comes in?" How will it feel when the milk comes in?" "Should I
give the baby water?" "What do I do about sore nipples?" "Is enough
of the areola in his mouth?" "Will my breasts hurt when I go back
to work and can't nurse for eight hours?" "What should I do if my
breasts leak on the job?" It is normal for a mother to have many
questions about nursing and about combining nursing and working,
especially if she has not done either before. She needs someone
who can instruct her in the mechanics of breastfeeding and who will
help her through difficulties should they arise.

The nursing instructor should be a woman who has nursed before and, preferably, a woman who has combined nursing and working. She can be the same person as the doula, or someone in addition who only assists with nursing. If the mother does not have a friend or relative of her choosing who can provide this service, she may turn to the La Leche League for advice.

The mother should be cautioned against expecting competent nursing assistance at the hospital where she delivers, even if that hospital has a rooming-in policy and a pro-breastfeeding attitude Staff performance on policy is always variable, and the mother cannot control who will be on duty when she delivers. The most realistic approach is to expect little or no help. If help comes, it is easier to modify low expectations to accept the help than to deal with the disappointment when the expectations of the hospital staff are too high. Rather than depend upon the medical staff, the mother should become informed and secure her own nursing instructor who can be on call to her at the hospital. She should make pre-arranged commitments to be able to call at any hour, day or night, when she might have a breastfeeding problem or anxiety.

Creating Working Mother's Support Groups

All human societies recognize the need that persons in transitional situations may have for "support." By "support" we refer to the combination of practical information about new role requirements, trouble-shooting in the process of identifying difficulties in making the transition, and the emotional aspects of sharing the feelings associated with such a transition.

The La Leche League, since 1956, has provided group support for mothers in both direct breastfeeding and general issues in child rearing. Relatively few members of the League are employed, however, in part because the League's philosophy supports full-time mothering. There is a great need for working mothers to find similar mutual support groups, because of the real or fantasized danger of criticism from both sides: from those who might criticize her as a mother because of her working, or might criticize her as a worker because of her commitment to her child. (This emphasis on avoiding criticism is not trivial; criticism is a stress, and during initiation of lactation it is the kind of stress which can inhibit letdown.) In most places, women interested in such groups will have formed them themselves. This is not difficult, and the benefits which can be gained from taking the initiative in organizing working mothers' breastfeeding and child rearing groups are considerable.

MANY WORKING WOMEN HAVE NOT TRIED TO BREASTFEED BECAUSE THEY THOUGHT IT WOULD BE IMPOSSIBLE. OTHERS, BREAST-FEEDING DURING THE FIRST WEEKS WHILE AT HOME, GIVE IT UP UPON RETURN TO WORK. IT IS POSSIBLE TO BOTH BREASTFEED AND WORK.

Managing the Return to Work

The preceding sections have talked about what the mother does with her infant to get the nursing relationship going before she returns to work. Now it is time to go back to work; it is assumed that the nursing relationship has had a good start in the optimal early nursing environment.

The most important concept a working mother should keep in mind as she returns to work is flexibility. There are many breast-feeding "lifestyles," or ways the breastfeeding relationship with the infant can be arranged. The baby nursing at the mother's breast is, after all, the model or "paradigm" of the personalized, mutually adapted relationship of mother to infant. And nowhere is the princi-ple of personalized, individualized mothering more important than in mother-infant relationships where a woman works outside of the home.

The flexible nursing style which the multiply-committed mother adopts must work for her and her infant; it must take into consideration the family, its financial circumstances, the infant's temperament, and her own occupational goals and priorities. A working mother who finds that a partial nursing relationship meets her needs should not consider herself a failure because she has not or cannot conform to rigid nursing standards. She may get a special satisfaction from being able to coordinate both her work and her nursing; this satisfaction is far more important than any single breastfeeding philosophy. The multiply-committed mother must be evaluated on her own terms: if she feels the nursing relationship is good and satisfying, it is a success.

Flexibility was exemplified by a professional woman who nursed her baby for 18 months, but who gave her baby glucose water during the hospital stay and depended upon formula supplements after returning to work two and one half months post-partum. Her breastfeeding lifestyle departed significantly from standard breast-feeding philosophy and was more liberal than many "flexible" pat-terns. Yet this woman's experience epitomizes the concept of flex-ibility. She maintained lactation for 18 months while working nearly

50 hours a week, and she and her child were a very relaxed, happy and satisfied pair. (It must also be noted that this mother-infant pair had a supportive family, and the breastfeeding began under optimal circumstances.)

Dealing With Separation

The nursing mother who returns to work will probably fall into one of the following three patterns as she begins to cope with the problem of working and mothering and the probability of temporary separation from her infant.

(1) A mother may take the baby to work or work in the home. A few women are fortunate enough to have this sort of flexibility with with their jobs and can thus entirely eliminate the separation problem. But until all women can nurse on the job and there are nurseries and day care centers in all places of work, most working women must find other solutions. In many cases there are health hazards at the place of work which would be detrimental to an infant -- the fumes of a chemical factory or the fiber in a textile plant, for instance. These issues of adequate child-care facilities and health and safety at the work-place must be dealt with in political ways; in the mean time women must find means of meshing their working and mothering needs and schedules.

(2) The baby sitter may bring the baby to the mother at work during her lunch hour or coffee breaks. This is a partial answer to the separation problem and may provide one or more nursings for the baby during the working day. However, there is no guarantee that the baby will nurse according to the mother's schedule.

(3) Substitute feeding of the infant may be provided by another person. This is the most probable solution for most working mothers. If the job does not permit nursing at work, or if the mother prefers to have the working day free from her infant, someone else will have to feed the baby. The father, a friend or relative or baby sitter might care for the baby, or the mother might choose to place the child in a day care center. The next problem to be considered, then, is the practical side of managing the return to work and separation.

Substitute Feeding

A major realistic concern of the nursing mother returning to work outside the home is, "Will I have enough milk to continue nursing once the number of feedings is reduced?" Although there are differences in the amount of suckling it will take for each woman to continue producing milk, and there are women who will be unable to do so, the answer for most women is "yes." However, it may require some degree of planning, commitment and discipline.

It is advisable for the baby to be fed its mother's milk during the substitute feedings, either from refrigerated milk expressed the day before or from supplies stored in the freezer. If this is not possible, a formula may be substituted. Unmodified cow's milk should not be used in infants under six months of age, as it is very hard to digest.

Fresh milk or milk refrigerated overnight is best for the baby. However, having a supply of frozen milk on hand is desirable as this is next best. The mother can begin to collect milk for freezing before her actual return to work. To freeze milk, she should express it into a cold sterile container (a dishwasher will adequately sterilize containers), securely fasten the cover, and label the container. Milk will last up to two years in a deep freeze, up to six months in a refrigerator freezer. Antibodies are stable in the freezer, although some other anti-infective properties are not.

The frozen milk besides being nutritionally sound is also psychological reassurance against lactation failure. It may give the mother a tremendous sense of potency when she sees her milk in the freezer and knows that if she has days when she is unable to produce fresh milk the infant will continue to have her frozen milk. She will not have to worry about manually expressing milk on a daily basis for the first several weeks after she returns to work, when she may be adjusting to new demands and schedules. It would be sensible to express the next day's milk at work and refrigerate it until use, reserving frozen milk for times when fresh is not available.

If the mother expresses milk at work, it is sometimes helpful to do this at the same time and place every day, thereby conditioning the milk to let down to a stimulus other than the infant suckling. Some women might find that expressing milk in the company of their co-workers during a break helps to relieve the monotony of the daily task.

The working woman should also be aware that she can turn leaky breasts to her advantage, especially in the early stages of lactation. She can collect the leakage for later use simply by wearing the Netsy Milk Cup, a plastic dome-shaped cover for the breast. The cup also holds the bra away from sore nipples, allowing air to circulate around them.[53] If this is done, it is important that the milk be refrigerated soon, since warm milk will rapidly spoil.

Planning for Substitute Feedings and Childcare: The "Rehearsal"

When mothers return to work, there are many concerns, especially how, and with what chance of success substitute feedings (of breast milk, cow's milk, or formula) can be initiated and carried out. If the father is available and willing, he is the ideal person to introduce the bottle to the baby as he and the baby are already acquainted. Once the bottle is introduced by the father, it should be easy to transfer bottle feeding to a sitter.

The person who will be the substitute mothering figure should be introduced to the infant before the time comes for the mother to return to work. That person should come and stay for increasingly longer periods of time. The first visits should be simply get-acquainted times for infant and sitter. Have the sitter make no attempts to feed the infant the first few times. Older babies, past six or seven months, may already be experiencing separation anxiety, and the introduction of the sitter and the actual separation should be more gradual with them.

Rehearsal separations should begin to take place once the infant is acquainted with the sitter. At first, the mother should go out for an hour or two (and remain within reach) having instructed the sitter to attempt a feeding about a half hour before the infant's usual feeding time. Since most breastfed babies are not on a regular schedule, an approximation should be made. Feeding the baby before it is really hungry gives time to deal with the bottle before the baby is acutely hungry. This helps prevent the escalating panic in an infant who has to cope both with an unfamiliar way of feeding and with extreme hunger.

The mother should not make predictions about how her baby will react to the bottle. Indicate to the sitter to gently insert the nipple in a back and forth manner, to subside if the infant becomes too upset and not to force the feeding, but to try again fifteen or twenty minutes later. A baby who has refused the bottle may respond to a little honey on the nipple. The NUK nipple is recommended because it functions similarly to the human nipple.

Most babies will accept a bottle when they are really hungry. Alternative techniques which can be employed after two or three failures with a bottle, include spoons, eyedroppers, and cups -- depending on the infant's age. Older babies, especially those receiving solid food (six months and over) may choose to wait up to six or seven hours for the mother to come home rather than take a bottle, and this should not be cause for concern.

The sitter should be advised that if the infant becomes really upset, she should call the mother back, and they should try again the next day. One need not make elaborate efforts to determine what went wrong; some babies just take more time.

In an emergency situation, if the mother, for example, unexpectedly has to leave town or enter the hospital, a baby might require substitute feedings without any chance for rehearsal. If this baby refuses the bottle or eyedropper, another nursing mother can feed the baby as a transition solution. Meanwhile, the mother can maintain lactation by manual expression.

Rejecting the Bottle or the Breast

An infant who refuses the bottle is often responding to the loss of the mothering person, not just the breast and milk. Therefore if an infant persists in rejecting the bottle the sitter should replace mothering as well as, or more importantly than, food. The baby should be cuddled, cooed, talked to, or given whatever stimulus it responds to. After "mothering" is offered and the baby is calmed, another feeding attempt can be made.

Some babies respond to the loss of the mother in another way -- by refusing the breast (rejecting the mother) when she returns to work. The baby's sense of loss of the mother and the mother's sense of rejection by the baby must be coped with. The mother in this situation must make a special effort at "extra" mothering: particularly prolonged and continuous tactile contact, stroking, cuddling, and holding. Every attempt should be made to maintain eye contact with the infant and to promote physical proximity and interaction between the natural mother and her infant.

The danger to be watched for if the baby refuses the breast is the withdrawal of the mother because she feels rejected, at a time when the infant is suffering most acutely from feelings of separation and loss (we refer to this as the "rejection cycle"). Signs that the mother is withdrawing include the feeling that she wants to avoid the infant, that she doesn't want to nurse, failure of the letdown reflex, and an expectation that the nursing relationship will fail. If not stopped in time, the vicious cycle of mutual rejection by the mother and infant can escalate to the point that the nursing relationship terminates. If the mother is able to maintain the close contact of "extra" mothering, the breastfeeding relationship can be maintained. If the baby rejects the mother, one technique to consider is offering the substitute feeding on a spoon or in another form that would significantly distinguish nursing from substitute feeding.

Maintaining the Milk Supply

Nursing

There is no substitute for nursing an infant to maintain lactation. Although hand expression stimulates about one third as much milk production as a suckling infant, the mother must allow the baby to nurse when she is home. Most nursing pairs do well if they maintain roughly four feedings a day. Both psychologically and physiologically, it is important to maintain a continuity of feeding at critical times: morning, evening after return from work, and bedtime.

1. Good Beginnings. Just as we emphasized a "good beginning" for initiating the nursing relationship, it is important to maintain good beginnings for each day. Even if the infant has fed during the night, the mother's milk supply is greatest after a night's rest. The infant is hungry and the mother's breasts need to be emptied. Both mother and infant will feel physically and psychologically gratified by a morning feeding, and it will stimulate the mother's milk production. We strongly urge working to get up an extra half hour early in order to have a relaxed nursing with the baby. A relaxed morning feeding can avoid the morning rush and the mother leaving with a sense of guilt, feeling she has not really "given" to her infant. The daily feelings of deprivation and guilt can initiate another vicious cycle, which, like the "rejection cycle" can end with the termination of the nursing relationship. Also, "good beginnings" is a sound practice to get used to each day for older children as well.

2. Good Reunions. The second critical time for nursing is upon the mother's return home from work. Mother and infant will be ready for each other. The infant may even be demanding to nurse when the mother returns, and the mother may feel the need to have her breasts emptied. Mother and infant have physiological and emotional needs for each other at this time.

It takes planning and foresight to assure a relaxed and comfortable reunion between the working mother and her infant, a time when they can each have their needs met. The mother needs to eliminate or minimize the demands of other family business and negotiations, and the immediate need to begin dinner. If other young children are at home she must plan for assistance in meeting and/or postponing their often pressing needs. This may be true of husbands, also.

The mother can make several practical arrangements to minimize stress for this reunion. She can arrange for all family negotiations to be postponed for at least half an hour after her arrival home. She could have a friend or another family member look after older children, or structure in advance an ongoing project which can be worked on during the "family hour." Other family members may assume dinner and other household responsibilities, or some may make some dinner preparations the night before. Another option, well worth the extra money, is to have the sitter stay to begin dinner preparations and to smooth the transition, or to hire someone else, perhaps a neighborhood teenager, to assist with dinner preparations. Friends should be asked not to call at this time.

3. Bedtime and Nights. Most nursing infants will continue to have nighttime feedings, which are very helpful in maintaining the mother's milk supply. The infant who has cut down on daytime feedings may make up for it at night. The simplest way of maintaining nighttime feeding is to take the baby to bed. The mother can roll over and nurse once or many times during the night, without fully waking up. The extra closeness to the baby, and the energy saved by not getting out of bed, are especially important to the working mother.

To be really comfortable with both the baby and its father, a king size bed is helpful. This still leaves some extra room if an older child has a bad dream and needs to crawl in for comfort.

 THERE ARE NO ARBITRARY DEFINITIONS OF SUCCESSFUL NURSING FOR THE WORKING MOTHER; IF THE NURSING RELATIONSHIP WITH THE INFANT BRINGS THEM JOY AND SATISFACTION, SHE HAS SUCCEEDED.

Success

The chances of carrying through breastfeeding successfully are excellent, once breastfeeding is established. If nursing has gotten off to a good start right after delivery and in the optimal early nursing environment, in which the working mother has had plenty of rest, relaxation and care, then it should be very easy to continue and to modify the nursing relationship once she returns to work. There will be days when the milk supply is down, and the mother should expect these days. Usually, some minimal curtailment of activity (postponing the return of one evening's phone call, having the husband or other family member take care of an older child for a couple of hours, or reducing other demands) will solve the problem.

If signs of stress approach a "caution" or "danger" stage, the mother should attempt to reduce that stress. Signals for "caution" include the "it's too much trouble" syndrome, excessive concern about the infant having enough to eat, preoccupation and worry about expressing the milk, and significantly reduced milk supply. If the source of stress is pressure to produce enough milk for substitute feedings, rather than give up nursing entirely, the mother may use formula for some of the feedings.

The mother knows when she has reached her stress tolerance if she is no longer able to nurse the baby when it's hungry. She should take a day off work, go to bed with the baby, and drink lots of liquids. It is rare for this not to stimulate enough milk production for substitute feedings. If a pattern of low milk production develops, the mother should spend extra time on evenings or weekends resting and nursing the infant.

The mother should remember that breastfeeding is not the only means by which the working mother can develop her relationship with her infant. Breastfeeding does stimulate emotional closeness by physical proximity -- skin contact, eye contact, rocking, cuddling, and holding -- but a mother cannot depend entirely upon nursing to develop her relationship with her infant. She must be conscious of mothering in other ways.

How Long to Nurse

Different mothers and different babies will want to nurse different lengths of time. The time to begin introducing other foods to the baby and the time to stop providing breast milk are two components of the "how long to nurse" question. There is usually no need to begin other foods before four to six months. In fact, there is some question whether younger infants can digest or utilize other foods effectively. At four to six months an iron-fortified cereal might be introduced, followed by other foods. Some infants will gradually lose interest in the mother's breast and milk as they reach a year of age. Others may continue nursing until 18 months or even two years. The duration of nursing is a continuum. There is no arbitrary point at which the working mother should stop giving milk.

There are risks and considerations in discontinuing nursing human milk at different times: (1) before it starts, (2) before the milk comes in, (3) in the early weeks, and (4) later on. Infants (and their mothers) who do not nurse, will receive none of the medical or psychological benefits of nursing. If nursing ceases before the milk comes in, the infant will receive some disease resistant factors from the colostrum, which will help it in the early weeks. The immunity conferred by the mother's milk may last longer than the actual time of nursing, so every drop of breast milk potentially helps the infant fight infection and decreases the likelihood of allergies developing. An infant who nurses for the first six weeks will have immune protection of its mother's milk as its own resistance begins to develop. The longer nursing is continued, the greater the protection against allergy and disease. This is an especially important consideration in families where there is a history of allergy.

Any amount of breastfeeding is important. A little bit helps; a mother should not consider her nursing a failure if she nurses for six weeks, then returns to work and discontinues breastfeeding. She has provided her infant with the best nutrition it could have in those early weeks of life. There are no arbitrary definitions of successful nursing for the working mother; if the nursing relationship with the infant brings them joy and satisfaction, she has succeeded.

Acknowledgements

The authors wish to acknowledge Estelle Marvel and Mary Gilmartin for manuscript preparation, Shiaomay Young for bibliographic research, and Carolyn Ashbaugh for editorial assistance.

We are grateful also to the founding mothers of La Leche League for all their contributions, but especially Marian Tompson and Edwina Froelich for their warm encouragement; and to Beverly Steinberg for flexible and personalized nursing instruction.

CITED REFERENCES

1. Schumacher, E., Small is beautiful: Economics as if people mattered, New York: Perennial Library, Harper & Row, 1975.

2. Klaus, M., and Kennell, J., Maternal-infant bonding, St. Louis: C.V. Mosby Co., 1976.

3. Janeway, E., Man's world, woman's place, New York: Dell Pub. Co., 1972.

4. Haller, J., and Robin, M., The physician & sexuality in Victorian America, Urbana: Univ. of Illinois Press, 1974.

5. Kellow, C., The Victorian underworld, New York: Schoken, 1972.

Cited References Cont'd

6. Cutright, P., The rise of teenage illegitimacy in the U.S.: 1940-71, in Zackler, J., and Brandstadt, W., (eds.), The Teenage Pregnant Girl, Springfield, IL: C.C. Thomas, pp. 3-46, 1975.

7. To...form a more perfect union... , Justice for American Women, Report of the Nat'l Comm. on the observance of Internat'l Women's Year, Washington, DC: U.S. Gov't Printing Office, p. 338, 1976.

8. Glick, P., Some recent changes in American families, in current population reports, Special Studies, Series P-23, No. 52, U.S. Dept. of Commerce, Washington, DC: U.S. Gov't Printing Office, pp. 1-11, 1975.

9. Bane, M., Marital disruption and the lives of children, J. of Social Issues, 32:103-117, 1976.

10. Bell, C., Age, Sex, marriage and jobs, Public Interest #30, pp. 76-87, Winter, 1973.

11. Newton, N., Interrelationships between sexual responsiveness, birth and breastfeeding, in Zubin, J., and Money, J., (eds.), Contemporary Sexual behavior: Critical issues in the 1970's, Baltimore: Johns Hopkins Univ. Press, pp. 77-98, 1974.

12. Seiden, A., Overview: research on the psychology of women. I. Gender differences and sexual and reproductive life. Am. J. Psychiat. 133:995-1007, 1976. II. Women in families, work, and psychotherapy, Am. J. Psychiatry 133:1111-1123, 1976.

13. Hoffman, L., and Nye, F., (eds.), Working mothers: An evaluated review of the consequences for wife, husband, and child, San Francisco: Jossey-Bass Publishers, 1974.

14. Nye, F., and Hoffman, L., (eds.), The employed mother in America, Chicago: Rand McNally & Co., 1963.

15. Howell, M., Employed mothers and their families (I). Pediat. 52:252-263, 1973. Employed mothers and their families (II). Pediat. 52:327-343, 1973.

16. Mostow, E., and Newberry, P., Work role and depression in women: comparison of workers and housewives in treatment, Am. J. Orthopsychiatry 45:538-548, 1975.

17. Hicks, M., and Platt, M., Marital happiness and stability: a review of the research in the 60's, J. of Marriage and the Fam. 32:553-574, 1970.

18. Campbell, A., et al., The quality of American life: Perceptions, evaluations, and satisfactions, New York: Russell Sage Foundation, 1976.

19. A statistical portrait of women in the U.S., in Current Population Reports, Special Studies, Series P-23, No. 58, U.D. Dept of Commerce, U.S. Bureau of Census, Washington, DC: U.S. Gov't Printing Office, p. 33, 1975.

Cited References Cont'd

20. Bricklin, A., Motherlove, Philadelphia: Running Press, 1976.

21. Kippley, Sheila, Breastfeeding and Natural Child Spacing: The ecology of natural mothering, New York: Harper & Row, 1974.

22. Sidel, R., Women and childcare in China, Baltimore: Penguin Books, 1973.

23. Cahill, M., Breastfeeding and working?, Franklin Park, IL: La Leche League Internat'l, Inc., 1976.

24. Alford, C., et al., Development humoral immunity and congenital infections in man, in Neter, I., and Milgrom, F., (eds.), The immune system and infectious diseases, Basel, Switzerland: Int'l Convocation on Immunology, 1975.

25. Goldman, A., and Smity, C., Host resistance factors in human milk, J. Pediat. 82:1082-1090, 1973.

26. Walker, W., and Hong, R., Immunology of the gastro-intestinal tract, J. Pediat. 83:517-530, 1973.

27. Kingston, M., Biochemical disturbance in bottle fed infants with gastroenteritis and dehydration, J. Pediat. 82:1073-1081, 1973.

28. Downham, M., et al., Breastfeeding protects against respiratory syncytial virus infections, Brit. Med. J. 2:274-276, 1976.

29. Wilson, T., Diseases of eye and ear in children, London: William Heineman, Ltd., pp. 29-38, 1955.

30. Beauregard, W., Positional otitis media, J. Pediat. 79:294-296, 1971.

31. Boat, T., et al. Hyper-reactivity to cow's milk, J. Pediat. 87:23-29, 1975.

32. Vaughn, V., and McKay, R., (eds.), Nelson Textbook of Pediatrics, Philadelphia: W.B. Saunders, p. 163, 1975.

33. Knowles, J., Excretion of drugs in milk, J. Pediat. 66:1068-1082, 1965.

34. Woodruff, C., et al., Iron nutrition in the breast-fed infant, J. Pediat. 90:36-38, 1977.

35. Hall, B., (untitled article), Lancet 1:779-781, 1975.

36. Miller, R., Pollutants in breast milk, J. Pediat. 90:510-512, 1977.

37. The absentism issue has been grossly distorted: However, female employees are absent an average of 5.6 days per year versus 5.5 for males according to E. Peterson in "Working women", Daedalus 93:671-699, 1976.

Cited References Cont'd

38. Ainsworth, M., et al., Infant mother attachment and social development: socialization as a product of reciprocal responsiveness to signals. The integration of the child into a social world, Cambridge: Cambridge U. Press, pp. 99-135, 1974.

39. Bowlby, J., Attachment and loss, Vol 1, Attachment, London: Hogarth Press, p. 24, 1969.

40. Brackbill, Y., et al., Effects of obstetrical medication on fetus and infant, Monographs of Soc. for Res. in Child Development, Serial #137, 35: 1-55, 1970.

41. Brazelton, T., Effect of prenatal drugs on the behavior of the neonate, Am. J. of Psychiatry 126:1261-1266, 1970.

42. Brackbill, Y., Psychophysiological reactions in the neonate. II. Effect of maternal medication on the neonate and his behavior, J. Pediat. 58:513-518, 1961.

43. Belsky, M., and Gross, L., How to choose and use your doctor, New York: Fawcett World Pub., 1976.

44. Pryor, K., Nursing your baby, New York: Harper & Row, 1963.

45. Newton, N., Lactation: its psychologic components, in Howells, J., (ed.), Modern perspectives in psycho-obstetrics, New York: Bruner-Mazel, 1972.

46. The womanly art of breastfeeding, Franklin Park: La Leche League Int'l, 1963.

47. Eiger, M., and Olds, S., The complete book of breastfeeding, New York: Worldman Publishing, 1972.

48. Raphael, D., The tender gift: Breastfeeding, Englewood Cliffs, NJ: Prentice-Hall, 1973.

49. Applebaum, R., The obstetrician's approach to the breasts and breastfeeding, J. of Repro. Med. 14:98-116, 1975.

50. Ahlenius, S., et al., Learning deficits in 4 weeks old offspring of the nursing mothers treated with the neuroleptic drug Penfluridol, Naunyn-Schmiedeberg's Arch. Pharmacol. 279:31-37, 1973.

51. Lundborg, P., and Engle, J., Learning deficits and selective biochemical brain changes in 4 weeks old offspring of jursing rat mothers treated with neuroleptics. Paper presented at Symposium on Antipsychotic Drugs, Pharmacodynamics, and Pharmocokinetics, Stockholm, Sept. 17-19, 1974.

Cited References Cont'd

52. Ahlenius, S., et al., Antagonism by d-Amphetamine of learning deficits in rats induced by explosure to antipsychotic drugs during early postnatal life, Naunyn-Schmiedeberg's Arch. Pharmacol. 288:185-193, 1975.

53. The Netsy Milk Cup can be obtained from The Netsy Company (Marianna Alstrom), 34 Sunrise Avenue, Mill Valley, California 94941. $3.50 each or $7.00/pair.

CHAPTER TWENTY EIGHT

A WORKING LAY MIDWIFE HOME BIRTH PROGRAM
SEATTLE, WASHINGTON:
A COLLECTIVE APPROACH

The Fremont Women's Clinic - Birth Collective
Miriamma Carson, Sharon Felton, Steve Gloyd, Sally Luehrs,
Marge Mansfield, Jackie Mertz, Suzy Myers, Susie Rivard

The original title of our chapter was to have been "Establishing a Safe, Legal Lay Midwife Homebirth Service with Physician
Back-up." We feel we can discuss "a safe lay midwife homebirth
service with physician back-up," but in Washington state, we are not
legal. This is not accidental. We want to discuss how and why
we've evolved as we have, what being "lay" means to us, what collectivity means, and why we feel it is important to remain lay people
whose primary accountability is to the people served. We want to
talk about lay medicine and professional medicine.

Right now we are experiencing a contradiction: On the one
hand, as lay practitioners, we want to continue to provide what we
see people want, i.e., an alternative to what United States obstetrics
is offering. But from our recent experience it seems we are meeting resistance from a political system where power and profit are
the dominant motivating factors, not only around childbirth, but in
health care in general, and in almost every aspect of our lives.

The Fremont Clinic

Fremont Women's Clinic was organized in 1971 by people in
the Fremont district of Seattle who recognized a need for a clinic in
their own neighborhood for people who had little access to high quality health care. The growing women's movement had raised issues
about the rights of women to more knowledge about and control over
our bodies and our sexuality. It had articulated for millions of
women that it was time to have control over our own health care.

FREMONT WOMEN'S CLINIC BIRTH COLLECTIVE is a group of midwives
and physicians engaged in home births in the Seattle, Washington, area.
The members of this collective are listed above as the authors of this article.

At that time there was also an active "free clinic" movement in Seattle, part of a national movement of people challenging the basis of the United States health care system, i.e., profit-oriented, hierarchical, expensive, and largely inefficient. These two trends came together in women's clinics, and Fremont is one of many.

The clinic began delivering health care in the areas of gynecology and pediatrics in 1972. Since then other areas have been added: an Older People's Clinic, a Lesbian Health Collective, extensive sexuality counselling, and most recently the Birth Collective. Fremont is a very full-time operation. Each week we have one geriatrics clinic, three gynecology clinics, two prenatal clinics, one pediatrics clinics, one gynecology clinic run for and by Lesbians, one business meeting and class for each of those groups, and prenatal and pediatric educationals and discussion groups for interested patients and/or members of the community.

All aspects of clinic work are done by lay paramedics who have been trained primarily at the clinic and have studied on their own. With one exception we have not attended professional schools; we are not certified or licensed. We share in medical practice, working in teams, and make preparation and presentation of educational material for ourselves. We share in community work and educationals, maintenance of the building and clerical office work.

Fremont is run by a collective of women, i.e., there are no bosses. All clinic policies are made by group discussion of the staff. There are doctors who donate time on a rotating basis in the geriatrics, pediatrics, and 1/3 of the gynecology clinics, including one gynecologist whom we consult frequently and who signs our charts. Currently the clinic has a paid staff of about 15, all of whom receive minimal wages of $100-350 per month for part- to full-time work, depending on amount of work and need. We receive some government funding to supplement the operation, including welfare medicaid (because we can use a doctor's name), but feel the bulk of the support should come from people who use the clinic.

We established the clinic to present a model of non-alienating, non-hierarchical relationships both between "patient" and health care worker and among health workers themselves. We feel it is imperative to work as a team together, using ourselves, lay people, as examples that our bodies and the practice of medicine don't have to be mysterious. We want people to "take their bodies back" through knowledge of preventive measures and understanding of problems that do come up, assume more responsibility and control over their health care and their lives, and be better able to demand good care and full rights when dealing with other institutions.

"COLLECTIVELY" MEANS TO US "EQUAL SHARING OF CHORES AND
RESPONSIBILITIES, DOCTORS PARTICIPATING IN CLEAN-UP,
EQUAL RESPECT FOR ALL MEMBERS OF THE GROUP REGARDLESS OF SEX
OR PROFESSIONAL STANDING, FLEXIBILITY IN SCHEDULES AND VACA-
TIONS, AND CONSENSUS DECISION-MAKING--I.E. FINAL MEDICAL DECI-
SIONS ARE NOT COMPLETELY IN THE HANDS OF DOCTORS, A DOCTOR'S
OPINION CAN BE OVERRULED BY OTHER MEMBERS OF THE COLLECTIVE."

The Birth Collective

The Birth Collective at Fremont cannot be viewed in isolation
from Fremont with its existing facilities, staff, and philosophy, or
from a similar clinic in Seattle, "Country Doctor," which had
created a prenatal and birth collective in '73. Five women had
studied with a doctor there to become skilled lay midwives and had
attended over 100 births in a 2-year period until that doctor left
town and the midwives' group disbanded. The experience of that
group, and specifically of one woman in it who also worked at Fre-
month, laid a lot of the ground-work for us.

Dreams of forming a birth collective materialized in February,
1975, when two family practice doctors expressed a willingness to
commit themselves to working with a group of midwife trainees.
Our initial meeting was open to any interested staff members at the
clinic and people of the community. During that meeting each person
expressed what she/he felt were her/his qualifications and commitments; we all shared our ideas of what the criteria for midwives
might be and what number would constitute a workable size group;
and we proceded to "self-select" a group of 5 women to be midwife
trainees and 2 men who were doctors who were all committed to
working collectively for at least a year.

Collectively means to us equal sharing of chores and responsibilities; it means doctors participating in clean-up; it means equal
respect for all members of the group, regardless of sex or professional standing; it provides for flexibility in schedules and vacations
for workers; it means decision-making which is done by consensus;
it means that final medical decisions are not completely in the hands
of doctors -- a doctor's opinion can be overruled by other members
of the collective.

In relationship to the people coming to us, collective working
aims toward breaking down the traditional focus and potential dependency on one practitioner and provides for exposure to different

styles and personalities and helps people assume more responsibility themselves. People meet all of us throughout the course of prenatal care.

Collectivity also provides a forum for constructive criticism of ourselves and each other and facilitates criticism from people we see as patients. We see this as a very necessary part of changing and growing. We've by no means perfected this, but it is a primary goal toward which we strive with varying degrees of success.

The group now consists of those same five lay midwives, one of the doctors, a childbirth education instructor, a midwife trainee from a neighboring island, and, periodically, other midwife trainees or interested and already skilled people.

WE FEEL THAT WORKING COLLECTIVELY IS SUPERIOR TO WORK-ING INDEPENDENTLY BECAUSE IT BREEDS MUTUAL RESPECT RATHER THAN COMPETITIVE, HIERARCHICAL ELITISM AND INVITES CONSTRUCTIVE CRITICISM BOTH WITHIN THE GROUP AND FROM OUTSIDE FOR OUR GROWTH AND IMPROVEMENT TO BETTER MEET PEOPLE'S NEEDS,

Our Training Program for Lay Midwives

We began our training by having weekly classes in obstetrics using first Myles' midwifery textbook and other material from the University of Washington Health Sciences Library. The woman who had worked at Country Doctor had had extensive home birth experience and was the primary teacher in the "home" aspects of childbirth. Both doctors had hospital experience and shared their knowledge. (Neither of them had attended any home births before we started.) By June we had acquired some basic theoretical knowledge of obstetrics and prenatal care. For four of us, having several years' experience as gynecology paramedics has been very helpful. Seeing women in prenatal clinic, starting in July, added tremendously to our knowledge. We started attending births in September, and again, this added another dimension to our study. After each birth the entire collective reviewed the labor and delivery in detail so it was a learning experience for all of us, even though only two midwives and one doctor typically attended each birth.

This style of learning has continued. Each person's medical progress and other relevant information is thoroughly reviewed after each clinic by the whole group. We meet weekly, in addition to the two clinics, for a three-hour business meeting and class or discus-

sion on various topics. Responsibility for preparing and presenting
material now rotates among all of us.

Our training goal is to become skilled midwives, offering high
quality prenatal care, both medical and educational to pregnant
women and people involved with them, identifying those who are unquestionably "high risk" and not candidates for home births, attending and monitoring normal labors and births, being skilled in identifying complications that would be referred to the hospital, and
dealing with complications which require immediate action. Among
those factors we consider sufficient to exclude a mother as a good
candidate for home birth are toxemia, multiple birth, breech, and
Rh sensitization. We feel flexible in many situations with increased
risks, and basically feel that if people understand those risks thoroughly and choose to take responsibility for the possible outcome,
we'll work with them to try to have the experience they want. When
a situation like this arises, our aim is to educate people about the
risks, discuss them objectively, and present our opinion about the
situation, making it clear that it is our opinion. We feel that when
people are armed with objective information and knowledge they can
make responsible decisions. We want to support people taking responsibility for themselves and their families. An example was a
41 year old woman having her eighth child and living on Vashon Island. She was objectively in a higher risk category and understood
those risks, but her diet, attitude, lifestyle, and obstetrical history
demonstrated that she was a very responsible and exceptionally
healthy person. (She had a great birth.)

WHEN THERE IS "INCREASED RISK" IN OUR OPINION, OUR AIM IS
TO EDUCATE PEOPLE, DISCUSS THE RISK OBJECTIVELY, AND PRE-
SENT OUR OPINION BUT MAKING IT CLEAR THAT IS OUR OPINION. WE
FEEL THAT WHEN PEOPLE ARE ARMED WITH INFORMATION AND KNOWLEDGE
THEY CAN MAKE RESPONSIBLE DECISIONS. WE FEEL FLEXIBLE AND BA-
SICALLY FEEL THAT IF PEOPLE UNDERSTAND THE RISKS THOROUGHLY AND
CHOOSE TO TAKE RESPONSIBILITY FOR THE POSSIBLE OUTCOME, WE'LL
TRY TO WORK WITH THEM TO TRY TO HAVE THE EXPERIENCE THEY WANT.

By February, 1976, we had attended 120 births. A doctor was
in attendance for the first 70-80, gradually moving more into the
background until the midwives had become adequately trained to
meet most complications and had the experience to advise in the
"management" (awful word!) of problems during labor. Working as

a team throughout pregnancy and labor, prospective parents, workers, midwives, attendants, whatever -- all share in the responsibility for the situation -- but the woman who is pregnant or in labor,
and her support people, are the ones who ultimately make the decisions about what to do, how to proceed.

Especially because we're not certified in any way, we're concerned that people analyze their level of comfort working with us.
We encourage people to educate themselves as much as possible,
consult the statistics we've kept, ask us lots of questions, talk to
others who have experienced obstetrical care in other settings, and
make conscious decisions -- to really think about what they want,
and make intelligent judgments. Our statistics are probably the
same as other home birth groups (see Appendix I.). We've had no
perinatal deaths or maternal deaths and have had good outcomes. A
doctor is not present at every birth now. Generally two midwives
attend -- occasionally a third, but never just one.

In addition to our internal training we have attended confer-
ences of people interested in home births, including licensed midwives, and of lay midwives and naturopaths in the Northwest. We
feel each group can benefit greatly by and learn from others' experiences, and that we must work together to strengthen our network.
We're trying to integrate the positive aspects of herbal medicine
with our knowledge of modern conventional medicine. Many lay
midwives rely solely on the former, partly because of lack of access
to the latter.

THE MONOPOLY OF THE MEDICAL PROFESSION EXTENDS NOT ONLY
TO PRACTICE, BUT ALSO TO EDUCATION WHERE THEY HOARD
KNOWLEDGE, MAKING IT DIFFICULT, IF NOT IMPOSSIBLE, FOR NON-
LICENSED PEOPLE TO GAIN THE KNOWLEDGE THEY NEED TO TRULY SERVE
THE PEOPLES' HEALTH.

Our Relationship with Hospitals and Support Physicians

We're also trying to develop relationships with hospitals and
alliances with people in the medical establishment. Country Doctor
had a less-than-optimal relationship with Seattle hospitals, and
many lay midwives are so underground as to have no relationship
with doctors or hospitals. We, too, have had bad experiences with
some hospitals, mainly in outlying areas, and as a result have approached several area hospitals to inform them assertively of what
we're doing via nurses' meetings, with the goal of improving rapport

and developing good back-up for complications before or during labor. This has had a favorable outcome at University Hospital where now, in addition to a woman's coach, one of the Fremont birth attendants can remain with a woman throughout labor and delivery in an "advocate" role for continuity and support. Although this was a somewhat risky move for lay midwives to make, we feel that developing hospital back-up is essential for safe home births and that it simultaneously keeps us in touch with the mainstream of hospital obstetrics and presents the medical community with the reality that people are seeking alternatives to what they are providing.

 WE ENCOURAGE PEOPLE TO PARTICIPATE ACTIVELY THEIR OWN CARE, CHECKING THEIR OWN URINE, WEIGHT, AND BLOOD PRESSURE, LEARNING AS MUCH AS POSSIBLE ABOUT PREGNANCY AND BIRTH.

Details of Our Prenatal Program

Our prenatal program includes the usual medical care, i.e., complete history, physical exam, pelvic exam, pelvimetry, and lab work; lots of discussion about nutrition (see Appendix II & III); the standard monthly checks until the eighth month, then bimonthly, then weekly until labor. We encourage people to participate actively in their own care, checking their own urine, weight, and blood pressure, learning as much as possible about pregnancy and the birth process (see suggested reading list, Appendix IV). Educationals and discussion groups, led by various prenatal and pediatrics staff, happen weekly and provide a forum for people to become acquainted and share questions and experiences (see Appendix V). A childbirth education instructor offers childbirth preparation classes for pregnant women and their coaches in their seventh month and follows through with postpartum groups after the births. We also feel it is essential that they know who we are and how we work together, so we distribute an introductory flyer to everyone describing the collective, which essentially contains the information presented in this chapter in the sections preceding this one. During the course of prenatal care, each person meets each of us, and sometime in the ninth month two midwives make a home visit. That decision usually grows out of mutual preference, and they are usually the ones who go on the birth when contacted through our answering service. Again, we rotate being on call. Parents choosing a home birth are given a list of preparations for the home, which is their responsibility to carry out (see Appendix VI).

Although we have some routines, e.g., checking blood pressure, listening to fetal heart tones, suggesting internal exams when they seem appropriate, etc., we operate from a non-interventionist point of view -- the less we do the better. We feel that people should be in control of their experience, and we'll fit in accordingly. That is, it's up to them where they want to have the baby, how many friends, relatives, children to have there, whether they want to bathe the baby, whether the father wants to catch the baby, etc. Of course, this is flexible, and if labor is prolonged or if complications develop, we all discuss together how we feel it would be best to deal with the situation.

We carry basic emergency drugs, IV's, and oxygen, in addition to a standard birth kit (see Appendix VII) but we very rarely see a need to use any of these.

After the birth, the midwives arrange to see the mother and baby on the first and third days postpartum; people come in at 10-14 days for PKU's and general rapping; and the clinic has pediatrics and gynecology clinics for later postpartum check-ups. We evaluate the newborn before leaving the house and put neosporin drops in the eyes, unless refused by the parent(s). We hand out a postpartum "instruction" sheet (see Appendix VIII) and encourage people to call either one of the midwives or the doctor via the answering service anytime if they have questions or concerns.

We ask at least $250 for what's been described above. This is flexible if people begin late or change midway in their prenatal care, but the fee is the same whether one stays home or ends up in the hospital, because we spend at least the same amount of time and energy when going to the hospital. As described, the money is pooled with clinic money, and workers are paid. We are also reimbursed by welfare and insurance companies, but usually a minimum of six months after the birth, and only because we can use a doctor's name.

Our Participation in Establishing Other Clinics

Another aspect of our work has been to be a resource for beginning rural clinics. Early in our existence people from communities as far away as 100 miles were wanting medical attendants at their home birth. Feeling this was unrealistic, and feeling that a dependency on Fremont, the established, experienced group, could be analogous to a doctor focus, which we were trying to break down, but recognizing that the medical establishment offered no support to people wanting alternatives, and that we had those skills and experiences to share, we talked with people from different communities about the necessity of organizing themselves to provide for their own needs and attempt to make home birth a safe and viable option.

This movement has taken various forms. In Olympia, a group of about thirty people got together and chose one woman to be their representative (barefoot doctor?) to come and work with us for three months. They're now working on establishing a clinic, but with slowly growing cooperation from the medical community. A similar set-up has been evolving in a rural community east of Seattle. A woman from Vashon Island near Seattle has been working with us for almost a year and acting as the island's midwife. We've limited our area to a 30-minute radius for our own sanity.

Summary of Main Points, and the Problem of Our Illegality

We feel that: (1) With difficulty, lay people, such as our-selves, can acquire good training both on their own and through alliances with people in the medical profession who have had easier access to scientific knowledge, and they can have a responsible attitude towards their training(2) Working collectively is superior to working independently, because it breeds mutual respect rather than competitive, hierarchical elitism and invites constructive criticism both within the group and from outside for growth and improvement to better meet people's needs; and (3) Accountability to the people is our foremost goal, and we try to achieve that by openly sharing the extent of our skills and experiences with them and asking them to consciously evaluate how they feel working with us in a team.

In spite of this, we are illegal. Our set-up is an alternative to what exists in and is approved by the medical establishment. Our training is not certifiable by their standards, and we are not licensed to practice midwifery and its associated "medicine." In Washington state, it is not only illegal for unlicensed people to practice mid-wifery, it's also illegal for licensed people to "aid and abet" those who do. Until recently the harrassment we'd been feeling had been only in the form of innuendos and slanderous comments. But recent-ly we've been experiencing harrassment in the form of an attack on the licensed doctors and paraprofessionals working with us. We've been able to be public and above ground partly because we were shielded for awhile by the direct involvement of those licensed people and partly because we've operated from a fairly accepted place in Seattle's alternative health care system, namely the Fremont Clinic. We see this as a distinct advantage we've had over other lay mid-wives who have experienced much less cooperation and much more harrassment from the medical establishment. We're into allying ourselves with other lay midwives and not using the advantage we've had to divide us.

So here we are -- out front, without licenses, and illegal. Licensing supposedly protects the public against misrepresentation and quackery. We wonder whose interests licensing really represents. In seeking an answer, we've found that a review of the rise of the medical profession is helpful in analyzing the situation from a historical perspective.

DESIRING TO ELIMINATE COMPETITION FROM THE "OUTSIDE" (I.E. MIDWIVES) AND CONSOLIDATE THE POWER WITHIN THEIR EXCLUSIVE GROUP, OBSTETRICIANS PUBLICALLY ARGUED THAT NORMAL LABOR WAS THE EXCEPTION AND THAT MIDWIVES WERE DIRTY, IGNORANT SPREADERS OF INFECTION, WHILE AMONG THEMSELVES, THEY ARGUED THAT DOCTORS AND HOSPITALS WERE LOSING MILLIONS OF DOLLARS AND MILLIONS OF BODIES ON WHICH MEDICAL STUDENTS COULD BE TRAINED.

History of the Disenfranchisement of Midwifery

In the eighteenth century, medicine in the United States was practiced by two groups: a small elite of mostly European-trained doctors whose clients were of the upper classes, and a variety of traditional healers who treated the majority of people. There were, of course, no licensing laws.

Most historians agree that neither group had claim to any great therapeutic benefit. At the time there existed no standard of training, in fact, no body of medical science to be trained in. Instead, the main therapeutic measures the university-schooled physicians used were so-called "heroic" measures, such as massive bleeding and calomel (a mercury-based laxative), which are now thought to have caused more harm than good, and which actually killed lots of people. Yet these people became known as "regular" physicians, while all the other practitioners (who, by and large, relied on herbs and dietary treatments which at least did no harm) became known as "irregulars."

The 1830's saw the first licensing fights, as the "regulars" made a grab for power. Thirteen states passed laws restricting the practice of medicine to the regulars alone. It was premature. There was no popular support for the idea of medical professionalism and no way to enforce the new laws. This inspired a mass movement, where lay practitioners came together with working people and the growing feminist movement to challenge (and nearly defeat) the notion of medical monopoly. This was known as The Popular Health Movement.

The Popular Health Movement represented a significant challenge to the regular doctors and offered a real alternative. "Ladies' Physiological Societies," teaching female anatomy, preventative care, etc., were started, as were many educational programs affirming people's traditional medicine. The structure of health care, its outrageous fees, its medical theories, and the way the regular healers were trained were all called into question, and these questions were raised on the basis of an analysis which saw the regular elite physicians as merely one manifestation of class privilege in a United States increasingly controlled by the wealthy.

The movement eventually lost its mass appeal, and consequently lost the fights against the licensing laws. Different factions of "irregular" practitioners emerged, competing with each other, imitating the "regulars'" structure, spawning a kind of non-regular professionalism. Some even joined forces with the regulars in their efforts to push through licensing legislation, on the promise that they, too, would be included as legal practitioners (the Homeopaths and Eclectics).

Following the demise of the Popular Health Movement, between 1880 and 1900, state legislatures again passed laws regulating the practice of medicine. But what finally sealed the medical monopoly of the regulars was the patronage of the Carnegies and the Rockefellers, the new ruling class.

This patronage came about at the same time that the germ theory (the first rational basis for disease prevention and control) was emerging in Europe. Now, for the first time there was a body of knowledge to be had, and the Carnegie and Rockefeller foundations had the money and power to decide who should have it.

The Carnegie Foundation hired Abraham Flexner to tour and evaluate American medical schools, and in 1910 he published his report. The famous Flexner Report proclaimed most schools totally inadequate and not worth funding. Most schools were forced to close without the financial backing to "come up to standard." These included six out of the eight black schools and the majority of "irregular" schools, which were the only ones that had accepted women. So medical training became available only through expensive university training. One group of healers had finally become the medical profession -- they were white, male and middle class.

IT IS A MATTER OF POLITICS AND POWER. WHO SHOULD CON-
TROL HEALTH CARE--PEOPLE, CONSUMERS, THE MASSES? OR A
SELF-SERVING ELITE? WHO SHOULD CONTROL CHILDBIRTH--WOMEN,
WOMEN HELPING WOMEN? OR A MALE, PHYSICIAN GROUP?

But there was one last holdout of the people's medicine --
midwives. The last vestige of autonomous women healers had to be
eliminated.

Two years after the Flexner Report was published, Dr. J.
Whitridge Williams, professor of Obstetrics at Johns Hopkins, made
his own report on the level of training in obstetrics in American
medical schools. He concluded that "poor schools with poor facilities and poor professors were turning out incompetent products who
lost more patients from improper practices than midwives did from
infection."

At a time when 50% of all registered births were delivered by
midwives (who were mostly immigrant, poor and black), Williams
and his professional colleagues had to sell the notion of the necessity
of medical expertise in childbirth, not only to a public which largely
viewed birth as an event controlled by nature, but to a dubious medical profession as well. Most regular doctors did not see attending
childbirth as "interesting pathology" or worthy of the skill of a
trained physician.

So publicly they argued that the normal labor and birth was the
exception, that midwives were dirty and ignorant, spreaders of infection to mother and baby. Among themselves, during the years
of the "midwife controversy," they argued that doctors and hospitals
were losing millions of dollars and millions of bodies on which
medical students could be trained.

There were some, the liberal "public health" advocates, who
argued for formal training of midwives, as had been done in Europe;
and a few cities even instituted such programs. But the obstetricians
won in the end. They built a popular appeal for a higher standard of
obstetrics, making the American woman not only respect, but fear
possible danger in childbirth.

By the 1930's most state legislatures had passed laws outlaw-
ing midwifery. The monopoly was sealed.

In summing up this history, we learned that the licensing fights
of the nineteenth century were of a political and economic nature.
The eventual exclusion of irregular practitioners and midwives was
a victory won by an elite group, but not without resistance from
masses of people. And historically the basis of the struggle be-

tween the regular and lay healers wasn't a matter of scientific superiority. It was only later, when a body of knowledge emerged that
the regulars horded it for themselves. So it isn't the science, but
the eiltism which must be fought against. We must not reject medical science, which can and should be a liberating force, giving people real control over their bodies and power over their lives. Part
of our work as lay practitioners should be to make every effort to
take hold of and share medical knowledge.

As we've shown, licensing was used to limit the types of health
care providers and sold to the public as a means to protect their
well-being. It was a tool used to consolidate power in the hands of
one exclusive group and to eliminate competition from the "outside."

Today we are also told that the function of licensing is to protect the public, to guarantee the expertise and professional standing
of the health care provider. But we must question the whole basis of
medical licensing. It seems to us that it protects not primarily the
public, but the medical profession itself, at the expense of the public.

If we examine the technicality of the law, we can see that license isn't really a guarantee of expertise: Anyone graduated from
medical school can legally deliver babies, even if they've had the
experience of only three or four deliveries. Yet we, with much
more experience, are barred legally. And if we spend the three to
four years of formal training -- nursing school followed by midwifery
school (in one of only ten schools in the country) -- then we come
under the control of the medical profession who dictates what is
proper obstetrics, the same people who have created the obstetrics
of today of which we are all so critical. Similarly, in California,
acupuncture, which for years has been practiced in the Chinese
community, has recently been restricted to licensed physicians
(Problems in Law and Medicine, University of California, Davis,
Law Review, Vol. 7, 1974, pp. 385-399). This takes the skill out
of the hands of experienced practitioners and centralizes it where
there is power, but not expertise.

This is a system that, with the power of the state, of the law,
allows the medical profession to maintain what amounts to a monopoly. It, in fact, denies people real choice in decisions affecting
their health care. In our view, medical licensing diminishes any
accountability to people, the "consumer," in favor of accountability
to a licensing board -- a group of medical professionals whose interests lie primarily in maintaining that power and monopoly and
only secondarily, if at all, in protecting the people's health.

THERE MUST BE A BASIS FOR ACCOUNTABILITY TO PEOPLE.
SOMEONE WHO HAS SEEN A FEW BABIES BORN AND DELIVERED
SOME GOATS CAN'T CALL HERSELF A MIDWIFE AND BE ACCOUNTABLE
TO PEOPLE.

Yet there must be a basis for accountability to people. Some-one who has seen a few babies born and delivered some goats can't call herself a midwife and be accountable to people. In practical terms, the medical profession's monopoly extends to the areas of medical education, making it difficult, if not impossible, for non-licensed people to gain the knowledge they need to truly serve the people's health.

This question of training, outside of the approved (and closed) channels, is an important one. We recognize the absolute necessity of training, of expertise outside of professionalism. We need teach-ers. For us, the teachers have been progressive medical doctors who themselves have rejected the system of elitism in which they obtained their training and who are committed to building an entirely different system of health care. And we'd like to emphasize this point: We don't feel the licensing factor alone should divide people working toward the same goals. There certainly are many progres-sive people who have licenses who are committed to sharing their knowledge. We're not opposed to all licensed individuals. What we are critical of is a system of licensing that controls who's trained, what they learn, and how they are able to use that knowledge.

MEDICAL LICENSING DIMINISHES ACCOUNTABILITY TO PEOPLE IN
FAVOR OF ACCOUNTABILITY TO A LICENSING BOARD--A GROUP OF
MEDICAL PROFESSIONALS WHOSE INTERESTS LIE PRIMARILY IN MAIN-
TAINING THEIR POWER AND MONOPOLY AND ONLY SECONDARILY, IF AT
ALL, IN PROTECTING THE PEOPLE'S HEALTH.

The Legal Consequences of Our Practice

Our movement needs renegades from the medical profession, as well as allies within it. But state licensing boards can and have targeted these people. Washington state law forbids "aiding and abetting" those practicing medicine or midwifery without a license, and we've lately seen some consequences of this law. Here are some examples:

(1) An M.D. known for his use of herbal medicine recently had his license summarily revoked, not only for so-called "improper treatment" of two of his patients, but also was cited for "aiding and abetting the practice of midwifery without a license."

(2) Another M.D., who both attends home births and has a clinic set up for birthing, had his hospital privileges restricted.

(3) In our own collective, one of the midwives is a licensed physician's assistant. Recently her supervision has come under close scrutiny by the State Board. She made a personal decision not to put her license in jeopardy by attending births or doing prenatal care (the latter which she was professionally trained to do but not licensed in our state to do).

(4) In response to a grievance we filed with the Ethics Committee of the Medical Society in Olympia, where a laboring woman with a problem was refused admission to the only hospital in two counties, members of that committee requested that the Medical Disciplinary Board, a part of the State Licensing Board, investigate our doctors' licenses.

(5) Stemming from the same incident (in March, 1977) the doctor working with us now is appearing before the Medical Disciplinary Board to discuss the "medical practices of the Fremont Birth Collective." We really don't know what the outcome of that will be.

Right now, it seems, the focus is on those of us who are licensed rather than on lay midwives.

The Chinese System

We might ask, can a system of health care be accountable to people, deliver proficient and skilled care, without being hierarchical and elitist?

We often turn to China's system of health care as an inspiring example that it can happen. In a society where everyone, on all levels, in all aspects of his/her life, is constantly combatting elitism, the medical system is of particular interest. A whole array of paraprofessional health jobs have been created. Neighborhood health centers and rural brigade clinics are staffed primarily by "Red Medical Workers" or "barefoot doctors," people who remain part of the community in their respective jobs, but who have special training to deal with common health problems and with health education. Most medical students in China today are chosen by their community to continue training, and most come from the ranks of these paraprofessional health workers.

Every health clinic in China bears the slogan "Serve the People." To the Chinese, this is no empty cliché. It is the basis of a way of life and for all human services. Because there exists no power or profit motive, and because everyone is struggling to break down hierarchies and elitism, serving the people becomes the motivation in training of health workers, in deciding who should receive this training, in the services health workers provide, and in medical research. China is attempting to blend the best aspects of traditional Chinese medicine, such as acupuncture and herbal remedies, with Western medicine and newer technology.

To return to our original point about licensing, it is not expertise, or even formal certification of expertise that we question. It is, rather, the institutionalization, in the law, of medical professionalism, elitism and monopoly, which operate, not to "serve the people," but rather to serve itself.

 IT IS NOT EXPERTISE OR EVEN FORMAL CERTIFICATION OF EXPERTISE THAT WE QUESTION. IT IS, RATHER, THE INSTITUTIONALIZATION, IN THE LAW, OF A MEDICAL PROFESSIONALISM, ELITISM, AND MONOPOLY WHICH OPERATES, NOT TO SERVE THE PEOPLE, BUT TO SERVE ITSELF.

Why Lay Midwives?

So, why is it important to maintain ourselves as lay healers, lay midwives?

We live under a system where profit and power are the motivating factors, where the health care system manifests its control through monopoly over medical education and monopoly through licensing. Our fight stems from the same fight waged by the Popular Health Movement. It's a matter of politics and of power. Who should control health care -- people, consumers, the masses (call them what you like), or a self-serving elite? Who should control childbirth -- women, women helping women, or a male, physician group?

Until such a political system is built in which people have real power and control over their health care, over their lives in all aspects, until that time, we see no reason to buy a piece of the medical profession for ourselves.

This is a position we have arrived at today, and it isn't an easy one to take. With it come many contradictions and many questions: How do we choose to meet resistance from the state? What principles are we willing to compromise? Can we change the law, become legal? Is legality something to aim for? We have not yet resolved these issues. We can't expect the state to sit idly by and allow us to continue breaking their law and perhaps even posing some real threat to a medical monopoly. An important question for us all is how we choose to meet the resistance from the state.

Perhaps it's time for a 20th century Popular Health Movement. We cannot wait until the 21st century. We are struggling for change, for the rights of mothers and babies, for the freedom of individual choice and responsibility Now!

APPENDICES

The following eight appendices give the information we hand out and our forms and our data. We also distribute a couple of sheets on the Fremont Birth Collective, itself, which is not presented in these appendices since this is essentially the same information presented in this chapter, pp. 507-510. What we actually hand out are simple regular-sized sheets duplicated by mimeograph, ditto spirit master, or regular machine copy. Appendices II, IV, and VI are simply facsimile reproductions (reduced) of what we actually use. The rest of the appendices present the content of our hand outs, but reset in the type of this book. The appendices are as follows:

Appendix I	Summary of Our Birth Experiences
Appendix II	The Information Forms that We Use
Appendix III	Nutrition During Pregnancy
Appendix IV	Suggested Reading List
Appendix V	Prenatal and Pediatric Discussion Topics
Appendix VI	Preparation List for Home Birth
Appendix VII	Supplies We Carry to Births as Midwives
Appendix VIII	Postpartum Suggestions for Mother and Baby

HISTORICAL REFERENCES

1. Altman, Kubrin, Knashik, and Logan, The peoples' healers: Health Care and class struggle in the U.S. in the 19th century, unpublished manuscript, 1974.

2. Ehrenreich, B., and English, D., Witches, midwives and nurses: A history of women healers, Old Westbury, NY: The Femenist Press, 1973.

3. Kobrin, F., The American midwive controversy: A crisis of professionalization, Bull. of the History of Med. July-Aug. 1966.

APPENDIX I

SUMMARY OF OUR BIRTH EXPERIENCES

Our data, like those of other home birth and lay midwife groups that have been published recently (e.g., Lewis Mehl's summary of Northern California midwife experience), suggests that home birth managed by midwives can be safe. Between September, 1975, through January, 1977, 114 pregnancies were followed to term. This "clientele" includes not only rural and urban "counterculture" folks and many working class people, but also professional people, including OB nurses and childbirth educators. Of these, 70 were first births, 28 second births, 11 third, 2 fourth, and 3 grand multiparas. Age ranges: 15 less than 20 years old, 95 between 20 and 35, and 4 women 36 or older. Of the 114 total, 8 were referred to the hospital before onset of labor for the following reasons: premature ruptured membranes at 36 weeks, herpes, toxemia, transverse presentation, suspected twins, prolonged gestation with falling estriols, and 2 with prolonged ruptured membranes and no labor by 36 to 48 hours. Of the remaining 106 women, 96 had home births and 10 were taken to the hospital during labor or in the immediate post-partum period. Of the hospitalized women, 5 were for first stage arrest, 2 for toxemia, 1 for premature labor, 1 for prolonged latent phase with ruptured membranes, and 1 for pain relief. 2 women were taken to the hospital shortly after birth, 1 for blood replacement and 1 for retained placenta.

We analyzed our outcome in terms of the 106 women who still had decided to have a home birth at the onset of labor or rupture of membranes. Of these 106, there were no perinatal or maternal deaths. The significant complications were the following: 5 with meconium staining (one with associated fetal heart rate drop, which was corrected by administration of O_2 to the mother), 5 with first stage arrest, 1 with second stage arrest, 2 with toxemia, 5 with premature rupture of membranes over 24 hours, 5 with postpartum hemorrhage estimated at 500 cc. or more, one requiring immediate IV replacement, 3 with retained placenta, 2 manually removed at home. All the women with hemorrhage were given oxytocics, and 9 more women were given oxytocics for less significant bleeds.

28 women had perineal tears requiring repair, 5 of these were episiotomies. There were 2 third degree tears, with 10 pound and 10 pound 14 ounce babies, both repaired at home.

Appendix I Cont'd

4 women developed a postpartum endometritis, and 4 developed mastitis (all but 1 treated with antibiotics).

Apgars were generally high, and only 5 were less than 7 at one minute, 1 of these less than 4. 2 babies required mouth-to-mouth resuscitation.

Of the 10 women who went to the hospital in labor, all the mothers and babies fared well. 4 had assisted deliveries, 3 forceps and 1 vacuum extractor. Of the remaining 6, 1 had a caudal, 1 had pitocin, 1 had both, 1 had $MgSO_4$, and 2 had nothing.

The overall impression we have come up with is that home birth seems relatively safe. Our complication rate is on the average less than one sees in a hospital population. Yet the critics of home birth often say that the favorable results only reflect the extremely low risk group we see, and that home birth is inherently unsafe.

We attempted to answer this criticism by developing a risk profile of our entire group and comparing it to a hospital-delivered group with similar risk. We assigned to each woman a risk score using the risk scoring system most currently used in this country and Canada (Goodwin, et al., Canadian Medical Association Journal, October 18, 1969, vol. 101, p. 459). The score is based on objective factors in previous obstetric and prenatal history such as parity, age, previous birth complications, gestation, and prenatal complications such as bleeding and premature membrane rupture. The score ranges from 0 to 10, highest numbers indicating highest risk. The following table lists our risk profile and compares it to the Goodwin group in Toronto. It seems to indicate that we have fewer low risk and fewer very high risk women. Furthermore, it seems that the Fremont group is slightly skewed toward higher intermediate risk.

Next, we calculated a predicted mortality and morbidity for our Fremont group based on the mortality/morbidity of the Toronto group for the women in each risk group. We simply took the mortality rates for each risk score between 0 and 10 and multiplied that rate by the number of women at Fremont in each of these groups, then added the products for a total predicted risk for the Fremont births. When this was done, we had followed 90 pregnancies, and this includes the women who had to go to the hospital in labor.

The results indicate our expected fetal death rate to be 2.10 and neonatal death rate to be 1.51, with a total perinatal mortality of 3.61 for 90 births given the characteristics of our population. It also predicts an APGAR rate less than 4 of 1.45. At Fremont we

Appendix I Cont'd

had no deaths and 1 APGAR less than 4. The difference between our death rate and the expected is significant statistically at a level of p<0.10 (Chi square method).

TABLE 1
RISK ANALYSIS

Risk Score	% at Fremont With Each Score	% at Toronto With Each Score
0	15.5%	24.0%
1	45.5%	28.4%
2	23.3%	18.0%
3	11.0%	9.0%
4	3.0%	6.0%
5	0	4.0%
6	1.0%	3.0%
7	0	1.0%
8	0	1.0%
9	0	<1.0%
10	0	1.0%

TABLE 2
COMPARISON OF CALCULATED AND ACTUAL
MORTALITY AND LOW APGAR

	Calculated Rates Based on Fremont Risk Profile	Actual Rates Based on 90 Fremont Births
Fetal Death	2.10	0
Neonatal Death	1.51	0
Perinatal Death	3.61	0
APGAR Less Than 4	1.45	1

TERMS: Fetal Deaths=between 28 weeks gestation and birth (including stillbirths).
Neonatal Deaths=between birth and one week of life.
Perinatal Death=fetal plus neonatal deaths.

Appendix I Cont'd

Of course our group is not the same as a group of hospital-delivered women in Toronto with similar risk scores. The attitudes of the Fremont women or any woman who chooses a home birth make them a qualitatively different group, and this makes comparison difficult. However, the above analysis does suggest that the criticisms of home birth outcomes on the basis of their being a low risk group may be exaggerated. We are now in the process of trying to get a better assessment of lay midwife-managed home birth safety by comparing our group with a matched group of CEA-trained women planning natural deliveries at the University of Washington Hospital in Seattle.

We believe that the answer to the question will probably never be adequate to everyone's satisfaction, particularly American obstetricians. However, there seems to be enough uncertainty about risks in the hospital as well as home to suggest that the decisions about where a woman has her baby should rest with her rather than the medical profession.

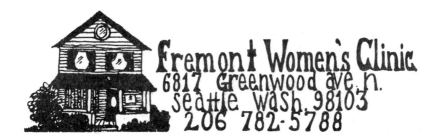

Fremont Women's Clinic
6817 Greenwood Ave. n.
Seattle Wash. 98103
206 782-5788

APPENDIX II

OUR INFORMATION FORMS

PRENATAL CHART

GENERAL INFORMATION

Name _____ Age _____ Primary person _____

Address _____ Relationship _____

Phone _____ Phone _____

Livelihood _____ Livelihood _____

_____

Why a home birth _____

Payment arrangement _____

FAMILY HISTORY Check if any of the following are in your family and indicate what and who, including self:

- Diabetes _____
- Twinning _____
- Genetic disorders _____
- Cancer _____
- Blood clotting problems _____
- High Blood pressure _____
- Heart problems _____
- Liver problems _____
- Kidney problems _____
- Varicose veins _____

MOTHER'S OBSTETRICAL HISTORY   G ___ P ___ M ___ Ab ___

Any problems with any? C-Sections? Toxemia? Stillbirths? Long labors? _____

PERSONAL HISTORY Check if you've had any of these: how treated, when, what:

- Urinary Tract infection _____
- Kidney infection _____
- Syphilis, gonorrhea, PID _____
- Vaginal infections _____
- Venereal warts _____
- Herpes _____
- Ovarian cysts _____
- Endometriosus _____
- Endometritis _____
- Uterine fibroids _____
- Cervical polyps _____
- Breast lumps _____
- Hepatitis _____
- Anemia _____
- Cervicitis _____
- Rheumatic fever _____
- Severe Headaches _____
- Water retention _____
- High/low blood sugar _____
- Severe emotional problems _____
- Asthma _____

Have you had any of the following? Describe.

- Allergies _____
- Hospitalizations _____
- Surgery _____
- Pelvic/back fractures _____
- Hemorrhage/blood transfusions _____

Do you have any ongoing medical problems? Are you taking any medications? _____
_____

Appendix II Cont'd

| PELVIMETRY | INLET: Diagonal Conjugata: felt   not felt | 11.5 cm |

INLET: Diagonal Conjugata: felt   not felt   11.5 cm
MIDPET: Sacrum: Anterior   posterior   concave   flat
         Ischial Spines: blunt   sharp   prominent
OUTLET: Bi-ischial Tuberosities: adequate   borderline
         Pubic arch:
         Coccyx: moveable   not moveable
ASSESSMENT: ADEQUATE   BORDERLINE

→ | PRENATAL CARE | ←

UA micro _____   UA micro _____
RH Titer _____   RH Titer _____

DATE												
WEIGHT												
BP												
URINE GLU												
PROT												
OTHER												
HCT												
UTER HT												
FHT												
PRESENT												
EDEMA												
CX EFF.												
DIL.												
STN												
INITIAL												
WKS GEST	12	16	20	24	28	32	34	36	37	38	39	40	41
MOS GEST	3	4	5	6	7	8		9					

LMP _____   GC _____   BLOOD TYPE _____
LMF _____   PAP _____   VDRL _____
DUE DATE _____   UA micro _____   RUBELLA _____

NOTABLE FACTORS:

PRENATAL VISIT NOTES

DATE		DATE	

Appendix II Cont'd

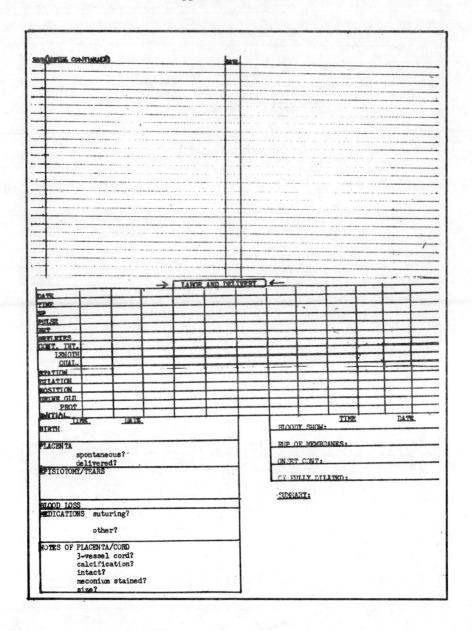

Appendix II Cont'd

PERSONAL BIRTH CONTROL HISTORY | Have you used any of the following?

	Type	When	Why stopped
Birth control pills			
IUD			
Diaphragm			
Foam/condoms			
Other			

PERSONAL OBSTETRICAL HISTORY   G____ P____ M____ Ab____   Baby's

	Date	Where	Wt gain	Wks gest.	Labor length	wt & sex	Problems
1.							
2.							
3.							
4.							

PRESENT PREGNANCY

LMP_____ Normal?_____ PMP_____   DUE DATE _____
Date of pregnancy test(s) and results _____
Date of bimanual(s) and results _____
Drugs/toxins exposure? Rx, drugs, X-rays, fumes_____

Disease exposure? Rubella? Toxoplasmosis? Vaccines?_____

Symptoms/problems as of first visit_____

PHYSICAL EXAM   Impression

HEENT

Heart

Lungs

Abdomen

Breasts

Thyroid

Neurological/Reflexes

Date _____ Initial _____
Height _____ Normal weight _____

Pulse _____

Cigarettes?_____

Nutrition: What have you eaten the past two days?
Breakfasts:

Lunches: Snacks:

Dinners:

PELVIC EXAM   BUS/VULVA _____   Date _____
Vagina _____   Initial _____
Cervix _____
Anus/Rectum _____
Hx Herpes _____
Other _____
Uterine Size _____ Date _____

Appendix II Cont'd

LABOR SUMMARY   length
    First Stage   latent
               active
               transition
    Second Stage
         position of
        delivery:
    Third Stage

    Comments:

NEWBORN EVALUATION   1 minute   5 minutes   Sex _____
        Heart
    Apgars   Breathing   Circumcision? _____
          Tone
          Reflexes
          Color

    Newborn: Length _____   Weight _____ Head Circ _____

    Physical Exam:
         Impression
         Head
         Heart
         Lungs
         Abdomen
         Congenital Abnormalities
         Hips
         Genitals
         Back
         Neurological

    Estimated maturity:

    Medications given:

FIRST DAY CHECK

THIRD DAY CHECK

OTHER   Jaundice   MOTHER Impression
        Nursing   Bleeding
        Elimination   Temperature
        Sleeping   Stitches
        pku   Hemorrhoids
        immunisations   Nursing-Breasts
        Cord

APPENDIX III
NUTRITION DURING PREGNANCY

Foodstuffs

This is the actual nutritive content of what you eat -- the stuff that provides the energy and substance for the baby to grow and develop. Foodstuffs include protein, carbohydrates, and fats; and you need all of them all the time, although in pregnancy the comparative requirements change both in regard to what and how you eat.

Most important is balancing one's dietary intake so the baby has fairly constant levels of nutrients. Eating one or two meals a day leaves long periods of time when the baby has low levels of nutrients. It is better generally to eat three to five smaller meals a day than one or two big ones. Furthermore, if you eat highly refined foods such as sugar, pastries, white flour, etc., the food is absorbed very rapidly causing a sugar "rush" which in turn the body reacts to violently, pushing the sugar levels down again. Not only is this a stress on the body's metabolic machinery, but it makes for very unstable nutrient levels for the baby. So coarse , less refined, whole grains or not-so-sugary or rich foods tend to be best. The essential foodstuffs are as follows:

(1) Carbohydrates (sugar chains). These are the main source of energy and body building substances. Generally 50-70% of one's diet are carbohydrates. To eat well you don't avoid carbohydrates; you eat the right kinds. Examples are: whole grains --they provide fiber for good bowel action and are a good source of vitamins. Vegetables, especially dark leafy greens, are great sources of the B vitamins and folic acid. The skins are especially high in vitamins, and vegetables stay more potent if not overcooked. Fruits are good bowel movers and good in vitamin C, especially citrus kinds. But they have a fairly high concentration of sugar and can be too caloric for those gaining more weight than desired. Honey is very concentrated, and although better than white or brown sugar, is pretty similar in its "rush" effect.

(2) Fats. We generally get more than enough fats in our diets to be enough for pregnancy needs, and although they are an excellent energy source, if that energy is not used, they can cause excess weight gain. The important thing is to eat fats in moderation and to get the right kinds. You should get two tablespoons of unsaturated oil (soy, safflower, corn, or peanut) each day. This should be

LAY BIRTH COLLECTIVE 534

Appendix III Cont'd

taken unheated, e.g., salad dressing. Unsaturated fats change chemically when heated, and in this form have been linked to cancer. It's better to use saturated fat (butter, lard) if you must cook with oils. Margerines have lots of additives, so better to stay away.

(3) Proteins. These are the major building blocks in pregnancy, and an adequate supply of protein is the single most important way you can insure the health of the baby and your own. High quality protein is found in meat, fish, milk, yogurt, cheese, eggs, brewer's yeast (nutritional yeast), and soy beans, especially tofu (soy bean curd). Other proteins, such as wheat germ, peanut butter, beans, and nuts are most useful to your body when mixed in certain ways. Diet for a Small Planet, by Frances Moore Lappe, has some suggestions. Powdered non-fat milk is a good thing to add dry to all baking for added protein.

Vitamins and Minerals

Vitamins and minerals play a role of helping the metabolic machinery digest and distribute the carbohydrates, fats, and proteins we eat. By themselves they are of no energy or building block value. Obviously then they cannot substitute for the foodstuffs. Certain ones are required in greater amounts in pregnancy, and here is a brief run-down:

Lecithin. To help absorb fats and break down cholesterol, we think it helps to take one to two teaspoons of powdered or liquid lecithin daily. Available in health food stores.

Calcium. Milk and soy products are the best sources. Pregnant and breastfeeding women need 2000 mg daily. One quart of milk supplies 1000 mg. Other good sources are dark green leafy vegetables. If you use a pill form supplement, such as Calcium Lactate, take it with meals, as it is better absorbed in an acid medium.

Magnesium. This is necessary for your body to use calcium, and for growth. You need 800-1000 mg daily, or 1/2 the amount of calcium. If this much is not in your diet, you should take a supplement, best taken between meals on an empty stomach, as it is better absorbed in the absence of acid.

Iron. The best food sources are organ meats (liver, kidney), brewer's yeast, wheat germ, blackstrap molasses, eggs, soy beans, dark green leafy vegetables, and dried fruit. B vitamins are needed to absorb iron efficiently, and they are found amply in brewer's yeast, wheat germ, and liver. We think iron is best obtained from

Appendix III Cont'd

food, and unless you develop a particular iron-deficiency anemia, a supplement is not necessary.

Iodine. Your thyroid gland, which needs iodine, grows 1/2 again as big during pregnancy, and your metabolism increases, so you need to use iodized salt, or sea salt, or kelp to provide adequate amounts.

B Vitamins. Supplement pills are not the best way to get B's because none of them have the perfect balance of all parts of the B-complex found naturally in food. Better sources are brewer's yeast, wheat germ, yogurt, whole grains and raw and lightly cooked vegetables. A deficient supply of folic acid, a part of the B-complex, can be a cause of anemia in pregnant women. B vitamins are water soluble and can be washed out of your body if you drink large amounts of water, coffee or alcohol.

Vitamin E. Little is known about vitamin E, but it is thought that not enough of E can cause anemia. It is relatively difficult to get this from food, so if you take a supplement we suggest capsules containing 100 IUs (d-alpha-tocopherol) at a meal with oil to aid absorption. If you're taking an iron supplement, take it about twelve hours before or after taking the E, because iron salts destroy E. More than 200 IUs of E is not recommended, especially in the latter half of pregnancy, as there have been problems with retained placentas.

Vitamin A. This is obtained from butter, cheese, egg yolk, It's hard to get enough from natural sources, but not impossible if you get lots of sunshine and don't wash your body's oils off for at least a couple of hours after exposure to the sun. Vitamin D is added to milk (400 units per quart). You should get 1000 IU daily. If you take a supplement take into account the milk you drink. A good source of both vitamin A and D is cod liver oil.

Vitamin C. This is found in fresh fruits and vegetables, especially in citrus fruits. If you want to take a supplement, 250 mg daily is fine. This is best taken after eating citrus fruit.

REMEMBER -- Taking a supplement is not a substitute for good food!

When food is impalatable, one way to get all the iron, protein, calcium, and B vitamins plus some other goodies is to drink (up to a quart a day) the following concoction, based on Adele Davis's pep-up drink:

Appendix III Cont'd

1/2 c. instant powdered milk	
1/2 c. non-instant powdered milk	Add a cup of water
1/2 c. wheat germ	to this and blend un-
1-2 Tbsp. brewer's yeast	til a smooth consist-
(gradually increase to 1/2 c.)	ency.
1/2 c. yogurt	
2 Tbs. vegetable oil	Mix with above ingre-
1 Tbs. lecithin	dients and blend with
1-2 raw eggs	an egg beater or in a
(yolks only if you have diarrhea)	blender til smooth.
1 tsp. vanilla	Then add 2 cups skim
1 c. mashed fruit (bananas, peaches,	milk and reblend.
pineapple, strawberries)	

The taste of this drink might take some getting used to, but is well worth the effort. If you're nauseated, try sipping 2-3 oz. at a time and build up gradually. It's probably the yeast that takes getting used to, so start out with just a little. You can also mix nutritional yeast with tomato juice which masks the taste quite well.

Things to Remember

* Babies of smoking mothers are smaller and more often premature. A good birth weight is important for baby's growth and development. So if you are a smoker, struggle with your habit. Any reduction in the number of cigarettes you smoke is good. Really try to quit now, for the sake of both your health and the baby's.

* Don't worry about weight gain if you're eating a good diet. This is not the time to diet. Just stay away from "junk foods." Choosing excellent foods is the best response to the stresses of pregnancy.

* "Adequate nutrition." here are some average figures the National Academy of Sciences has set as standards. Remember, almost nobody is average.

      Calories - 2200 for average height/weight

      Protein - 65-75 grams

      Fats - up to 1/4 of total calories, or 60 grams per day

Breastfeeding requires 1/2 again the amount of pre-pregnant food intake. That is, 3000 calories and proportional increases in protein, fat and liquid intake.

Appendix III Cont'd

* Exercise is real important to develop your cardiovascular system and get these nutrients and oxygen to your cells. Being in good shape will help you meet the extra demands of pregnancy and labor, not to mention having a child around. Women find swimming to be great exercise. Walking lots and running are good, too.

APPENDIX IV

SUGGESTED READING LIST

We have compiled this list to encourage people to read as much as they can. Of course, we don't expect you to get to everything on this list. The starred (*) titles should be a basic reading for everyone. A good place to find most, if not all of these books is the Childbirth Education Association Supplies Center located on the X NW corner of 70th and Alonzo NW in Ballard. Also use the library!

A CRITICAL VIEW OF U.S. OBSTETRICS
*Arms, Suzanne Immaculate Deception
Haire, Doris The Cultural Warping of Childbirth
Shaw, Nancy Stoller Forced Labor

ON HOME BIRTH
*Lang, Raven The Birth Book
Sousa, Marion Childbirth at Home
Ward, Charlotte and Fred The Home Birth Book

ON PREGNANCY, CHILDBIRTH PREPARATION AND POSTPARTUM
Bean, Constance Methods of Childbirth
Bing, Elizabeth Six Practical Lessons for an Easier Childbirth (Lamaze)
*Hazel, Lester Commonsense Childbirth
Karmel, Marjorie Thank You, Dr. Lamaze
Kitzinger, Sheila Experience of Childbirth
Nillson, Ingelman-Sundberg and Wirsen A Child is Born (photos)
Rozdilsky, Mary Lou and Banat, Barbara What Now? A Handbook for Parents
     (Especially Women) Postpartum

BREAST FEEDING
*Pryor, Karen Nursing Your Baby

NUTRITION
*Davis, Adelle Let's Have Healthy Children
               Nourishing Your Unborn Child

CHILD DEVELOPEMENT
Brazelton, T. Berry Infants and Mothers-Differences in Developement
Caplan, Frank The First 12 Months of Life
Klaus and Kennell Maternal-Infant Bonding
Spock, Benjamin Baby and Child Care

GENERAL- ON HEALTH AND POLITICS
Boston Women's Health Book Collective Our Bodies Our Selves
Ehrenreich, Barbara and English, Deidre Witches, Midwives and Nurses and
     Complaints and Disorders - The Politics of Sickness
Illich, Ivan Medical Nemesis

APPENDIX V

PRENATAL & PEDIATRIC DISCUSSION TOPICS

The following is a typical series of discussions we offer free every Saturday morning from 10 am until noon at the Clinic.

1.   Slides of Home Births
2.   Responsibility--issues we feel everyone should be thinking
        about in regard to having a home birth with us. We
        strongly urge you to attend this one.
3.   Exercises and relaxation techniques for pregnancy and labor
4.   People discuss their labor experiences
5.   Mechanics/physiology of labor and delivery (we encourage men
        wanting to catch the baby to attend this one)
6.   Newborns--baby care the first few days
7.   Nursing and breast care
8.   Fetal development
9.   Baby's food and nutrition
10.   Dealing with discipline
11.   Child development--infant to 2-year old
12.   Common child ailments and remedies

Discussions are led by various clinic members. We feel they are a valuable forum to discuss subjects we can1t adequately cover at medical check-ups. Most folks have the same questions and we feel it's better and easier to deal with them in a group than individually.

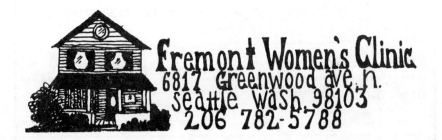

Fremont Women's Clinic
6817 Greenwood ave. n.
seattle wash. 98103
206 782-5788

APPENDIX VI

PREPARATION LIST FOR HOME BIRTH

Have the following together several weeks before due date:

1. Clean home, free of dust, particularly birth room.
2. Plastic covering for bed (old shower curtain). Be sure bed dosen't sag.
3. Small table for sterile kit, preferably at bed level.
4. Room should have outlet near bed for lamp, or have an extension cord.
5. At least 4 pillows for support.
6. 2 sets of clean sheets
7. 6-8 clean towels
8. Clean wash rags
9. Fleets enema
10. Several plastic garbage bags
11. Oil for massage (vegetable oil id fine).
12. 2 straight back chairs
13. Covered pan of water, boiled 20 minutes and cooled to tepid temperature.
14. Sanitary pads and belt
15. Thermometer-to take your temp. during postpartum period. A rectal thermometer is a good thing to have, too, for taking baby's temp.
16. Baster or plastic squeezer, so you can spray water when you pee, should you have uncomfortable skin splits from delivery.
17. Light food for you during labor-- honey, yogurt, ice cubes made from raspberry leaf tea, fruit juice, other drinks rich in carbohydrate
18. Munchies for us
19. For baby: 4-6 clean receiving blankets, diapers, pins, loose fitting shirts or gowns.
20. Baby bath tub, large basin or something suitable for giving baby a warm bath following the birth,if you want.
21. Mirror, if you think you'll want to watch baby emerge.

Just in case we don't make it, you should have the following material ready:
    Gauze- about 3" sterile 4x4 sponges
    Gloves - can be bought sterile

    sharp scissors   } boil for 20 minutes to sterilize <u>or</u>
    2 shoe laces   wrap in paper bag and seal, put in 250°
    infant ear bulb syringe   oven for 1 hour, with pan of water so
                            bag won't burn. Contents will remain
                            sterile till you open the bag.

Call us if you have any of the following signs that labor is starting or imminent:

-Contractions that get stronger and closer together

-Loss of mucous plug, often blood tinged

-Breaking or leaking of bag of waters

      <u>ANSWERING SERVICE #</u> 522-8700

      (one of us is always on call)

APPENDIX VII

SUPPLIES WE CARRY TO BIRTHS AS MIDWIVES

Sterile Delivery Pack

clamp
scissors
infant ear syringe
mucous trap
cord clamps or ties
4x4 gauze sponges
towels

Sterile Minor Surgery Pack

needle holder
tissue forceps (pickup)
clamp
10cc glass syringe and needles
scissors
3-0 chromic suture
4x4 gauze sponges
towels

Sterile Speculum Pack

Graves speculum
2 ring forceps
4x4 gauze sponges

Medicines

$MgSO_4$
Pitocin
Methergine
Ergotrate
Neosporin opthalmic solution
1 litle D5W
1 liter Ringer's Lactate
Xylocaine HCl 1%

Other

BP cuff and stethoscope
fetal stethoscope
Uristix
sterile gloves
lubricating jelly
syringes and needles
Betadine surgical scrub
Nitrazene paper
I.V. infusion set
O_2 tank
infant scale
tape measure
alcohol wipes
blood collection tubes
Blood Bank Forms
Woman's chart
post-partum instructions
birth certificate forms

APPENDIX VIII

POSTPARTUM SUGGESTIONS

For Mother

1. Bleeding should smell like your period, not foul or like pus. If at any time you soak more than 2 pads in 1 hour, call us. The lochia or discharge should be bright red for the first few days, changing to pink, tan, yellowish over the first weeks.

2. Uterus must be massaged as often as you can (at least every 1/2 hour) during the first 12 hours. It should feel firm like a grapefruit in the middle of your abdomen. If it's soft, massage till it firms up. Nursing helps the uterus naturally clamp down and return to its pre-pregnant size (you may even need to do some breathing with these cramps while nursing). Just after birth the uterus is about 3 finger widths below your umbilicus. After 24 hours it has risen to the umbilicus, then continues to shrink down until by the end of the first week you probably won't be able to feel it when you press on your belly. It will be at its pre-pregnant size by 6 weeks postpartum.

3. Take your temperature 4-6 times daily for the first 5 days. You may have a rise in temperature when your milk comes in. This should go down within 12 hours. If it doesn't, or if you have a rise before or after the milk is engorging your breasts, call us. This could mean you have an infection.

4. When nursing, limit baby's sucking to 3-5 minutes on each breast for the first few days, nursing frequently on demand. Gradually build up to longer sucking periods. It's good to nurse from each breast at each feeding. Air dry your nipples. Avoid soap on nipples, but keep them clean. For dry, cracked or sore nipples, try pure lanolin (ask for it at any drugstore) or Masse cream. Wear a good-fitting nursing bra for support. You may want to use nursing pads (not ones with plastic lining) to soak up leakage (this stops after you and baby adjust to nursing). A cheaper method is to cut up some diapers to put inside bra cups. These can be washed out. It would be helpful to have a book on breastfeeding to answer questions and concerns. We recomment Karen

Appendix VIII Cont'd

Pryor's <u>Nursing Your Baby</u>. Or, contact the La Leche League (their number is in the phone book) for specific questions and support, or call us.

5. <u>Urinating may sting</u>. Try pouring some warm water over pubis as you pee to dilate urine. Or try straddling the toilet, standing over it rather than sitting so stream of urine comes straight down and doesn't touch tender skin. Another technique is to cut one egg holder from an egg carton, punch a small hole at the bottom and hold this up to your urethra (where the urine exits) as you pee. The urine will come out the hole and not touch your skin. Peeing in the shower has helped too. You may not have a bowel movement for a few days. Eat plenty of whole grains, prune juice and bran to keep stool soft and bowels moving. If you need a stool softener, let us know.

6. <u>If you have stitches</u>, an ice pack on the area for the first 12 hours will help reduce swelling. For stitches or hemorhoids, gauze pads soaked in witch hazel and applied are very soothing.

7. <u>Rest and fluids are essential</u>. Try to sleep whenever the baby does for the first few days. Take as much help as your friends will give. Diaper service is a big help, especially in the beginning. Arrange for someone else to buy food, cook, wash dishes, etc. Leave almost all your time for yourself and your baby. If you have other children, arrange some childcare for the first few days, but also plan "good" time to spend with them. Try to drink 10 or more glasses of fluids daily. It's also important to keep your nutrition up. You need more protein, more good calories now than when you were pregnant.

8. <u>Exercise, intercourse, resumption of normal activity</u>, is mostly a matter of personal preference and common sense. As a general rule, don't do anything that doesn't feel right. Keep things out of your vagina until all bleeding stops and tenderness in vagina is gone. No douching till 4-6 weeks postpartum. Bathing in a clean tub is OK. This is a good time to think about birth control. You can get pregnant even when you're breastfeeding and even though you may not menstruate. Make a postpartum check-up appointment with us or someone else for 4-6 weeks following delivery. If you have intercourse before that time, you should use a condom to be protected against pregnancy.

Appendix VIII Cont'd

For Baby

1. <u>Watch the cord.</u> Dab it with alcohol several times daily. Keep it clean and dry. Fold diaper so it's under umbilicus. Call us if you notice:
   *substantial bleeding from cord
   *pus at any time
   *foul smell
   *red area on belly around base of stump (a red line at juncture of cord and future belly button is OK)

2. <u>Baby should breathe through nose.</u> If it seems clogged, use bulb syringe to gently remove mucous.

3. <u>Note time of first pee and shit.</u> If urine is dark, baby may be dehydrated. Give water if so. First shits are greenish, tar-like (called meconium). After the milk comes in they are loose and yellow.

4. <u>Baby has a very inefficient heat-regulating system at first.</u> Keep baby warm! If hands and feet are cool and body is warm, she/he is a good temperature. No need to bathe immediately or frequently.

5. <u>It's better to lay baby on his/her side or belly to sleep.</u> Mucous and/or milk can't go down the wrong tube. Even newborns can move their heads from side to side when on their bellies.

6. <u>Don't use mineral oil on your baby's skin.</u> It absorbs all oil-soluable vitamins. Use vegetable oil if you want, but wiping baby's bottom with warm water during diaper changes is sufficient. Use cornstarch (put it in a salt shaker for easier use) instead of talcum (ground rock).

7. <u>It's normal for babies' skin to peel and flake</u>, especially around wrists and ankles during the first week.

8. <u>Newborns' genitals are normally enlarged.</u> Don't be alarmed if there is some blood-tinged discharge. If you have a boy and want him circumcised, or just want to discuss it, let us know.

Appendix VIII Cont'd

9. Baby is not fully capable of fighting infections, though he/she receives some protection from mother's milk. Avoid exposing him/her to people with colds or other illnesses. Probably a good idea not to expose baby to crowded places at all during the first week or two.

10. Let baby decide his/her own feeding schedule. Let him/her sleep as long as he/she wishes. Try to get a burp up after each feeding, though breastfed babies don't always need to after each feeding. Again, it takes awhile for you and baby to get breastfeeding together. Relax. Call us if you have questions.

11. It is normal for some babies to become slightly jaundiced (yellow) between the second and fifth day of life. This is one thing we will check for on our return visits.

12. Baby should be immunized starting at about 4-6 weeks old. A physical exam will be done at that time, too. Fremont Women's Clinic can do this in the Pediatric Clinic (call for an appointment). If you'd rather go elsewhere, choose a doctor or clinic for your baby's care now.

13. A screening test for PKU, a rare (1 in 10,000) metabolic disorder causing mental retardation, can be done on the baby between the sixth and fourteenth day of life. It involves pricking the baby's heel to obtain a small blood sample. There is no effective cure for PKU, though it can be controlled through diet. If you wish to have your baby screened, please let us know, or call the clinic for a pediatric appointment.

CALL US IF YOU HAVE ANY QUESTIONS... WE WILL MAKE A HOME VISIT ON THE FIRST AND THIRD DAYS

ENJOY YOUR NEW BABY!

***For us, for other pregnant people: Write us an account of your birthing experience -- how you felt, what your labor was like, whatever you think would be helpful to others who are preparing for their own deliveries. Include photos, if you have any. Thank you.

CHAPTER TWENTY NINE

A WORKING LAY MIDWIFE HOME BIRTH CENTER
MADISON, WISCONSIN

Thya Merz

I am part of a home birth program in Madison, Wisconsin. I have no guidelines or formulas as to how to begin a successful birth center. I want to share with you the thing that is most important to me, the intimate process of a group of women coming together through the shared ideals of serving pregnant women and their families. We strive to create a milieu that is safe and supportive in which individuals can discover for themselves what it means to give birth. To open themselves on physical, emotional and spiritual levels to another person -- to become parents.

Birth is a beautiful and primal physical experience demanding not only sensitive hearts but skilled hands as well. We recognize that it is our responsibility to provide people with tools with which they can build and maintain their health. It is also our responsibility to train ourselves to recognize potential problems and work with the parents to correct them. When we have reached our limits it is our responsibility to seek help from those more skilled. By doing these things we are responding not only to our own inner promptings but also to the demands of people seeking to have more control over their own experience. People come to us not so that we will care for them but so that we will help them care for themselves.

Right now we do our work without the support of the established medical community. We do maintain loose contact with a couple of resident physicians who are willing to come out to the home and do stitching in the event of severe lacerations, but we have no formal back-up system. We ask each woman to make arrangements with her physician, if she has one, for back-up in the event that it is needed. I feel that an open exchange with the medical community would be beneficial in that it could provide for a more fluid transition between home and hospital. Such cooperation could also eliminate some of the duplication of services that people receive now seeing both physician and midwife for prenatal care. Though I do not feel as if lack of formal support in any way compromises the safety of what we are doing.

THYA MERZ is a practicing lay midwife with the Madison Birth Education Association, Inc., Madison, Wisconsin.

THERE ARE LAWS AGAINST MIDWIFING. I FEEL I CANNOT SUPPORT THESE LAWS AND THE WOMEN I SERVE CANNOT WAIT FOR THEM TO BE CHANGED. NO ONE HAS THE RIGHT TO DICTATE WHERE A WOMAN MAY GIVE BIRTH AND WHO SHE MAY HAVE ATTEND HER DURING BIRTH.

Many people are concerned with the legal aspects of midwifing at this time. Naturally it is also a concern of mine, though one I feel is totally unresolved. There are specific statutes in the Wisconsin law against midwifing. I feel that I cannot support these laws and the women I serve cannot wait for them to be changed. No one has the right to dictate where a woman may give birth and who she may have attend to her during birth. In my eyes, that is a direct violation of our civil rights. This struggle brings to my mind the struggle of the popular health movement that was taking place around the turn of the century, where lay people fought for the right to care for themselves since the self-proclaimed, wealthy, "regular" doctors were not. I have no solutions to this problem and realize that my beliefs may be challenged. I accept that risk.

As lay midwives in America in the 1970's we have no strong traditions on which to draw. We are carving our own. We are actively seeking sound medical knowledge to blend with our intuitive understanding of birth, life and death. We constantly question established birthing patterns and draw from within ourselves integral teaching and healing skills. We have no desire to replace old patterns with our own beliefs, rather provide the environment for people to explore the meaning of birth in their own lives. Before I go on to paint our group portrait, to talk about our training and the ways we work, I would like to share some of the things we are learning about the dynamics of being in a group.

We are in a very early point in our development, trying simultaneously to bond ourselves together and provide a much needed service for the community. The most positive element of forming a group or collective is for the amount of support it offers, as well as the continual impetus for self criticism and growth. In challenging institutional traditions we are also demanding change from the social beings within ourselves. This takes strength, support and constant attention. Group efforts move much slower at times than individual efforts at creating change. They can be frustrating at best, and therefore it is important, once there has been a decision, to act collectively. Mechanisms must be outlines for the resolution of interpersonal conflicts. Limits must be understood.

PEOPLE COME TO US, NOT SO THAT WE WILL CARE FOR THEM, BUT SO THAT WE WILL HELP THEM CARE FOR THEMSELVES.

Our group consists of three lay midwives and a few women seeking to be trained. Of the three midwives, we have all been in Madison for less than a year, and we all acquired our skills before coming to town.

My initial training was in a Boston hospital where I worked as a somewhat glorified nurse's aid. I had what I consider to be a very solid three month factual crash course in the physiology of pregnancy, labor and birth, and learned minimal crisis intervention skills. There are advantages and disadvantages to this type of training. I was training in crisis intervention, and the focus was quantity not quality. I was forced to draw on my own resources, that part of ourselves that is "untrainable," to make my contact with laboring women positive and supportive. I did see a number of complicated labors and births which opened my eyes to the reality of potential problems and showed me a number of ways of resolving them. The entire time I felt the need to question and determine for myself what were iatrogenic problems, where were we failing to meet people's needs, and what were the really invaluable, indispensible tools of modern obstetrics. When the situation became too draining and I felt I had absorbed all I could, I went to work with a physician who was doing home births. I was challenged to put my ideals into practice and found I had much to unlearn from my hospital experience and much to unlearn about giving up my own insights and powers to a man/physician. My independent midwifing work began with my move to Madison.

Carol Brendsel and Paula Murphy, the other two midwives in our group, both came from Santa Cruz, California. I'm unsure of what the format for training midwives was in Santa Cruz, or if there was one. Carol first came in contact with the birth center through the birth of her child, which was attended by midwives from the Santa Cruz birth center. After her birth, about three years ago, she started attending study groups, open birth center times, and prenatal sessions, and then began attending births with one woman. Shortly after she began attending births. She was asked to do one alone, to which she hesitantly agreed. From that point on she was more or less on her own, with back-up from the more experienced midwives at the center. Carol has said a number of times that she does not feel that going out on your own so early is a solid way to learn midwifing. There are too many uncertainties. She did not put herself out to be a midwife right away when she was on her own, rather she went as a friend and helper. It is important to be honest about your level of skill when agreeing to help someone.

Paula apprenticed to Carol in Santa Cruz about a year and a half ago, after Carol had attended to her during her pregnancy and birth. At first her apprenticeship involved a lot of watching, listening, and receiving, during prenatal session, classes and birthings. Gradually she felt herself opening into a place where she could give back much of what she had learned and started working on equal terms with Carol. Unlike Carol and myself (Carol is an R.N.) Paula has no formal medical training. To me, she maintains a purity of spirit and skill that points to what we can teach ourselves and one another.

No matter how it is that a person acquires midwifing techniques, there is an element to being a midwife that cannot be taught. It is a gift, and one that must be shared to truly come to life.

Carol and Paula came to Madison specifically to share their knowledge and experiences and to help us form a birth center out of which we could provide services to the pregnant community and begin to pass on midwifing skills. Carol will be leaving Madison in July, and it is the relationship between Paula and I that is forming the nucleus of the Birth Center.

In the initial phases of our group, our desire for openness overshadowed our ability to focus. There were no clear lines as to who was training who, what was involved in training and no clear ways to work out our differences. At that time the group consisted of a resident physician, myself and two women, both R.N.'s seeking to expand their knowledge of birth. We tried to focus on parent education and held three good series of prenatal classes that started during early pregnancy and continued through birth. We covered such topics as normal physiologic changes during pregnancy, nutrition, exercise and movement, risks and responsibilities of home birth, fears, breath awareness, physiology of labor and birth, complications and how to deal with them, postpartum, newborns and breastfeeding. These classes accomplished a vast number of things. We were able to become known to the community at large, to pass on our knowledge and to become more aware of what people wanted and needed from us. The issue of training still remained a problem for us, however. When Paula and Carol arrived the physician who was working with us slowly faded out of the picture, and we began working woman to woman, trying to decide what our teaching/learning relationships would be and how we would offer ourselves to the community.

IT IS IMPORTANT FOR YOU WHO ARE ATTENDING BIRTHS TO BE HONEST ABOUT YOUR LEVEL OF SKILL WHEN AGREEING TO HELP.

I have taken on an apprentice, and Paula is considering doing the same. I find that as I am developing my skills as a teacher, it is easiest for me to work on a one-to-one basis. Sue is not someone who was part of the original group. I was her midwife. Everyone in the group understands and respects my choice.

We are preparing to offer two different kinds of classes to the community. Paula will be teaching a class that is open to anyone. The theme of the class will be Birth Consciousness, with special emphasis on home birth. Some of the areas to be covered are: Why couples choose home birth; The sexuality and spirituality of birth; Sensitivity to the newborn; Preparation for conception and pregnancy; and Woman's body/birth rituals. I am planning a class that is specifically for people preparing for home birth very similar in content to the kinds of classes I mentioned earlier.

In addition to classes, we offer prenatal care and attendance at birth. Much of our teaching is accomplished on a one-to-one basis during prenatal sessions. Though most of the women coming to us are also seeing physicians, we feel it is important to follow a woman prenatally for a number of reasons. First, if we are willing to take responsibility for helping a woman at the time of her birth we must know that she is caring for herself. We must get to know her physically, emotionally, and spiritually.

For most women prenatal visits with their physicians are very unsatisfactory. They have very little opportunity to talk about the things that are most important to them.

With respect to the established medical profession for giving us guidelines by which we might determine a pregnancy at risk, we include standard tests, including: blood pressures, urine tests, measuring the growth of the uterus, listening to fetal heart tones, pelvic measurements, as well as taking full family, medical and obstetric histories. We encourage each woman to see a physician in order to obtain essential bloodwork as well as to establish individual emergency back-up. The major point of emphasis for our prenatal counselling is nutrition. Each woman keeps a record of what she ate for a week and then goes over it in detail with her midwife to check for adequacy of protein, vitamin and mineral content, as well as amounts and combinations. We respect the influences of unconscious emotions and psychic forces on the physical body and encourage mothers and fathers to share dreams, fears and fantasies.

We have no agreement about what constitutes a pregnancy at risk, and therefore not viable for home birth. Each situation is handled individually as a negotiation between parents and midwife. Parents are educated as to possible risks and the limitations of their midwife. Ultimately the decision is theirs. The midwife must then establish for herself whether or not she can take responsibility for supporting them. The problem has confronted us a couple of times with breech presentation and, most recently, with an incidence of transient hypertension during the last six weeks of pregnancy. In this situation there was no indication of developing preeclampsia. The parents closely monitored blood pressure and urine for protein. After consulting a couple of physicians about reasons the condition may have developed, risks, and possible solutions, they chose chiropractic treatment. The decision to give birth at home was considered in depth, and they decided that it was what they wanted. Their midwife supported them, and just a couple of weeks ago they gave birth to a beautiful healthy son, with no problems for mother and baby.

As a collective, we were in disagreement as to what should be done, but the final contract was between parents and individual midwife. We are experiencing not only the growth and eventual birth of a new person, but the birth of a new consciousness for all of us involved.

Each birth carries its own ritual. The most beautiful and satisfying experience for me as a midwife is watching the ceremony unfold from the relationship of parent and child and to share in that ceremony as an invited guest.

Whenever I receive a call I will go out to the home. For me it is never too early. I do not encourage parents to be dependent on my presence, but I know that simply being in the next room can give parents enough confidence to relax into the events together.

Upon receiving a call, I gather together my birth kit, which includes: blood pressure cuff, stethoscope, fetoscope, watch, bulb syringe, a few kelly clamps, a few cord clamps, blunt-end scissors, green soap, a few pair of sterile gloves, some gauze pads, a special bags of herbs, and some medications to handle a postpartum hemorrhage. When I arrive at the house I usually go and sit with the mother for a while to see how she is doing. Just being with her and observing the way she moves through her contractions often gives me all the information I need to determine her stage of labor. I'll do a vaginal exam if she wishes. Then I'll take her blood pressure, listen to the baby's heart, and tour around to make sure everything is set and ready to go.

One of my first trips is to the kitchen to put on the herbs for the postpartum tea. It is never too early to do this, since once prepared it can always be strained and set on the back of the stove until it is needed. Sometimes I laugh when I compare this little ritual of mine to the act of the hospital OB nurse who goes into the delivery room and draws up the oxytoxic medication she knows the physician will want immediately after birth. Though our actions vary and the elements with which we work differ in the quality of life force, I wonder how deeply ingrained this ritual of preparation is in our psyche.

Here I must stop with my description of repeated rituals, because there is no repetition from birth to birth. Each birth is a unique process that cannot be duplicated.

In closing I will reiterate that what I have shared with you is a growing and changing process, not a static program. I have goals and ideals for the form I would like to see us take on. These include finding a physical space in which to house our Center, taking steps toward bridging the medical/lay gap, and having our group become close and fluid enough so that I personally can take on one or two people a year from parts of the country where there is no opportunity to work with a skilled midwife.

I seek more skill, humility and strength. I affirm the power within each one of us to enter into a new, cooperative relationship between parents, midwives and physicians.

CHAPTER THIRTY

THE LAY MIDWIFE: A CURRENT PERSPECTIVE
Cedar Koons

It is impossible to look at alternatives in American childbirth today without noticing the return of the lay midwife. Who is she? What is her calling? What are her goals? What is her background, her training? Why is she appearing wherever couples are seeking alternatives to mechanistic hospital birth? Is there a movement of midwives? Everyone is asking questions about midwives; midwives are asking questions of themselves.

Midwives have been with us in most cultures as far back as we have record. Midwives are respected today as the guardians of normal childbirth throughout most of the world. By and large these are and have been women working independently with no medical training and guaranteed income. In most parts of the U.S. this heritage of midwifery has been lost. Only a few grannies remain. "Midwifing is answering a call; you got to have a mission to midwife," said Flossie Harris, 65, a midwife from Berea, North Carolina. "I learned from my mother; she learned from her grandmother. I hate to see it die out..." said Tessie Vaughan, the most active midwife left in that state. In the communities of these midwives most women are now hospitalized for childbirth. The hospitals are impersonal; medication and separation are routine; the government picks up the tab. Infant mortality remains shockingly high as it always has been throughout the rural South. No one bothers to compare statistics or consider alternatives. The eventual demise of the midwife is anticipated by many as an advance for medical science.

But for those alert to the signs, it is clear that the midwife, far from dying, is being reborn. The "call" continues, and many are answering it. Midwife is a consciousness of support and steadiness, a role of tireless presence and protection to the birthing woman and her family. As such it lives in husbands, nurses, doctors, nurse-midwives and countless others in every imaginable birth setting. Midwives are needed, and so the call is strong. Increasingly it is being answered by people hesitant to call themselves midwives but ready to make their own path through the brambles of unmet needs and unclear policies.

CEDAR KOONS is Editor of the NAPSAC NEWS; a childbirth educator; and is active in the national lay midwife movement.

THE NEW MIDWIVES ARE MEETING NEEDS THAT HEALTH CARE PROFESSIONALS ARE EITHER UNWILLING OR UNABLE TO MEET.

Most of these people are women, mothers themselves, and non-professionals. They are self-established and by and large independent. Their training is of the "however-I-can-get-it" variety, from apprenticeship, through some medical training, to on-the-job. They operate by word of mouth, and if they charge fees at all, they are generally low. Many see themselves as spiritually and politically oriented. Often they work illegally or under laws that are vague or archaic. In all of the above characteristics they are not unlike the grannies. But these midwives are largely young, educated and white, though many are in some way in touch with cultures that diverge from the American mainstream. Again, like the grannies, the new midwives are meeting needs that health care professionals are either unwilling or unable to meet. Levels of knowledge, skill, experience and sensitivity vary tremendously. No established, accredited training programs exist to teach these special skills. No real control of the competency of these midwives exists or will ever exist until effort is being made to meet the need of every woman for personal, thorough prenatal care, support and security during labor, birth in the place of her choosing, and friendly help through the postpartum months.

Suzanne Arms has called the midwife, "the conscience of the doctor." The new midwives, unlike the grannies, are making themselves heard. The fact of their very existence is already being felt in the maternity practices of the hospitals that refuse to acknowledge them. They intend to help turn the tide away from increased intervention, mechanization, medication and separation in American childbirth. For many of them their own experiences in childbirth are fresh and recent in their minds, increasing their sensitivity to the birthing public and allowing them to think and function as consumers as well as providers. Coming into the homes of the families they serve, midwives cannot avoid interpersonal relationships as is possible in the hospital. Within these relationships the issues of responsibility and control are faced more openly. Birth becomes a shared experience of work and wonder, never routine, and more often a true culmination for mother, father and newborn, less often a "delivery" performed.

None of the above is always true. In the rebirth of the midwife there have sometimes been problems, stresses and complications. Many expectations and concepts have been challenged. Some midwives are men; some are medically trained; some nurse-midwives and physicians regularly act as midwives in the home. Many people have been justifiably concerned about untrained people representing themselves as midwives after attending only a few home births. Disasters have occurred at home with midwives attending. Some people, calling themselves midwives, "manage home deliveries" with the same objectionable dominance deplored in the hospital. Tempers have flared, and polarization has occurred between many midwives and the professional care providers and institutions to which they must occasionally turn. Walls go up; rumors proliferate.

Like any newborn, the movement of midwives has real adjustment, growth and potential ahead. Attempts to control or direct its development have been unsuccessful to this point, but an intrinsic direction has been in effect, bringing midwives together to share their struggles and goals. The First International Conference of Practicing Midwives, held in El Paso, Texas, in January, 1977, brought about a tremendous sense of unity among the midwives attending, many of whom had harbored fears and animosities toward what they thought a movement of midwives might be.

Plans had been made to actually form a national organization and elect midwives to represent shared goals of midwifery and birthing women to the public. Tensions mounted as the conference approached. Many midwives felt that organizing to set standards and make pronouncements was premature and could only serve to entrench an elite over what was a grass roots movement. Other midwives believed that only through a national organization could the pressures from well-organized professionals and governmental bureaucracies be countered. The conference was truly a first of its kind. From well-known California midwives to women who wanted to know how to get started, from Ina May of "the Farm" in Tennessee, to Dorothea Lang, President of the ACNM, many, many viewpoints were shared. Instead of conflict there was harmony; not agreement on particular issues, but a sense of oneness of purpose. During the last plenary session of the conference, chairs were pushed back and the attendees made a giant circle filling the entire ballroom. The circle was an expression of spiritual strength beyond political power. It remains a unique image for the birth of a movement, a good beginning.

 SOME PEOPLE, CALLING THEMSELVES MIDWIVES, "MANAGE HOME DELIVERIES" WITH THE SAME OBJECTIONABLE DOMINANCE DEPLORED IN THE HOSPITAL

The unity forged at El Paso was experienced again at the 1977 NAPSAC Conference in the informal session on lay midwifery. Once again the intrinsic direction within each participant allowed midwives to share helpful information, deep concerns and support and inspiration without hierarchy or contention. While the midwives talked and laughed together in the penthouse ballroom overlooking O'Hare, well-known speakers from the plenary sessions the day before sat quietly listening.

Statistical studies, controlled programs and scientific inquiry, as important as these things are, are not what midwives talk about when they get together. The topics they do discuss are at the cutting edge of change in American childbirth -- sensitivity and simplicity in birth, people accepting responsibility for their own bodies and souls, the limits of medical science and their own limits as practitioners, the privilege that it is to serve **people**. Many people are unready to hear what the "lay" midwife has to say, accustomed as they are, perhaps without realizing it, to only giving credence to truth which comes professionally wrapped. But the message is being made, quietly, like roots in good soil.

SENSITIVITY AND SIMPLICITY IN BIRTH, PEOPLE ACCEPTING RESPONSIBILITY FOR THEIR OWN BODIES AND SOULS, THE LIMITS OF MEDICAL SCIENCE AND THEIR OWN LIMITS AS PRACTITIONERS, THE PRIVILEGE THAT IT IS TO SERVE PEOPLE . . . THESE ARE THE TOPICS DISCUSSED BY LAY MIDWIVES TODAY.

CHAPTER THIRTY ONE

CHILDBIRTH AND THE LAW:
HOW TO WORK WITHIN OLD LAWS, AVOID MALPRACTICE,
AND INFLUENCE NEW LEGISLATION IN MATERNITY CARE

George J. Annas, J.D., M.P.H.

This brief article is about the law as it relates to childbirth and how to either work within existing laws or attempt to change them. It appears in this collection for one primary reason: the perception by many that the obstacles to progress in the implementation of alternative childbirth modalities are legal, rather than medical, cultural, political or economic. As seductive as this suggestion is, especially in the post-medical malpractice "crisis" era, I will argue that this perception is false. The law in this area, as in most others, acts as a mirror of the public's desires and, in matters medical, is highly supportive of "standard medical procedures." Those who view it as obstructionist usually fail either to understand its content or its purpose.

The foundations for the current law are based on a long tradition of protecting the public against medical quacks and a more recent desire to protect children from abuse by their parents. Since both licensure laws and child abuse statutes have ample rationales, independent of childbirth, neither is likely to be abandoned. The challenge for those desiring change is therefore to work for modifications within the framework of these laws. To do this, it is essential to understand the current state of the law regarding childbirth.

In a previous paper on this topic, I make three major points: (1) the law is very conservative, and is likely to reflect standard medical practice; (2) the law varies from state to state; and (3) the law is outcome-oriented, generally getting involved in situations like homebirth only if some tragedy has occurred.[1] Specifically,

GEORGE J. ANNAS is Director, Center for Law and Health Sciences, Boston University; Vice-Chairperson, Massachusetts Board of Registration and Discipline in Medicine; Author of books, Rights of Hospital Patients, Law and Genetics, and Informed Consent.

it was noted that no lawsuit filed against a hospital to change its maternity practices has ever been successful, and that none was likely to be given the present "hands off" posture of the courts regarding hospital by-laws. It was next noted that the legislative trend is toward licensing only nurse-midwives who have had some additional qualifications, with no specific mention of homebirths. Finally, the paper examined the potential liability of all the participants in a homebirth in the unlikely event that the child died because the birth took place at home, and concluded that while potential liability was real the risk of it was minimal. This article reviews the current law to determine why it is as it is, and uses these reasons as a basis for suggesting ways to both work within it and to change it.

The Present Law

An Overview

While the answer to the question "what is the law?" varies from state-to-state, some generalizations about childbirth can be made. The first is that no state either requires a woman to have her child in a hospital or forbids homebirth. The second is that given certain minimal due process requirements have been met, hospitals can establish and enforce their own procedures with regard to obstetrics within their walls, and courts will generally not second guess their policies.[2] Third, in many states delivering a child is considered the "practice of medicine," and in those states only licensed physicians can lawfully hold themselves out to the public as competent to attend births. Fourth, parents are obligated to provide their children with necessaries, including medical care, and neglect in this area can result in a child abuse charge.

What does all this mean to a couple that wants to give birth a certain way in a hospital, or have their child at home? To the hospital-bound couple, it means that they and the physician they choose must follow hospital policy in regard to deliveries (including such things as the presence of the father and/or others, method of delivery, etc.). The woman, however, does have the right to refuse any particular medical procedure or drug offered (e.g., anesthesia, episiotomy).[3] Control is thus reactive only since the patient cannot demand that things happen in a certain way, but can merely refuse certain things that are offered. Given the proper hospital environment and a cooperative physician, this may be entirely satisfactory. If it is not, the only current viable alternative is to give birth outside of the hospital, in a birth center or at home.

THE WOMAN DOES HAVE THE RIGHT TO REFUSE ANY PARTICULAR MEDICAL PROCEDURE OR DRUG OFFERED (E.G., ANESTHESIA, EPISIOTOMY). HOWEVER, THIS CONTROL IS REACTIVE ONLY SINCE THE PATIENT CANNOT DEMAND THAT THINGS HAPPEN IN A CERTAIN WAY, BUT CAN MERELY REFUSE CERTAIN THINGS THAT ARE OFFERED.

Homebirth

The initial question one probably asks about a homebirth is, who shall attend the birth? While one might want to answer, "whoever the parents wish," the state has an interest in the outcome of the birth, and thus in the qualifications of the attendant. In the abortion decisions, for example, the United States Supreme Court noted that while a woman had a right to have an abortion before viability, the state had such a strong interest in protecting the life of a viable fetus, that after viability it could constitutionally forbid abortion altogether except in cases where the woman's life or health was at stake.[4] Thus while women have a "right to privacy" that prohibits the state from interfering with their use of contraceptives or pre-viability abortions, "the right to privacy has never been interpreted so broadly as to protect a woman's choice of the manner and circumstances in which her baby is to be born."[5] In fact, the abortion decisions specifically hold that a state can constitutionally require that abortions, at any stage of pregnancy, be performed only by licensed physicians. No state has ever attempted to pass such a statute regarding childbirth, however, and no current law prohibits couples from having unattended homebirths.

As for physician attended births, the analogous case of Dr. Kenneth Edelin presented, among others, the issue of the physician's duty to an unborn but potentially viable fetus. Three of the six justices involved concluded that physicians owed no duty to such a fetus. The other three, however, thought that if the fetus could be saved, the physician had a duty to it to attempt to save it.[6] The issue, therefore, remains unresolved in the abortion arena. It is worth noting that after delivery, even in an abortion setting, all six justices agreed that the physician owed a duty to treat the potentially viable child. In the area of childbirth, where all parties are seeking the birth of a healthy child, the pregnant woman's physician has a duty toward the fetus to provide it (through its mother) with adequate medical care both before and during the delivery. This duty will generally not prevent a physician from participating in a home delivery, but does require the physician to perform standard screening tests for high-risk pregnancies, and to take some steps to encourage such couples to make use of hospital facilities for birth.

Physicians' fear of the potential of increased malpractice liability for participation in homebirths is probably based on a combination of ignorance of the law of medical malpractice in general, and the climate of fear that has been created in many states.[7] This ignorance has led to an increase in so-called "defensive medicine," in which physicians allegedly perform certain procedures (like skull x-rays in emergency wards) not because they think they are medically indicated, but because they think that they may be necessary to disprove negligence to a jury should the patient later decide to sue. One type of "defensive" posture would be to refuse to do home deliveries on the grounds that hospital births, while unnecessary, are standard medical practice, and failure to hospitalize could look bad to a jury and could be taken as de facto negligence. Indeed, at least one physician -- himself a specialist in medical malpractice -- has argued in a book on malpractice written for the public that a physician-attended homebirth in New York City is de facto evidence of physician negligence.[8] This is simply wrong. So long as the decision to have a homebirth is made by the woman after she has been fully informed of the potential risks and complications, and so long as all generally-accepted medical steps have been taken concerning screening the woman and emergency back-up facilities, it is highly unlikely that any malpractice action against a physician would be successful. Indeed, I would conclude that, because of the absence of things like general anesthesia and the presence of a well-informed and participating woman, that a physician is less likely to be sued for malpractice in the homebirth setting than he or she is to be sued for malpractice in the hospital-based birth setting.

> PHYSICIANS' FEAR OF THE POTENTIAL OF INCREASED MALPRACTICE LIABILITY FOR PARTICIPATION IN HOMEBIRTHS IS PROBABLY BASED ON A COMBINATION OF IGNORANCE OF THE LAW OF MEDICAL MALPRACTICE IN GENERAL AND THE CLIMATE OF FEAR THAT HAS BEEN CREATED IN MANY STATES.

If for whatever reason the couple does not want or cannot obtain the services of a physician, the next choice would be a licensed midwife. Statutes and qualifications vary, but in states that have specific legislation providing for the licensing of midwives, it is likely that courts would find that any non-physician, or non-licensed midwife who held themselves out as experts in childbirth and attended a childbirth would be guilty of the crime of practicing either medicine or midwifery without a license. The court's reasoning in reaching this conclusion would probably parallel that of a recent California Supreme Court decision which found that the legislature had an "interest in regulating the qualifications of those who hold themselves out as childbirth attendants ... for many women must necessarily rely on those with qualifications which they cannot personally verify."[9] The rationale is that the legislature can reasonably find that the only way to protect the health of the public in the matter of childbirth is to insure that those who hold themselves out as experts to the public are required to pass certain standards and to be licensed. And once this finding is made by the enactment of such a statute, anyone practicing outside of its limitations is guilty of a crime (practicing without a license).

As to the parents themselves, their primary duty is to the child, but so far only <u>after</u> it is actually born. No state has yet attempted to require pregnant women to take any affirmative action to safeguard their fetuses. However, all states have passed child abuse statutes that forbid parents from abusing their children, and require them to provide their children with necessary medical attention. Parents may thus in general make a decision to have a home-birth with impunity. If they have reason to know that complications are likely to develop that will require hospital care to save the child from death or permanent injury, however, and the child dies or is permanently injured because of the homebirth, it is possible that a zealous prosecutor could bring a criminal complaint against the parents. The charge would be child abuse in both cases, and possibly manslaughter (depending on the cause of death and its predictability) if the child dies.[10] This possibility is intended to discourage parents from attempting to manage homebirths by themselves, and encourage them to seek a licensed attendant at the homebirth, and to seek hospitalization when it is indicated to protect the health of the child.

UNDER THE LAW, THE PRIMARY DUTY OF PARENTS IS TO THE CHILD ONLY AFTER IT IS ACTUALLY BORN. NO STATE HAS YET ATTEMPTED TO REQUIRE PREGNANT WOMEN TO TAKE ANY AFFIRMATIVE ACTION TO SAFEGUARD THEIR FETUSES.

NO CURRENT LAW IN ANY STATE PROHIBITS COUPLES FROM HAVING AN UNATTENDED HOMEBIRTH.

Summary

In summary, states have required members of certain professions, like physicians and midwives, to be licensed to protect the public from quacks. In states that provide such licenses for midwives, only those qualifying under the statute can practice midwifery legally. In states that do not, midwifery will usually be governed by the medical licensure statute, and the legality of non-physicians attending childbirth will depend on whether or not the medical licensure statute encompasses childbirth attendance in its definition of the practice of medicine. In all states, parents are forbidden by law from abusing or neglecting their children, and are required to provide them with necessary medical care. While they can put themselves at risk with impunity, they cannot neglect the medical necessities of their children. If the presence of a physician or a hospital is reasonably predictable to be necessary to safeguard the life of the newborn due to some specific prenatal condition or finding, failure to properly care for the child after birth could constitute abuse. The child abuse statutes are, of course, designed to protect the child and to encourage parents to take medically-indicated steps for the child's benefit.

 A PHYSICIAN IS <u>LESS LIKELY</u> TO BE SUED FOR MALPRACTICE IN A HOMEBIRTH SETTING THAN HE OR SHE IS TO BE SUED FOR MALPRACTICE IN THE HOSPITAL-BASED BIRTH SETTING.

Changing Laws

Reasons for the Current Laws

Common to both of the licensing and child abuse statutes, and at the heart of the homebirth and alternative birth debate, is the issue of health and safety.[11] Since this is a legitimate state interest, and since it has special application to children who could become wards of the state and may be otherwise defenseless, it is (other than ignorance) the primary issue that must be dealt with to broaden the alternatives available for childbirth.

Put another way, in the absence of extremely strong public opinion, the only way a legislature is likely to widen the scope of a midwifery statute, for example, is based on a showing that midwives with qualifications can deliver children <u>as safely</u> as either previously-licensed midwives or physicians. No other argument is likely to be persuasive. Likewise, the only way parents who have suffered the loss of a child in a homebirth setting are likely to prevail in a criminal action of child abuse or homicide (such an action is extremely unlikely, but not out of the question), is to persuade the jury their homebirth decision was "reasonable" based on its safety for the infant.

Burden of Proof on Those Proposing Change

We now come back to the beginning. The law has been established to protect the "health and safety" of the public in general, and children in particular. No one favoring alternative modes of childbirth is likely to seriously argue that their alternatives are less healthy or more unsafe than standard hospital-based births. The issue then becomes one of proof. In matters affecting the health and safety of the public, it is traditional to put the burden of proof on those who want to change. This, of course, makes things somewhat difficult for the homebirth movement, since ample statistics cannot be gathered in many states because of the low incidence of homebirth, the fear of reporting them due to misunderstanding of the law or local medical society pressures, the unavailability of the option, or a combination of reasons. While the way out of this may ultimately involve changes in the law, I would suggest that such changes are not likely to take place until the safety and reasonableness of homebirths can be adequately demonstrated to the lawmakers. The medical profession has succeeded in medicalizing birth to such an extent that some courts now consider it to be "comparable to other serious hospital procedures."[12]

 IN MATTERS AFFECTING THE HEALTH AND SAFETY OF THE PUBLIC IT IS TRADITIONAL TO PUT THE BURDEN OF PROOF ON THOSE WHO WANT CHANGE.

A Proposed National Demonstration Project

The establishment of safety is, of course, a non-legal matter. I do, nonetheless, have a suggestion as to one possible approach. Congress has indicated that it is interested in programs that reduce medical costs and improve quality.[13] This goal was enunciated in the PSRO provisions of the 1972 Social Security Amendments, but to date no programs have been found (with the exception of reducing unnecessary operations) that can meet both goals simultaneously.

The thesis of much of the alternative childbirth movement is that the proposed alternatives are not only reasonable, but would be both safer and cheaper. One way to attempt to prove this is through a national demonstration, funded by the Social Security Administration or the National Institutes of Health. It would identify and follow pregnant women, and match all those having homebirths with similar women having hospital-based birth (birth centers could also be used as a third grouping). Special provisions should be made to insure that all participants in the homebirth group study have physicians or licensed midwives in attendance if they so desire, that relevant screening tests are conducted and recorded, and that no woman is required to use any setting or birth attendant not of her own choosing as a condition of participating in the project. Only through such a large demonstration project are we likely to generate the quality and quantity of data that will lead to such things as the inclusion of midwives on the list of future federally-licensed health practitioners, and the inclusion of birth centers and homebirths as alternatives under any future national health insurance plan.

While generally viewed as a negative influence, it is entirely possible that the trend toward regionalization of maternity facilities for "high-risk" infants could actually serve to foster homebirths and birth-center births.[14] If methods can be devised to screen "high risk" cases from "normal" cases, and if the facilities for high-risk cases are relatively expensive, there will be considerable economic pressure (at least in a system run by the federal government rather than local obstetricians) to make more economical alternatives available for the "normal" pregnancy.

 WHILE GENERALLY VIEWED AS A NEGATIVE INFLUENCE, IT IS ENTIRELY POSSIBLE THAT THE TREND TOWARD REGIONALIZATION OF MATERNITY FACILITIES FOR "HIGH-RISK" INFANTS COULD ACTUALLY SERVE TO FOSTER HOMEBIRTHS AND BIRTH-CENTER BIRTHS.

Conclusion

The law is an obstacle to progress in alternative childbirth experiments primarily to those who misunderstand it. It is reflective of currently held medical and societal beliefs regarding home-birth, primarily concerned with protecting the public in general, and the newborn in particular. Courts are likely to continue to bow to "standard medical procedures" and properly adopted hospital by-laws rather than mandate changes demanded by consumer groups. Legislatures are also unlikely to change either their licensing posture in the health care field or to abandon their concern with the health of newborns. Changes in legislation regarding birth alternatives are likely only after enough persuasive data can be mustered to demonstrate that the proposed alternatives are not only wanted by the public, but are reasonable and safe for the newborn. Establishing safety will probably require a national demonstration project, but if the results are favorable to alternatives, they will be included in any national health insurance plan, and provisions are likely to be made for national licensure of qualified midwives.

CITED REFERENCES

1. Annas, G. , Legal aspects of homebirths and other childbirth alternatives, Stewart, D. , and Stewart, L. , (eds.), Safe Alternatives in Childbirth, 2nd edition, Chapel Hill: NAPSAC, pp. 161-181, 1977.

2. Id. , and see, e.g. , St. Vincent's Hospital v. Hulit, 520 P. 2d 99 (Mont. 1974) Fitzgerald v. Porter Mem. Hospital, 523 F. 2d 716 (7th Cir. 1975); Fahey v. Holy Family Hospital, 336 N. E. 2d 309 (Ill. 1975); Khan v. Suburban Comm. Hospital, 340 N. E. 2d 398 (Ohio 1976); and Sosa v. Bd.of Managers of Val Verde Mem. Hospital, 437 F. 2d 173 (5th Cir. 1971).

3. Annas, G. , The rights of hospital patients, New York: Avon, 1975.

4. Roe v. Wade, 94 S. Ct. 705 (1973), and Doe v. Bolton, 93 S. Ct. 739, 1973.

5. Bowland v. Municipal Ct. for Santa Cruz City, 134 Cal. 630, 638, 1976.

6. Commonwealth v. Edelin, 1976 Mass. Adv. Sheets 2795 (Mass. 1976).

7. Annas, G. , Katz, B. , and Trakimas, R. , Medical malpractice litigation under National Health Insurance: Essential or expendable, 1975 Duke L.J. No. 6, 13335-1373.

Cited References Cont'd

8. Gots, R. , The truth about medical malpractice, New York: Stein & Day,
    p. 48, 1975.

9. Bowland v. Municipal Ct. for Santa Cruz City, 134 Cal. 630, 638 (1976). see
    also Magit v. Bd. Medical Examiners, 366 P. 2d 816 (Cal. 1961); Sanfilippo
    v. State Farm Mutual Automobile Ins. , 535 P. 2d 38 (Ariz. 1975).

10. See State v. Sheperd, 255 Iowa 1218, (1973), and discussion in Robertson, J.
    Involuntary euthanasia of defective newborns: A legal analysis, 27 Stan-
    ford L. Rev. 213, 1975.

11. See, e. g. , Births at home create debate on safety, The Nation's Health, Feb.
    p. 12, 1977.

12. E. g. , Judge John Paul Stevens in Fitzgerald v. Porter Mem. Hospital, 523 F.
    2d 716 (7th Cir. 1975). And see Note, Family Law - Constitutional Right
    to Privacy: The father in the delivery room, 1976 N. Car. L. Rev. 1297.

13. "Quality assurance in hospitals: Policy alternatives, Monograph of Boston
    University's program on public policy for quality health care," April,
    1976, Springer International, p. 4, 1976. Decreasing length of stays for
    childbirth can also cut costs. See Yanover, et al. , perinatal care of the
    low risk mothers and infants: Early discharge with home care, N. Eng. J.
    Med. 294:702, 1976.

14. See, e. g. , Ryan, G. Improving pregnancy outcome via regionalization of
    prenatal care, JOGN Nurs. 3:38, July, 1974.

CHAPTER THIRTY TWO

THE CULTURAL UNWARPING OF CHILDBIRTH: HOW CAN IT BE ACCOMPLISHED?

Doris B. Haire, D.M.S.

One has only to look at our track record on infant mortality and morbidity in the U.S. to see why there is a sweeping movement toward out-of-hospital births in the United States.

Dr. Stanley James, neonatologist and former Chairman of the American Academy of Pediatrics' Committee on Fetus and Newborn, recently stated,

"In our own institution, and I believe in others across the country, approximately one-third of the admissions to the newborn intensive care unit come from mothers who are completely normal at the beginning of labor."

Dr. Roberto Caldeyro-Barcia, President of the International Federation of Obstetricians and Gynecologists, has stated publicly,

"Iatrogenia is the main cause of fetal distress." "In the last forty years many artificial practices have been introduced which have changed childbirth from a physiological event to a very complicated medical procedure in which all kinds of drugs are used and procedures carried out, sometimes unnecessarily, and many of them potentially damaging for the baby and even for the mother."

In a personal communication to this author anesthesiologist Dr. Nicholas Greene of Yale University cautioned,

"Anesthesia during labor and delivery constitutes a demonstrable and significant contributory factor in neonatal brain dysfunction."

There is growing evidence that these effects, once assumed to be temporary, may indeed have permanent consequences.

DORIS B. HAIRE is President, American Foundation for Maternal and Child Health; former President, International Childbirth Education Association; Author of numerous works including book, Implementing Family Centered Maternity Care, and the best-selling booklet, The Cultural Warping of Childbirth.

According to our most reliable organizations and resources,

* An infant born in Japan or in the Netherlands is 3 times more likely to survive the first day of life than is an infant born in the U.S., despite the fact that in Japan and the Netherlands there is no strong inclination, as opposed to the U.S., to save infants who cannot be expected to participate in society to a reasonably normal degree.

* One out of every 35 American children will eventually be diagnosed as retarded (75% of these cases there is no genetic or sociological predisposing factor).

* One out of every 8 American children has some form of minimal brain dysfunction or significant learning disability. Learning disability appears to be primarily an American problem.

* Forceps may have formerly unrecognized long-term deleterious effects that do not manifest until young adulthood. The incidence of initial gran mal seizures in young adults between the ages of 20-25 is apparently on the increase in the United States. Neurologists hypothesize that intra-cranial hemorrhage resulting from forceps delivery causes the process of gliosis to occur. As the glia cells (scar tissue) continues to accumulate over the years eventually the glia cells thicken to the point where they interfere with the normal functioning of the brain.

* One out of every 4 American graduates from high school is functionally illiterate, unable to read beyond the fifth grade reading level.

We are producing a generation of subnormal Americans. The statistical disasters described above are not limited to the poor but cut across the entire socioeconomic and ethnic strata of the United States.

Those who like to blame our high incidence of defective children on prematurity fail to take cognizance of the fact that the Boston component of the Collaborative Perinatal Study [1] found that 80% of the 7 year old children who were diagnosed as having abnormal or suspect central nervous system functions were within the normal range of gestational age and weight at birth.

LEARNING DISABILITY APPEARS TO BE PRIMARILY AN AMERICAN
PROBLEM. WE ARE PRODUCING A GENERATION OF SUBNORMAL
AMERICANS.

Resuscitation of drugged newborn infants resulting from central nervous system depression is so commonplace in the United States that such a condition is no longer considered by many to be a cause for alarm. Blue hands and feet are so common among our newborn infants an hour after birth that expectant parents are now told that such a condition is normal. Dr. Albert Huch, German obstetrician-physiologist, described the problem very well when he recently replied to an American neonatologist,

"Yes, you Americans consider blue hands and feet after the first few minutes of life to be normal, but we do not consider a baby in that condition to be in optimal condition."

Therein lies the difference! While American health professionals tend to be satisfied with the "average" or "normal" baby, health professionals in countries such as Japan and the Netherlands, which have a far better infant outcome than we do, tend to put their efforts into seeing that every baby is in optimal condition at birth.

Obviously, the causes of mental deficiency are multi-factorial, but there is no doubt that commonly employed obstetric procedures and drugs which interfere with the normal progress of labor and birth and the immediate sustained respiration of the newborn infant contribute to the skyrocketing incidence of mental retardation and learning disability in the United States.

Two national perinatal studies,[2,3] one carried out in the United States and the other in the United Kingdom, involving many thousands of mothers and their offspring, have shown fetal hypoxia and a delay in respiration to be major correlates of low IQ and neurologic impairment. Research by Ucko [4] in England also suggests that fetal hypoxia and a delay in respiration at birth can interfere with the child's later ability to cope normally with stress, even though that child demonstrates a normal IQ.

In this day of machines and technology, I propose the use of a device which I feel could do more to change obstetric care in the United States than forceps or fetal monitors or anything else we have. It is a stopwatch. If we could give every couple who goes into a delivery room a stopwatch, and have the couple announce to the obstetrician during labor that they are going to time how long it takes their newly born baby to breathe and to have pink fingers and toes, I am sure they would get a better baby. So, let's put aside the mechanical fetal monitor for low-risk mothers and give every mother a stopwatch to take into the delivery room.

While it is important to reduce the incidence of prematurity and low birthweight, Hoffman [5] found these factors as causes of infant morbidity to be comparatively minor when compared to the incidence of difficult delivery, cyanosis and prolonged labor. Prolonged labor and cyanosis occurred 20 times more often among the children who were failing in school. Difficult delivery (breech delivery was a separate category), which can be precipitated or aggravated by the administration of common obstetric drugs, occurred 16 times more often among the births of those children who were failing in school.

 THERE IS NO DOUBT THAT COMMONLY EMPLOYED OBSTETRIC PROCEDURES AND DRUGS CONTRIBUTE TO THE SKYROCKETING INCIDENCE OF MENTAL RETARDATION & LEARNING DISABILITY IN THE U.S.

It is interesting to note that Dr. Hoffman found that induced labor put the baby in the same category of risk as those babies who were products of prematurity, breech delivery and post-maturity, conditions one would hardly inflict on a baby if at all possible to avoid.

Two additional studies carried out in different areas and along the same line as Dr. Hoffman's study have since shown almost identical data.

There is no question that medically indicated obstetric drugs have saved thousands of lives. But that does not excuse the fact that millions of unborn children in the United States have been exposed during their intrauterine existence to the risks and hazards of unnecessary avoidable drugs.

My article published in the 1976 book, [6] Safe Alternatives in Childbirth, a NAPSAC publication, (pp. 13-22) goes more thoroughly into the risks, hazards and areas of uncertainty regarding the immediate and delayed effects of obstetric-related drugs. The essential fact to be stressed here is that, according to the American Academy of Pediatrics' Committee on Drugs,

> There is no drug, whether over-the-counter remedy or prescription drug, that has been proven to be safe for the unborn child. [7]

THE FDA DOES NOT GUARANTEE THE SAFETY OF ANY DRUG WHICH IT APPROVES AS "SAFE AND EFFECTIVE."

The FDA does not guarantee the safety of any drug which that agency approves as "safe and effective." According to Dr. Richard Crout,[8] Director of the Bureau of Drugs of the FDA, the FDA has no specific definition for "safe." It is a pathetic situation indeed when you have a Federal agency, charged with the responsibility for deciding on the safety of a drug without that agency's having a specific definition of "safe."

An investigation [9] carried out by the General Accounting Office into the functioning and dysfunctioning of the Food and Drug Administration came to the following conclusion:

"The Food and Drug Administration has neither adequately monitored new drug tests nor adequately enforced compliance with testing requirements. Consequently, it lacks assurance (1) that the thousands of human subjects used in such tests annually are protected from unnecessary hazards of new drugs or (2) that the test data used in deciding whether to approve new drugs for marketing is accurate and reliable."

Unfortunately, this statement also holds true for those "old" drugs already on the market.

If you have any doubts or questions about any specific prescribed drug for you or your family, don't just ask your doctor, ask your pharmacist as well. Many pharmacists know a great deal more about the effects of drugs than doctors. It is perfectly legal for a pharmacist to share such knowledge with you and many are quite willing to do so when asked.

Data from animal research published in the July 1976 issue of Scientifie American [10] strongly suggests that artificial hormones administered to pregnant and parturient women may alter the neurological development of the fetus with resultant alteration in sexual behavior in the adult offspring. According to the Health Research Group in Washington, 500,000 prescriptions for hormone therapy were prescribed for pregnant women in 1976.

 INDUCING LABOR PUTS THE BABY IN THE SAME CATEGORY OF RISK AS THOSE BABIES WHO ARE PRODUCTS OF PREMATURITY, BREECH DELIVERY, AND POST-MATURITY--CONDITIONS ONE WOULD HARDLY INFLICT ON A BABY IF AT ALL POSSIBLE TO AVOID.

There is currently a concerted effort by many health professionals to push epidural blocks as the "Cadillac" of anesthetics. At
a 1976 conference in Seattle, Washington, sponsored by the International Childbirth Education Association (ICEA), Daniel Rosen [11] of
Harvard Medical School reported on a paper by Tronick and his colleagues, published in Pediatrics (July 1976) which concludes that
epidural anesthesia has no adverse effects on "highly selected" infants.

What the authors did not discuss in their paper is that in order
to get this "highly selected" group of infants, they excluded from the
study group (i.e., they did not test) any infant who had a problem in
the delivery room, such as a delay in respiration, marked acrocy-
anosis, hypothermia, mid-forceps delivery or high-forceps delivery
-- all conditions which can be precipitated or intensified by the use
of drugs used during epidural blocks.

Furthermore, any deviations from the accepted standard of
normal newborn behavior or condition in the nursery were further
grounds for exclusion. The investigation's conclusions, drawn from
such a pre-screened sample of infants, is somewhat analogous to
saying,

> "Having limited our study to a 'select group' of healthy
> soldiers, who survived the war without trauma or injury,
> we found that none of the 'highly select group' demon-
> strated any adverse effects from having been in combat."

Those who would justify the routine use of drugs during labor
and birth on the grounds that the external fetal monitor using ultrasound will identify deviations in normal fetal physiology should be
reminded of the fact that Barrett and Andersen [12] have demonstrated
that diagnostic levels of ultrasound have been shown in animal studies to disrupt the spleen's ability to produce antibodies, the body's
primary defense mechanism against infection. No one knows the
delayed, long-range effects of electronic or ultrasonic fetal monitoring on the offspring exposed to these procedures in utero. Gabbe
et al. [13] have demonstrated in animal studies that rupturing the
amniotic membranes, which is necessary in order to screw the
electrode into the fetal scalp, is a procedure which can, in itself,
cause a slowing of the fetal heart. The loss of the amniotic fluid
elminiates the hydraulic cushion which serves to equalize the uterine pressure over the fetal body mass and permits the compression
and occlusion of the umbilical cord which carried oxygenated blood
to the placenta. [18]

WILL ULTRASOUND BE THE DES OF THE NEXT GENERATION? WHAT WILL BE THE LONG-RANGE CONSEQUENCES OF ROUTINELY IRRADIATING, WITH ULTRASOUND, THE DELICATE, VULNERABLE OVUM OF THE FEMALE FETUS? IT WILL TAKE AT LEAST A GENERATION TO FIND OUT.

Will ultrasound be the DES of the next generation? It will take at least a generation to find out. In October 1976 I attended the International Congress of Obstetricians and Gynecologists in Mexico City and heard Dr. Susuki from Japan, who is one of the world's most prominent specialists in irradiation, being questioned about the safety of ultrasound. Dr. Susuki said he did not feel that exposure to ultrasound would harm the fetus, although there was no proof of safety in regard to the delayed, long-range effects of ultrasound. Dr. Susuki did express his concern over the possible delayed, long-range effects of ultrasound on the <u>ovum</u> of the female fetus. What will be the long-range consequences of routinely irradiating with ultrasound the delicate, vulnerable ovum of the female fetus? No one can possibly know the long-range effects of such exposure until the next generation is born years hence.

If the members of the American College of Obstetricians and Gynecologists are truly concerned with the safety of the unborn and newborn infant, then the officers of District II of the ACOG who so adamantly oppose out-of-hospital birth (see Chapter 5, Vol. 1) must call for a state-wide computerization of all prenatal, intrapartal and postpartal records over the past year in the State of New York. By such collective data we can see what were the factors which immediately preceded the low-risk fetus becoming the high-risk fetus and neonate. Then, let's look again at those children at the age of seven to see if there are correlates between obstetric practices and low IQ or learning disability. Surely the ACOG would want to know.

Unfortunately, at present it seems that in most states the only way mothers will have the possibility of getting their obstetric records will be if they have an out-of-hospital birth. It is interesting to note that in the State of Illinois -- where the headquarters of the American College of Obstetricians and Gynecologists, the American Academy of Pediatrics, the American Medical Association, the American Hospital Association, the American Society of Anesthesiologists are located -- these groups have chosen to be noticeably silent regarding the fact that <u>in the State of Illinois a hospital can destroy the mother's prenatal and intranatal records as soon as the</u>

bills are paid.   All of the aforementioned organizations are fully
aware that preservation of these records is essential if we are to
ever properly evaluate the safety or hazards of common obstetric
practices.   For those of you who are interested, the International
Childbirth Education Association, P.O. Box 20852, Milwaukee, WI,
53220, has a record of all U.S. state regulations which affect hospital preservation of maternal and infant records -- (a) how long the
records must be preserved by the hospital, (b) how soon the records
may be microfilmed and the original records destroyed, etc.

 IN THE STATE OF ILLINOIS, HOME OF THE MAJOR AMERICAN
MEDICAL ASSOCIATIONS SUCH AS THE ACOG, AMA, AAP, AND
AHA, A HOSPITAL CAN DESTROY THE MOTHER'S PRENATAL AND INTRA-
NATAL RECORDS AS SOON AS THE BILLS ARE PAID.

In regard to microfilm, microfilmed records are not considered proof of what actually went on during the patient's hospital stay.
The information in the original records can be distorted by making
changes (deletions and additions in the text, new pages added, etc.)
before the original records are microfilmed.   If the Federal Bureau
of Investigation wants an absolutely accurate account of a record,
that agency does not rely on microfilmed records.   FBI document
experts advise me that when they have really important records they
do not microfilm them.   They keep the original records.

So, I think it would be a protective measure if every woman
who plans to give birth in a hospital -- and there are still going to
be many women who must go into hospitals to have their babies because there are no alternative systems available to them -- be prepared to write in "Signed but not read" above her signature on the
hospital admission consent form and that she bring along a previously
prepared signed directive which reads:

> "I hereby direct that neither I nor my baby shall be used
> as a teaching or research subject unless I am so advised
> in advance and my informed consent obtained. All medi-
> cations, therapy and/or treatment procedures must be
> approved in advance by me or my chosen companion
> _____ (name of designee) after consulta-
> tion with my personal physician or midwife."

Presenting this directive after the mother has been admitted
to the hospital creates less resistance from the hospital staff because no hospital administrator in his or her right mind is going to

turn a laboring woman out of the hospital with a newspaper just waiting for a story. The mother should be prepared to be coopera- tive on admission, then just call the nurse over and say, "I would like this note to be attached to my hospital record."

Such a directive is not an absolute guarantee that the mother's wishes will be honored; however, most hospitals are extremely leery of going against a specific written directive from a patient.

In many hospitals today, if someone wants a copy of his or her hospital medical records, it is given the patient because smart hos- pital administrators know that an angry patient is much more likely to sue than a curious patient.

A growing number of hospitals now allow patients to have a copy of their complete medical records. The nurse-midwives at Grady Memorial Hospital in Atlanta allow patients to work with the assigned midwife in preparing their own records.

HOSPITALS CAN MAKE THEIR SETTINGS MORE HOME-LIKE. BUT A GROWING NUMBER OF EXPECTANT PARENTS WANT MORE THAN A HOME-LIKE SETTING. THEY WANT THE SENSE OF CONTROL THAT COMES ONLY WHEN BIRTH OCCURS AT HOME.

The Maternity Center Association's Childbearing Center in New York (see Chapter 21, Vol. 2) is an outstanding example of what can be done to improve the environment for a family-centered birth. The Alternative Birth Centers developed at San Francisco Medical Center and Mr. Zion Medical Center in San Francisco and at Henne- pin County Medical Center and Golden Valley Health Center in Min- neapolis are fine examples of what hospitals can do to make the hos- pital setting more homelike for birth. But a growing number of American expectant parents want more than a homelike setting. They want the sense of control that comes only when birth occurs at home. As long as hospital-based health professionals will not trust the couple to make wise decisions based on truthful information about the risks and hazards of routine obstetric practices then the couple will not trust the hospital-based personnel.

AS LONG AS HOSPITAL-BASED HEALTH PROFESSIONALS WILL NOT TRUST COUPLES TO MAKE WISE DECISIONS BASED ON TRUTHFUL INFORMATION ABOUT THE RISKS AND HAZARDS OF ROUTINE OBSTETRIC PRACTICES, THEN COUPLES WILL NOT TRUST HOSPITAL-BASED HEALTH PROFESSIONALS.

How to Unwarp Childbirth in the United States

There are many ways we can bring about improvements in
U.S. maternity care. Let's discuss some of the things a consumer
can do and list some of the agencies, committees, organizations and
media people who would benefit from the input of knowledgeable consumers and courageous health professionals who will speak out for
the patient.

I.   Health Systems Agencies (H.S.A.) Call the administrator of
     your local hospital for the name and address of the Chairperson
     of your area H.S.A. or consult the National Health Directory
     [15] in your library which lists all officers of all H.S.A.'s in
     the U.S. (H.S.A.'s were formerly called Comprehensive
     Health Planning Board). These federally mandated groups, by
     law, must be comprised of more than 51% consumers. If there
     is no opening on the H.S.A. board when you call, ask to be
     sent a list of the present H.S.A. members and the date their
     respective memberships expire. Ask to have your name placed
     on a list of possible candidates for forthcoming vacancies.

II. Perinatal Regionalization Review Committees. These agencies
     tend to lean heavily in favor of consolidation as a means of
     regionalizing perinatal care. (There is no evidence that big-
     ger is better for the low-risk mother and her baby, and con-
     solidation of facilities can mean great inconvenience for the
     obstetric patient and her family.[14]) These committees
     should have the input of informed, assertive consumers who
     are concerned with both the psychological aspects as well as
     the technical aspects of regionalization.

III. Local Council on Maternal and Child Health. Form a state or
     local council made up of knowledgeable consumers, psycholo-
     gists, ethicists, sociologists, clergymen, teachers of learn-
     ing disabled children, and courageous health professionals.
     Such a Council could have a great impact on both local and
     state obstetric practices by holding public hearings and "speak
     outs" on obstetric care. The Council could hold press confer-
     ences and issue press releases to alert the media to the pre-
     sent state of obstetric care. But remember, do your home-
     work well and know your facts. Health professionals can make
     a concerned but inaccurate consumer look foolish and irre-
     sponsible. Listen to opposing views, seek out the weak points

in their opposition and be well prepared to defend your position. Make sure your council stationery looks impressive, and in keeping with the dignity of your concern. Contact the chief administrative officer of each local hospital and request permission to tour the obstetric department, including the labor and delivery area. Politely request scientific data which justifies those regulations which parents find objectionable (95% of obstetric practices are based on folklore!).

IF YOU WANT TO KNOW WHAT HAS GONE WRONG IN OBSTETRICS, READ THE PEDIATRIC JOURNALS!

IV.   Consent Form. Request a copy of the consent form required to be signed by obstetric patients prior to their being admitted to the hospital. After reviewing the consent form with a sympathetic physician and attorney the Council could then ask to meet with the hospital administrator, the hospital attorney and the chief of obstetrics, in order to develop a consent form which will not only protect the patient but also protect the hospital and doctor. (A consent form which deals honestly with the risks, hazards and pertinent areas of uncertainty, as well as the benefits of a treatment or procedure can help to protect everyone.)

V.   Patient Acquisition of Hospital Medical Records. Some hospitals destroy the medical records shortly after the patient leaves. Others keep them for a limited period of time and then dispose of them.

      If you would like to obtain a copy of your hospital medical records it is more effective if the letter below is sent to the chief administrator of the hospital. To get his name call the hospital and ask for the "Administrator's Office." Tell the secretary that you would like to address a letter to the chief administrative officer and would like his name and official title. Such information is usually readily given.

      Make several copies of the letter you send. Send a follow-up copy of your letter in two weeks if you have not received a reply.

      If you have not received your medical records or a satisfactory reply within one month of sending the first letter you may choose to send the second, less friendly letter.

      The word "authorize" in the letter below is essential.

FIRST LETTER

Address
Date

Chief Administrative Officer
_____ Hospital
Our Town, U.S.A. 00000

Dear Sir:

    I hereby authorize the administration of (name of
hospital) to release directly to me a copy of my and my
baby's complete hospital medical records, including nurses'
notes, pertaining to our stay in_____ Hospital
from   (date)   to   (date) .   I will pay an appropriate fee
for the reproduction of our records and for first class
postage.

    I realize that the physical records belong to the
hospital; however, I am aware that the information contained in our records belongs to me.   I therefore authorize
the administration of _____ Hospital to send a complete copy of my and my baby's complete records, including nurses' notes, directly to me, not to my doctor. I wish
to maintain a copy of my and my baby's complete hospital
medical records in my own files and would appreciate a
frendly compiance with my request.

                              Sincerely,

                              Ms. Jane Smith

    In the event that the hospital proposes to charge you
more than 10¢ or 15¢ a page ask the hospital's Medical Record
Administrator what the copying charge is per page when hospital records are requested by a physician. There is no justification for the charges to be different -- a patient's retention of a

SECOND LETTER

Address
Date

Chief Administrative Officer
_____Hospital
Our Town, U.S.A. 00000

Dear Sir:

In my letter of __(date)__ (see enclosed copy) I requested that you release directly to me a copy of my and my
baby's complete hospital medical records, including nurses'
notes, pertaining to our stay in_____Hospital from
_(date)__ to __(date)__. I have authorized the release of
our records directly to me (not to my doctor) and have offered
to pay an appropriate fee for their reproduction and mailing
by first class mail. Your refusal to comply with my request
indicates either that you and your hospital have something
to hide or that I have not stated my authorization properly.
If the latter is the cause for the delay, I would appreciate
your advising me as to the proper procedure for securing the
records I have requested.

If I do not receive a complete copy of our hospital
medical records (I do not wish a summary or extract) within
two weeks then you will force me to bring legal action
against the hospital to obtain our records.

It would be foolish indeed if the hospital forces me
to take legal action when mere compliance with my request
would solve the problem in an amicable way.

Sincerely yours,

Ms. Jane Smith

copy of his or her hospital records insures continuity of care.
If the hospital persists in charging you a higher rate, contact
your local newspaper's health editor and suggest that the newspaper publicize this obvious effort to place obstacles in the
way of patients' access to their own medical records.

VI. <u>Hospital Board of Trustees.</u> Write a letter to the President of the Hospital Board of Trustees of your local hospital(s) and to the chief administrative officer (the title varies from hospital to hospital). The letter need not be typewritten, but it must look neat and organized. Tell the President of the Board of Trustees that you would like to serve on the Board. If he or she tells you that all positions on the Board are filled then ask for a list of the present members of the Board and the dates their respective memberships expire. Ask to be placed on a list of prospective candidates for the Board. Few hospital boards have a fair proportion of women members -- the same proportion of women on the Board as the proportion of women cared for in that facility (a subject that should be brought to the attention of the media in your area).

VII. <u>Media: Science, Health and Education Editors of Local Newspapers, Radio and Television Stations.</u> Do your homework and have your scientific facts straight, because most journalists working in the life sciences are quite knowledgeable and learn fast. In most cases you may offer an important perspective that the journalist can appreciate and promulgate. If you are rebuffed there is usually a bias in the journalist's own perspective. Find out why!

VIII. <u>Medical Journals, Newspapers and Reference Books.</u> Read the obstetric and pediatric journals whenever possible (if you want to know what has gone wrong in obstetrics read the pediatric journals!). If your public library does not carry medical journals such as the <u>American Journal of Obstetrics and Gynecology</u> or <u>Pediatrics</u> ask the Director of the library to subscribe to the journals. Goodman & Gilman's basic book, <u>The Pharmacological Basis of Therapeutics,</u> published by Macmillan, is an excellent resource on drugs. The <u>Physician's Desk Reference</u> is usually more readily available; however, the information is prepared by the manufacturers of the drugs listed in the book, and many drugs are not listed. Another valuable reference for learning where to initiate actions in appropriate places is the current (published annually) <u>National Health Directory,</u>[15] which lists 363 pages of current addresses and phone numbers of literally thousands of health officials, including federal and state congressmen and senators on health related committees, directors of H.S.A.'s, the various health branches of each individual state as well as the innumerable health related branches of the U.S. Government. Directors of libraries usually have funds to obtain newly requested educational materials. If your local library refuses to subscribe to the journals request permission from the administrator of the local hospital to use the hospital's medical library. Any reluctance should be followed by a reminder that the hospital is funded by public taxes and financial gifts and that, therefore, the hospital medical library should be open to citizens who use the library properly and quietly.

IX. Institutional Review Committees (I.R.C.). Hospitals and medical schools involved in any type of human research should have an Institutional Review Committee (I.R.C.). This committee is responsible for deciding whether patients in that facility may be used as research subjects. While the U.S. Food and Drug Administration recommends that consumers be included on such committees the FDA has no power to enforce such a recommendation. A recent federal investigation of such committees found that the vast majority were heavily weighted with individuals who were pro-research and tended to be more concerned with the status of the research grant than the well-being of the research subject.[17] "Consumers" on the I.R.C.'s were frequently employed by the health facility in which the research was being carried out.

To insure the safety of patients in your state write to your governor and recommend that in order to protect the public, the credentials of every Chairman of every Institutional Review Committee in your state be reviewed and, if appropriate, approved by the State's Department of Health, in order to be sure that the Chairperson has the expertise and lack of bias necessary for such a responsible position.

In addition, recommend that the Chairperson of every I.R.C. in the state be registered with:

1) the U.S. Food and Drug Administration in Washington, and
2) the state and county medical boards in the areas in which the research is being carried out, and
3) the state and federal Offices of Consumer Affairs, wherein the information can be made available to the public.

X.   Commission for the Protection of Human Subjects for Bio-
     medical and Behavioral Research, U.S. Department of Health,
     Education and Welfare.   Write to this agency in Washington
     and ask for information regarding the use of pregnant women
     as research subjects.   (U.S. Department of H.E.W., Office
     for Protection from Research Risks, West Wood Bldg.,   5333
     West Bard Ave., Bethesda, MD, 20014, (301) 656-4000.) The
     Commission has recommended that pregnant women may be
     used as research subjects if, in the opinion of the research
     investigator and his or her I.R.C., there is "little or no risk
     to the fetus."   This is an outrageous decision, for how does
     the I.R.C. know what the risks to the fetus are if the proce-
     dure or drug is in its experimental phase. The Commission's
     position regarding research and pregnant women opens wide
     the possibility that a disaster equally as tragic as that caused
     by the administration of diethylstilbestrol (DES) to pregnant
     women over the past three decades may be repeated.[16]
     When will we learn!

          This laxity on the part of federal regulation of research
     on human subjects is only made worse by the laxity of the
     medical research community itself where, according to a re-
     cent survey of the attitudes of medical researchers,[17] only
     6% showed anything that could be classified as "ethical con-
     cern for the research subjects."

XI. Question Everyone.   Don't waste your time trying to convince
     hospital-based health professionals that what you want is right.
     Demand proof, scientifically controlled data, which proves that
     the individual obstetric practices carried out in the hospitals
     in your area are in the best interests of both low-risk mothers
     and their babies.

 "95% OF OBSTETRIC PRACTICES ARE BASED ON FOLKLORE!"
                          DORIS B. HAIRE, DMS

CITED REFERENCES

1. Niswander, K., and Gordon, M., Women and their pregnancies: The collaborative perinatal study of the National Institue of Neurological Diseases and Stroke, Philadelphia: W.B. Saunders & Co., 1972.

2. Broman, S., et al., Preschool IQ: Prenatal and early developmental correlates, Hillside, NJ: L. Erlbaum, 1976.

3. Chamberlain, R., Chamberlain, G., Howlett, B., and Claireaux, A., British births 1970: Vol I, First week of life, London: Medical Books, Ltd., 1975

4. Ucko, L., Comparative study of asphyxiated and non-asphyxiated boys from birth to five years, Dev. Med. Child Neurol. 7:643-657, 1965.

5. Hoffman, M., Early indicationf of learning problems, Academic Therapy, 7:23-35, 1971.

6. Haire, D., Maternity practices around the world: How do we measure up? in Stewart, D., and Stewart, L., (eds.), Safe Alternatives in Childbirth, 2nd edition, Chapel Hill, NC: NAPSAC, pp. 13-22, 1977.

7. Am. Acad. of Pediatrics, Committee on Drugs, Pediat. 51:297-299, 1973.

8. Crout, R., personal communication, 1977.

9. Comptroller General of the U.S., Federal control of new drug testing is not adequately protecting human test subjects and the public, Report to Congress, General Accounting Office, Washington, DC, July 15, 1976.

10. McEwen, B., Interactions between hormones and nerve tissue, Sci. Am., 235:48-58, 1976.

11. Rosen, D., Effects of obstetrical medication on newborn behavior and subsequent mother-child interaction, in Simkin, P., and Wallace, V., (eds) Proc. of 9th Bienniel Conv. of the Internat'l Childbirth Ed. Assoc., Seattle, WA, June 13-17, 1976, Seattle: Childbirth Ed. Assoc. of Seattle, pp. 161-170, quoting Tronick, E., et al., Regional obstetric anesthesia and newborn behavior: Effect over the first ten days of life, Ped. 58:94-100, 1976.

12. Anderson, D., and Barrett, J., Immunosuppression of I.G.M. by ultrasound, Dept. of Microbiology, Columbia, MO: Univ. of MO (in press), 1977.

13. Gabbe, S., et al., Umbilical cord compression associated with amniotomy: Laboratory observations, Am. J. Ob. Gyn. 126:353-356, 1976.

Cited References Cont'd

14. Haire, D., Birth Related mortality rates by size and type of hospital, in Stewart, D., and Stewart, L., (eds.), Safe Alternatives in Childbirth, 2nd edition, Chapel Hill, NC: NAPSAC, pp. 89-90, 1977.

15. Seay, J., National Health Directory, 1740 N Street, NW, Washington, DC: Science & Health Publications, Inc., (published annually), 1977.

16. Am. Acad. of Pediatrics, Committee on Drugs, Stilbestrol and adenocarcinoma of the vagina, Pediat. 51:297-299, 1973.

17. Barber, B., The ethics of experimentation with human subjects. Sci. Am. 234:25-31, 1976.

18. Schwartz, R., and Caldeyro-Barcia, R., et al., Pressure exerted by uterine contractions on the head of the human fetus during labor, Perinatal factors affecting human development, Science Pub. #185, Washington, DC: Pan Am. Health Org., pp. 115-126, 1972.

CHAPTER THIRTY THREE

BIRTH AS THE FIRST EXPERIENCE OF MOTHERING

Michelle Harrison, M.D.

Why does it matter how birth happens? It matters because we relate to our children by way of their history as well as their present, and birth is their history. It exists as an event in which they have taken part.

In the standard American birth a woman has little part in the birth of her child. She is a mere item excluded from the process and is allowed to reappear after technicians have certified her and her child "ready" to see each other.

Life has become sterile. Sterile walls and penicillin resistant staphylococcus are the background. Human instinct is "dangerous." The birthing woman is "inept."

I recently witnessed a birth that seemed to characterize all that is wrong with the American System of Birth. I was the house physician. I was called in the night to deliver a woman whose doctor had not arrived, although he had been called several times. I arrived to meet the family first, standing at the door, grateful a doctor would be there. I remembered meeting them early in the evening. We had chatted in the snack room when I had stopped in for a can of Tab. They were talking of the girl in labor, the daughter and sister of the two women present. I remembered them because they were calm as they talked of the birthing woman, and I had the feeling the woman herself was doing well. I stayed out of the labor rooms because I had been told not to volunteer.

I arrived in the delivery room. The patient, a seventeen year old, was doing well, mildly pushing, groaning, but not screaming. Nurses were saying anesthesia was on the way. I asked the patient if she had had any classes or preparation. She had not. I was looking forward to this delivery because the woman was in control. She had already successfully labored many hours alone and I thought would enjoy the rest. The delivery itself, faced without panic, is far more rewarding, or more immediately rewarding, than the hours of laboring.

MICHELLE HARRISON is a Fellow of the American Academy of Family Physicians; and instructor, Department of Family Medicine, Rutgers University School of Medicine.

I gowned, gloved, checked her. She was fully dilated and would deliver quickly. I draped her according to patterns learned many years ago and repeated many times since. My hands always remember.

Then the anesthetist arrived -- a young man, arrogant -- and seated himself at her head. He placed a mask over her face and told her to breathe deeply. He reassured her it was almost all over. She had only two or three contractions to go. I asked him what he was giving her. He ignored my question. I knew he was ignoring me -- it's one of those sexist moments. I was the "doctor in charge," but he was male. Minutes later he decided to answer, but I couldn't hear what he mumbled.

It didn't matter, though, because at that moment the obstetrician arrived. The anesthetist deepened her sleep to await the scrubbing and gowning of the OB. I stood at the perineum, disappointed I would be stepping out. The OB stepped in, ignoring my presence.

He and the anesthetist began to speak to each other. The patient was now choking on the tubes in her throat. Her labor had stopped; the table had been tilted further so the OB could look down on the spreading lips.

Then they spoke with contempt. The anesthetist saying angrily that the woman was gagging. The OB that she had stopped being any help to them -- she wasn't pushing, her uterus wasn't contracting.

Forceps were unwrapped, applied, and with deepened anesthesia the infant was lifted up and out of his mother's womb by the iron clamps about his head. He was blue and listless, but soon recovered, with oxygen and some slapping

The obstetrician and the anesthetist went on talking while the patient was sewn up. They spoke of partners, Puerto Rico, vacations, weather, etc. The event of birth was lost to standard male locker room talk. It was a standard American birth, but with one ironic loss. A student nurse had gone out to tell the family of the birth of a son. The doctor was angry. The nurse in charge was stern. It is the doctor's privilege to tell the family. It is part of the "delivery" to announce what he has delivered. His show had been stolen.

Much was lost in this delivery, though it is far from a bad one by our standards.   LOST:

(1) This woman has now been re-enforced in her belief that she could not birth herself, and that is a loss since she did so well for so many hours.

(2) This woman and her family are now ever more grateful that the doctor arrived to remove the baby with forceps, since the patient couldn't deliver. They do not know that the need for forceps was created by the use of anesthesia.

(3) This woman was treated with contempt while in a light state of anesthesia, and so was capable on some level of hearing.

(4) This woman missed a chance to know her baby, touch and hear her baby at birth. They will already be strangers when she wakes.

(5) This blue born infant ought to have been born pink and active. He had been sedated. We do not know what effects will be seen in his future.

(6) This patient, her family, her child will all be grateful she delivered in a hospital where all this help was available.

WHY DOES IT MATTER HOW BIRTH HAPPENS? IT MATTERS BECAUSE WE RELATE TO OUR CHILDREN BY WAY OF THEIR HISTORY, AS WELL AS THEIR PRESENT, AND BIRTH IS THEIR HISTORY.

CHAPTER THIRTY FOUR

SOCIAL IMPACTS OF UNNECESSARY INTERVENTION AND UNNATURAL SURROUNDINGS IN CHILDBIRTH

Ashley Montagu, Ph. D.

We live in a time when we are experiencing the not quite final consequences of the Industrial Revolution--a revolution which commenced in the middle of the eighteenth century in England to attain its maximum effect in the second third of twentieth century America. Today we flatter ourselves that we can make machines that can think like human beings, while overlooking the fact that for many years we have been making human beings who can think like machines.

Civilization has become identified with technology to such an extent that technologically undeveloped societies are denied the status of civilization, and are called "primitive," when, in fact, they may, in many ways, be more complex, advanced, and better adapted to their various environments than many so-called "civilized" societies. Technologically developed peoples may conquer technologically undeveloped ones, but that does not necessarily render the conquerors superior to the conquered in anything other than their superior technology. The gun happens to be a more murderously effective weapon than the hunter's bow and arrow. With the gun the white man has destroyed innumerable cultures that had far more to offer him than he had to offer them. Redefining patriotism to serve their own self-seeking ends the imperialist flag-wavers, armed with their jingoistic slogans, sought to establish their place in the world by making technological success the measure of superiority, of innate merit. This technological jingoism has invaded virtually every aspect of modern life, to such an extent that we, in the western world, have come to believe that if you can take anything out of human hands and the human heart and have a machine do it instead you have made progress.

ASHLEY MONTAGU is former Chairman, Department of Anthropology, Rutgers University; former Regents Professor, University of California; and Author of 23 books, including Touching, Prenatal Influence, Life Before Birth, On Being Human, The Natural Superiority of Women, and others.

WE HAVE COME TO BELIEVE THAT IF YOU CAN TAKE ANYTHING OUT OF HUMAN HANDS AND THE HUMAN HEART AND HAVE A MA- CHINE DO IT INSTEAD, YOU HAVE MADE PROGRESS.

Technology, indeed, has become the measure of progress. In many areas of life the more a man resembles a highly efficient machine, whether he be an executive in a large corporation or a worker on the assembly line, the more highly is he valued. Unfortunately, one of the professions most severely afflicted with this technological disorder is that of medicine.

The disaster begins with the medical school. The first evidence of its disorder is its admissions policy. Admission to medical school is highly correlated with success in what is called "doing well" in college. Hence, the best examination-passers stand the best chance of getting into medical school. Being a good examination-passer is usually evidence of little more than an ability to regurgitate rote-remembered facts on to blank sheets of paper. It isn't even a measure of a good mind, and it certainly isn't an evidence of the student's interest in human beings. Students in whom the latter interest predominates, and who do not excel at examinations, are likely to find themselves rejected by medical school admission committees.

The second disaster to which the admitted medical student is caused to succumb is the method by which he is taught. He is exposed to a large number of different subjects, which are taught in normative ways, with the emphasis almost always on disease and the blessing of technology. In this maze of subjects and techniques the constant pressure under which the student labors the human being he may once have been, together with any notion of the patient as a human being he may once have had, gets lost, and he graduates from medical school equipped with a battery of technical skills and accumulated knowledge relating almost exclusively to disease.

The third disaster to which our victim is exposed is the internship year, a year in which he learns from his "betters" how patients suffering from every kind of disease should be treated -- not so much as human beings, but as disease-entities. During this year he extends and intensifies his knowledge of the uses of the various technological devices and special procedures, and learns that the technology is there to be used, or rather that the technology is to be used because it is there.

Throughout his medical training seldom, it would appear, does anyone ever tell our developing doctor that the care of the patient begins with caring for the patient, that at the very least one of the most important parts of the treatment is the doctor himself. Indeed, the human relations aspect of the practice of medicine seems to have been virtually entirely displaced by the pre-eminent importance assigned to technology.

DURING TRAINING, THE PHYSICIAN LEARNS THAT TECHNOLOGY IS THERE TO BE USED, OR RATHER, THAT THE TECHNOLOGY IS TO BE USED BECAUSE IT IS THERE.

We have all, to a greater or lesser extent, been victimized by the prevailing values of our society, and, as a consequence, the tragedy for most of us lies in the difference between what we were capable of becoming and what we have in fact been caused to become. And this is true of most doctors as it is true of most other people. Because, among other things, the main focus of the doctor's training has been upon disease he may, in certain situations, constitute the greatest threat to the patient's health. Because of his failure to understand the human needs of those who come under his control, he will be especially dangerous to the human development of both mother and child in the momentous event we call childbirth.

Most obstetricians behave as if they understand neither the social meaning of labor nor the dramatic and socially important event that childbirth is; while most pediatricians altogether fail to understand what the reciprocal social needs of mother and child are following birth. A lack of understanding on the part of these two kinds of specialists results in practices that add up to a considerable amount of behavioral damage to mother and child, to the family, and to society as a whole.[1]

BECAUSE THE MAIN FOCUS OF THE DOCTOR'S TRAINING HAS BEEN UPON DISEASE HE MAY, IN CERTAIN SITUATIONS, CONSTITUTE THE GREATEST THREAT TO THE PATIENT'S HEALTH.

The unfortunate social impacts of unnecessary intervention and unnatural surroundings in childbirth are largely, if not entirely, due to ignorance of the human requirements, not only of mother and infant, but also of the needs of the other members of the family -- husband, siblings, and significant others. If this were comprehended, labor would be understood to be not only a physiological preparation for birth but also a readying for postnatal functioning of the infant as a social being, for babies at birth have a great many social communications to make, principally to the mother, and secondarily to the father, as well as to siblings and others. Any interference with the baby's ability to make these communications by debilitating it through the administration of drugs to the mother during labor is likely to reduce or suppress the ability of the infant to communicate these very necessary messages, and thus retard the physical as well as psychological recovery of both.   There are now many research reports on the damaging effects of such interference on the newborn, as well as their effects on behavior in later life.[2] When confronted with a sluggish baby the mother suffers in many ways from the loss of benefits that a normally active baby provides.[3] The deprivation from which she suffers is akin to that other deprivation induced by obstetricians: the separation of the baby from the mother. And this brings us, before we consider that separation, to a brief discussion of two of the malpractices of most contemporary obstetricians: drugs and the induction of labor.

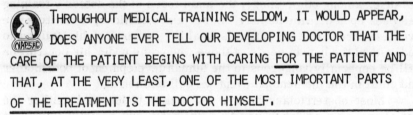

THROUGHOUT MEDICAL TRAINING SELDOM, IT WOULD APPEAR, DOES ANYONE EVER TELL OUR DEVELOPING DOCTOR THAT THE CARE OF THE PATIENT BEGINS WITH CARING FOR THE PATIENT AND THAT, AT THE VERY LEAST, ONE OF THE MOST IMPORTANT PARTS OF THE TREATMENT IS THE DOCTOR HIMSELF.

Drugs

Virtually all drugs, no matter when or by whatever route administered, are known to have a detrimental effect upon the fetus, not to mention their often ill-effects upon the mother. It took the thalidomide tragedy to bring the danger of administering such drugs to the pregnant woman to the attention of the public. Nevertheless, to this day many anesthetists and obstetricians blithely continue on their unrestrained way assaulting the fetus and mother with drugs, ignoring the literally hundreds of researches which prove beyond any question that such drugs are damaging.[4] The consequences to the individual, to the family, and to the society resulting from such professional irresponsibility are so serious that the time is now long overdue for government intervention. It was the refusal of a government official, Dr. Frances O. Kelsey, Director of the scientific investigation staff of the Bureau of Food and Drug Administration, to license the drug thalidomide in the United States, on the ground that it had been insufficiently tested, that prevented untold numbers of tragedies from occurring. One can well imagine what would have happened had their been no Food and Drug Administration to ensure that such drugs should not be commercially exploited. I would suggest that the time has arrived for us to have a medical branch of the FDA to regulate the administration of drugs to pregnant women.

Dr. Kelsey, in a recent discussion of the effects of drugs in pregnancy attributes some 80 percent of congenital abnormalities of unknown causation to the uncontrolled administration of drugs. Everything from cleft-palate and harelip to various degrees of mental retardation has been traced to the administration of drugs to the pregnant mother. The facts are now fully documented, and it is therefore quite inexcusable for anyone, let alone alleged specialists, to go on disregarding them.[5]

While some physicians may interpret their license to practice medicine as the freedom to do so licentiously, we must see to it that the physician of the future is trained to be professionally responsible. We must all of us recognize our responsibility to the unborn child to do everything in our power to see to it that it is born free of physical and mental handicap. Freedom, as Lord Acton remarked, is not the liberty to do what we like, but the right to be able to do what we ought. To the obstetrician that should mean, at the very minimum, the freedom to do the very best that can be done for the unborn child and its mother. And that requires of the obstetrician that he keep abreast of the latest research findings in the furtherance of those ends. For what is the purpose of obstetrics -- which means "standing by" -- unless it be to secure the best possible outcome for the unborn child and its mother?

Induction

"Elective induction," as it is sometimes miscalled -- for it is not the mother who usually "elects" to be induced, but the obstetrician -- is the technique whereby labor is started by drugs, usually oxytocin, the trade name of which and by which it is often called is "Pitocin." Oxytocin is also used to stimulate or speed up labor. Another technique for inducing labor is by rupture of the membranes. More than 35 percent of all hospital deliveries are now induced, and in some hospitals induction has become a routine procedure. As Dr. Caldeyro-Barcia has stated, labor should be stimulated only when uterine contractions are too weak or infrequent to achieve the normal progression of the infant through the birth canal. Labor should never be induced, except in such conditions as Rh sensitization of the mother, severe pre-eclampsia, severe diabetes,

or other threatening conditions. According to Caldeyro-Barcia, restricted to such contingencies induction would be performed in no
more than 3 percent of cases.

The practice of induction today is responsible for medically
produced prematurity which is in most cases the cause of neonatal
damage.[6]

The intensification of labor by drugs results in stronger uterine contractions which are faster paced, but with shorter relaxation
periods between contractions. This results in a decrease in oxygen
supply to the fetus. Such deprivation can result in more or less
severe brain damage.

Drug-induced babies show a 50 percent increase in neonatal
depression as c o m p a r e d with non-induced babies. The induced
babies tend to be blue in color at birth, to have breathing difficulties,
and to lack muscle-tone. Induction through rupture o f the membranes may result in increased pressures to the fetal head, dis-
placement of the skull bones, with resulting brain and scalp hemorrhages.

Since in induced labors the mother often experiences unusually
severe pain owing to the stronger uterine contractions, she is generally given pain-relieving drugs during labor and delivery. The
effect of these is a further assault upon the fetus and a depression
of its respiratory abilities.

As a vigorous editorial in the esteemed British medical journal,
The Lancet, put it in November, 1974, "Induction on the grounds of
social convenience is a pernicious practice which has no place in
modern obstetric care. The mother's holiday, the calls of the obstetrician's private practice, must not influence, for the sake o f
even a few days, an event which for the child may affect the outcome
of his entire life." And that, it should be added, holds true for many
other obstetrical practices.

 WHILE SOME PHYSICIANS MAY INTERPRET THEIR LICENSE TO
PRACTICE MEDICINE AS THE FREEDOM TO DO SO LICENTIOUSLY,
WE MUST SEE TO IT THAT THE PHYSICIAN OF THE FUTURE IS TRAINED
TO BE PROFESSIONALLY RESPONSIBLE.

Mother-Infant Separation

I have for years endeavored to draw attention to the fact that
at birth mother and infant need each other as no two creatures can
need each other again. It seemed to me reasonably clear that at

birth the infant is looking forward to a continuation of the life he had enjoyed in the womb, in other words, that he is looking forward to a womb with a view. This is something more than a merely metamorphic way of saying that both the newborn and his mother are designed to continue their symbiotic relationship postnatally without the slightest interruption.

The mother has been beautifully prepared throughout pregnancy to meet the requirements of her dependent infant, and the infant has also been marvellously well readied to adapt to his mother. By "adapt" I mean not merely prepared to derive all the benefits she is capable of conferring upon him, but his ability to confer many benefits, physical and psychological upon her, too. I refer to the contractions of the uterus upon contact with the baby's body, the continuing contractions generated by the infant's suckling at the mother's breast, the stimulation of secretion of maternal pituitary hormones such as oxytocin, which helps the uterus to return to normal size, and prolactin, which stimulates lactation. Oxytocin, by producing uterine vasoconstriction as well as contraction of the uterine musculature, results in arresting the postpartum bleeding, plus the completion of the third stage of labor: the detachment and ejection of the placenta. These are only a few of the benefits conferred by the suckling infant upon its mother.

The enduring immunogenic benefits conferred by the mother's colostrum upon the baby are well known -- or perhaps they aren't as well known as they ought to be, in which case it should be said that the gammaglobulins contained in the lemony-yellowish substance secreted by the mother's breast during the first several days after birth of the baby confer a passive immunity upon the baby against all viral infections, help to clear its gastrointestinal tract, and probably stimulate to greater efficiency the genitourinary tract, for as McCance and Otley have shown, if rats are removed from their mothers immediately after birth their kidneys remain functionless.[7] The fact is that if the newborn non-human mammal is removed from the mother before she has licked it, it is very likely to die of a failure of function of the gastrointestinal and genitourinary tracts.[8]

 EARLY MOTHER-INFANT SEPARATION, FAILURE-TO-THRIVE, OR CHILDREN SEPARATED BY HOSPITALIZATION FROM THEIR MOTHER ARE DISPROPORTIONATELY AT RISK OF BEING BATTERED, NEGLECTED, OR OTHERWISE ABUSED BY THEIR PARENTS.

In the dog removal of the puppies from the mother immediately after birth results in a listless mother, who often hemorrhages badly, and who recovers slowly even after the puppies are returned to her.[9] In human mothers similar effects are only too often produced as a consequence of removing the baby from the mother to the nursery. The nursery is so-called, presumably, because nursing has in the past been discouraged in it. In addition to that, other series of offenses are committed against the baby beginning with abandoning it to a prison-like structure appropriately called a crib, which is surrounded on all sides by perpendicular bars and white surfaces, and where it is often not fed for 12 to 24 hours or more. And this in the face of all the published evidence showing how important it is for mother and newborn to be together from the moment of birth.[10]

A number of independent investigations have shown that starving the newborn is harmful to it. It is natural for the baby to lose some weight following birth, but not as much weight as customarily supposed. A good proportion of the weight loss is due to the sudden and prolonged withdrawal of nutrition which the baby has factitiously been caused to suffer after birth. Quite as importantly, if not more so, it should be noted that the same holds true for prematures, who are generally not fed for two or three days. Virginia Smallpiece and Pamela Davies have shown that the feeding of prematures of low birth weight (2 lb. 3 oz. to 4 lb. 6 oz.) with undiluted breast milk virtually eliminated the iatrogenically caused neurological symptoms of hypoglycemia and also reduced the incidence of hyperbilirubinemia.[11] In a later study Pamela Davies and Hazel Russell confirmed this and found also that there was a more rapid return to birthweight.[12] Similar results have been obtained with either oro-esophageal gavage or bottle.[13] Intravenous feeding is not recommended because what the infant needs is milk.[14]

Starvation of the newborn, premature and full-term, appears to have been first advocated in the 1940's. The hazards of aspiration, edema, breathlessness, and other possible ill-effects were cited for delaying the feeding. It was also believed that the infant's own stores of fat and protein could be catabolized without extra calories being necessary. But the fact is that edema is not associated with an excess of chloride and sodium, aspiration is no longer a hazard when skilled feeding techniques and supervision are available, while breathlessness and other possible ill-effects are purely imaginary.

The separation of mother and baby creates separation anxiety in both of them, the effects of which are the immediate suffering in each, a suffering which we know to have long-enduring effects in the mother, and highly probably also in her offspring. The position of helplessness in which the mother is placed when the baby is separated from her is exceedingly depressing. Well over 80 percent of women giving birth in hospitals in the United States suffer from postpartum blues, and the principal cause of postpartum blues is separation of the baby from the mother. When all her drives are directed toward satisfying the needs of her baby she is denied that satisfaction, with the result that she may come to look upon the baby as a stranger, a foreign object, and eventually to maltreat it because its demands interfere with the fulfillment of her own newly developed needs.[18] It is not without significance here that early mother-infant separation, failure-to-thrive, or children separated by hospitalization from their mother, are disproportionately at risk of being battered, neglected or otherwise abused by their parents. [19, 20, 21]

In the case of prematures, infant-mother separation may lead to complete loss of self-confidence on the part of the primiparous mother and a gnawing self-recrimination.[22] Mothers from whom the baby has been separated tend to be noticeably hesitant and clumsy when they assume the infant's care. In the hospital, when the baby is eventually returned to her, she often greets it with some such remark as, "Hello, little stranger," while some freely confess that had the baby not been returned to them they would not have missed it.

As Kennell has remarked, "Drastic things are done to mothers and healthy babies in hospitals." Solutions are put in the baby's eyes that blur its vision, swell its lids, and sometimes close its eyes, thus interfering with the important eye-to-eye contact which is so early established between mother and child. Excessively bright lights are for the same reason contraindicated. The baby's skin is washed and wiped, as are the mother's nipples, which probably changes the odors. Drugs given the mother during labor dull her perceptions and cause amnesia during a period when, as Kennell emphasizes, heightened responsiveness is needed for attachment between mother and infant to occur.[23] Such drugs may have exactly the same physical effect as physical separation.[2

 I SEE MUCH OF WHAT MANY AUTHORITIES REFER TO AS "THE BREAKDOWN" OF THE FAMILY AS, IN LARGE MEASURE, DUE TO THE WAY WE START THE FAMILY OFF--IN THE UNNATURAL SURROUNDINGS OF THE HOSPITAL.

IT IS VERY IMPORTANT THAT THE FATHER BE PRESENT DURING THE BIRTH OF HIS CHILD, AND IT SHOULD BE TAKEN FOR GRANTED THAT HE WILL BE THERE.

The Maternal Sensitive Period

Observation has determined that the period most crucial for the bonding of mother and child is the first thirty minutes following birth. Klaus and Kennell have called this "the maternal sensitive period."[25] It is the period also crucial for bonding between mother and husband and father with child.

It is very important that the father be present during the birth of his child, and it should be taken for granted that he will be present during labor, in the accomplishment of which he shall be the principal support of his wife and unborn child, and that as soon as the mother has shared herself with the baby the father will do his part in becoming actively involved with his offspring. There is already some evidence that when the father does this, the early bond established between himself and his child results in permanently enduring beneficial effects upon their subsequent relationships.[26] The same would probably hold true for siblings were they early involved with the new member of the family.

One of the most serious effects of the unnecessary intervention and unnatural surroundings of childbirth by overtrained and over-specialized exponents of the doctrine of patriarchal coercion, has been the impact upon the family. I see much of what many authorities refer to as "the breakdown" or "disintegration" of the family [27] as in large measure due to the way in which we start the family off -- in the unnatural surroundings of the hospital. The natural place for the welcoming of a new member into the family should be the home. Why in the world should such a dramatically binding family event take place in a hospital? Is the birth of a baby a disease? For some conditions a hospital may be a better place than a home. Major surgery is better done in a hospital than at home, and some serious illnesses are better dealt with in a hospital than at home. But childbirth does not usually require major surgery, nor is it an illness that requires overspecialized treatment. It is usually a perfectly healthy normal event. Most babies get themselves born naturally, when allowed to do so.

A mother in labor, however, needs help -- human help, not technological devices. There are some hospitals that have realized this, and have converted to Family Centers. These represent considerable advances. However, my own strong feeling is that we should work toward a return to home birth for the reason that from every possible point of view, with the rare exceptions in which the hospital may provide the better service, everyone involved stands to benefit from the experience. Covering all possible emergencies, a well ordered society could provide mobile units equipped with virtually everything necessary to take care of the mother or child or both either at home or in hospital. Good prenatal care should reduce the number of such cases to a very small proportion, and predict long before parturition a goodly number of those cases that may become emergencies.

WE SHOULD WORK TOWARD A RETURN TO HOME BIRTH FOR THE REASON THAT FROM EVERY POSSIBLE POINT OF VIEW, WITH RARE EXCEPTIONS WHERE THE HOSPITAL MAY PROVIDE THE BETTER SERVICE, EVERYONE INVOLVED STANDS TO BENEFIT FROM THE EXPERIENCE.

Even from the purely medical standpoint the hospital compares unfavorably with the home as a place in which to have a baby. Mortality and morbidity rates are significantly higher in hospital deliveries than in home births.[28, 29, 30] In the supportive familiar surroundings of the home labor is likely to be less difficult and prolonged than it is in the strange and often frightening surroundings of the hospital; moreover, it is much less likely to be interfered with. The very fact that it is a hospital renders the whole childbirth situation one of abnormality, of unnaturalness, anxiety, and mystery; a place in which babies are not born to mothers but are delivered to them by obstetricians. Whereupon the fragmentation of human relationships immediately proceeds apace. Not only are mother and child separated, but in many hospitals the father is still not permitted in the delivery room, so that husband and wife are kept apart during a period when they should both be together for that bonding to occur between them, which nothing else can ever replace.

In this technologized environment is initiated the process of dehumanization which terminates in a dehumanized society. For where one begins learning the fundamentals of humanity is at one's mother's breast within the bosom of the family. I do not hold obstetricians or pediatricians responsible for the ills of society. I am simply saying they are one of its effects. I do believe, however, that by their blinkered ignorance of what the human requirements of the childbirth experience really are they do considerable damage to the human development of those involved, not excluding the obstetrician and the pediatrician himself, and that this damage has an immediate and long-term effect upon our society. The obstetrical and pediatric treatment of childbirth sets the pattern for that fragmenta- tion, that atomization, and disengagement, that characterizes re- lationships in our society. One of the results of this is that most people, in common with most obstetricians, have no idea of what the human requirements are of the experience of childbirth. Most women today still freely choose to have their babies in hospital, and most women freely choose not to breastfeed their babies, but to bottle-feed them. Such women have been forced into the position of having to accept the direction of professionals. They have never been told that a professional is one who should know, that, as Bernard Shaw said, all professions represent a conspiracy against the laity. Hence, it becomes the moral obligation of the layperson to question the authority of the professional, to question the bases of his views and practices, for what is humanly wrong cannot be professionally right. Such questioning should, of course, be extended to pediatri- cians, and, indeed, to every medical practitioner whose opinion the layperson seeks.

BY THE BLINKERED IGNORANCE OF OBSTETRICIANS AND PEDIATRI- CIANS OF WHAT THE HUMAN REQUIREMENTS OF THE CHILDBIRTH EXPERIENCE REALLY ARE, THEY DO CONSIDERABLE DAMAGE TO THE HUMAN DEVELOPMENT OF THOSE INVOLVED, NOT EXCLUDING THEMSELVES, AND THIS DAMAGE HAS AN IMMEDIATE AND LONG-TERM EFFECT UPON OUR SOCIETY.

Speaking of pediatricians, it was the leading New York pedia- trician, Luther Emmett Holt, Professor of Pediatrics at the New York Polyclinic and Columbia University who, through his book The Care and Feeding of Children, first published in 1894 and in a 15th edition in 1935, influenced several generations of mothers to substitute the stationary crib for, as he called it, the "unnecessary and vicious" "and sometimes injurious" habit of rocking the child to sleep in a cradle. And so one of the best and pleasantest inventions for the baby's comfort ever devised was consigned to the attic or lumber room, and that modern atrocity of the stationary prison-like crib installed in its place.

Rocking cradles are not only good for babies but, in the form of rocking chairs, good for human beings of all ages, and especially for nurses on baby wards, as well as nursing mothers. Rocking chairs have been introduced into some hospitals. They should become standard equipment in all. Rocking, in both babies and adults, increases cardiac output and is helpful to the circulation; it promotes respiration and discourages lung congestion; it stimulates muscle tone; and it maintains a feeling of relatedness. A baby, especially when it is rocked, knows that it is not alone. A general cellular and visceral stimulation results from the rocking. Again, especially in babies, the rocking motion helps to develop efficient functioning of the baby's gastrointestinal tract. The rocking assists the movements of the intestine like a pendulum and thus serves to improve its tone. The intestine always contains liquid chyle and gas. The rocking movement causes the chyle to move backward and forward over the intestinal mucosa. The general distribution of chyle over the whole of the intestine undoubtedly aids digestion and probably absorption. Infants who are rocked after nursing as a rule have less colic, less intestinal spasm, and become happier babies than those who are incarcerated in a crib. Zahovsky, to whom I am indebted for most of these facts, states that he had several times availed himself of this physical therapy to relieve the dyspeptic baby.[31]

It was Dr. Luther Emmett Holt who was responsible for causing mothers not to pick up their babies when they cried, because, he said, it would spoil them if that were done. He was also responsible for persuading mothers not to feed the baby on demand but by the clock; too much handling of the baby was to be avoided; and while breastfeeding was recommended, bottle-feeding was not discounted.

It seemed to me so astonishing that anyone could make the kind of recommendations that Holt did, I thought it would be of interest to discover what kind of person he was. Fortunately, I was able to locate a biography of him published in Pediatric Profiles in 1957, written by his last assistant and the latter's collaborators, Drs. Edward A. Park and Howard A. Mason. They write of Holt that, "He appeared a highly efficient, perfectly coordinated human machine. He seemed to us austere and unapproachable." He is not known to have said, "Good Morning," to his secretary in the many years she worked for him, nor was he ever known to praise anyone or anything. Finally, of Holt's The Care and Feeding of Children the authors write, "It is only fair to point out that in recent years some pediatricians have felt that through its rigid philosophy of upbringing the booklet had had a harmful influence." (p. 53).[32]

 IS IT POSSIBLE THAT THERE ARE PEDIATRICIANS WHO DON'T LIKE CHILDREN AND OBSTETRICIANS WHO DON'T LIKE WOMEN?

ALL PROFESSIONS REPRESENT A CONSPIRACY AGAINST THE LAITY. HENCE, IT BECOMES THE MORAL OBLIGATION OF THE LAYPERSON TO QUESTION THE AUTHORITY OF THE PROFESSIONAL, TO QUESTION THE BASES OF HIS VIEWS AND PRACTICES.

What this suggests is that pediatricians, and certainly obstetricians, ought to be required to submit to examinations in the qualities of their humanity before they are permitted to enter into contact with such sensitive creatures as parturitive mothers, babies, and children. Is it possible that there are pediatricians who don't like children, and obstetricians who don't like women? It may seem unkind to ask such questions, but in view of the issues that are at stake the time has arrived for us to begin to do so. The laity, it is clear, need to be protected against the alienation of the overtrained technologist.

Holt died in 1929 at the age of 69, but his booklet went marching on in new editions, edited by his son of the same name and the same profession, until 1935. By that time the behaviorism of the psychologist at Johns Hopkins, John Broadus Watson, had already been working its influence for some twenty years. Influenced, I have no doubt, by the atmosphere that Holt and his followers had created the behaviorists insisted on treating children as if they were mechanical objects that could be would up any which way one pleased. Children were considered to be at the mercy of their environment, and parents could by their own regulatory conditionings make them into anything they desired. Sentimentality was to be avoided because any show of love or close physical contact made the child too dependent upon its parents. What one should aim for, urged the behaviorists, is the encouragement of independence, self-reliance, and any avoidance of dependence on the affection of others. One must not spoil children with affection.

It was through his book, Psychological Care of Infant and Child, published in 1928,[38] that Watson and his disciples were able to compound the blunders of Luther Emmett Holt. Mothers were enjoined to keep their emotional distance from the child, to desist from kissing, coddling, or fondling it. They were not to respond too readily to their children's cries for food or attention. The capacities of children, Watson said, should be trained toward conquering the world. In order to do so children must be taught to master their feeding schedules, toilet training, and other tasks, according to a strict regimen. It is problem-solving techniques and boundless absorption in activity with which the child must be prepared that will enable him to cope with the demands of American society. Such a child will be "as free as possible of sensitivities to people and one who, almost from birth, is relatively independent of the family situation."

It is perhaps not altogether surprising that with such beliefs it was not long before Watson was offered a lucrative post in the advertising world, which he quickly accepted and remained in to the end of his life.

Psychology and pediatrics were greatly influenced by the teachings of the behaviorists, as may be judged from the mechanistic regimens recommended by pediatricians to parents. Pediatricians advised parents to maintain a sophisticated aloofness from their children, keeping them at arm's length, and managing them on a schedule characterized by both objectivity and regularity. They were to be fed by the clock, not on demand, and only at definite and regular times, preferably at four-hour intervals. If they cried during the intervals of three or four hours between feedings, they were to be allowed to do so until the next feeding time. During such intervals of crying they were not to be picked up, since if one yielded to such weak impulses the child would be spoiled, and therefore any time he disired anything he would cry. And so millions of mothers, and often fathers, sat and cried along with their infants, for as genuinely loving parents they were obedient to the "best" thinking on the subject, they bravely resisted the "animal impulse" to pick up their infants and solace them in their arms. Most mothers felt that this could not be right, but felt themselves hardly in a position to question the advice of their pediatricians.

A mother of that time poignantly recalls that dismal period:

> They told me babies should not be held;
> It would spoil them and make them cry.
> I wished to do what is best for them,
> And the years went swiftly by.
>
> Now empty are my yearning arms;
> No more that thrill sublime.
> If I had my babies back again,
> I'd hold them all the time.

Alas, in the period of which this mother writes, the combined efforts of obstetricians and pediatricians had made of the home an unnatural and disturbing environment in which the tender, loving care of which the child is so much in need was deliberately withheld because the "authorities" on the subject said that to do so was best for the child. The result was the production of many problem children who grew into problem adults who required the attention of a burgeoning army of psychotherapists, and who continue to do so to this day. The inability of such individuals to relate themselves warmly in a healthy, creatively enlarging human manner toward others has resulted in personal and social disorganization of incalculably disproportionate dimensions. The cost in disorganized lives, broken marriages, damaged children, and other social consequences of such dehumanized socialization processes is beyond calculation. Confused parents, in a confusing social environment, have produced confused children who have become problems in search of a solution.

There are pediatricians who have not discouraged breast-feeding. But most have not encouraged it, nor have they discouraged the disaster that bottle-feeding is. Had pediatricians really understood what is involved in breastfeeding, both its physiological and human meaning, they would have encouraged it and strongly discouraged any attempt at bottle-feeding. That they have not done these things can only be attributed to their profound ignorance of the facts which it should have been their moral obligation to have understood.

 A PLASTIC BOTTLE WITH A RUBBER TIRE AT THE END IS NO SUBSTITUTE FOR THE MOTHER'S BREAST AND ITS CONTENTS, ALL OF WHICH ARE PERFECTLY ADJUSTED TO THE BABY'S DEVELOPING NEEDS.

I have already touched upon some of the physiological benefits of breastfeeding, but there are innumerable others that I have not mentioned. Morphologically the face, jaws, and occlusion of the teeth develop far better than they do in bottle-fed infants.[34] Speech is clearer in the breastfed,[35] and general developmental rate is accelerated.[36] The breastfed tend to feel more secure in later life than the bottle-fed.[37] But what is most important is the humanizing effect that breastfeeding has upon the adequately loved infant. It has been said that breastfeeding is the first way to tell the truth to a baby, and keep a promise. What greater promise can there be of good things to come than the experience that the loved baby enjoys at his mother's breast. We may be quite certain that the psalmist who wrote the words, "I will lift up mine eyes unto the hills: From whence cometh my help,"[38] could not possibly have been a bottle-fed baby.

WE MAY BE QUITE CERTAIN THAT THE PSALMIST WHO WROTE THE WORDS, "I WILL LIFT UP MINE EYES UNTO THE HILLS: FROM WHENCE COMETH MY HELP," COULD NOT POSSIBLY HAVE BEEN A BOTTLEFED BABY.

However that may be, the evidence that has accumulated during recent years concerning the interchange that goes on between mother and infant during breastfeeding is basic not only for the human development of the baby but for the further human development of the mother, for each time a baby is born a mother is born, too. It is the exercise of all the infant's senses in contact with his mother's body and in communication with her eyes, her facial expressions, the sounds she utters, the caresses and cuddlings she gives him, and much else that is both tangible and intangible that passes between them, that is so important for their reciprocal human development. Touch, and taste, and vision, and hearing, and pressure, and warmth, are all part of the experience which, together with that tender loving care that the mother bestows upon her child, enables him to grow in his own abilities for tenderness, love, and caring. It is at his mother's breast that the child commences to learn how to relate to another as a warm, loving, human being.

This kind of learning can nowhere nearly be as well communicated to the bottle-fed baby. A glass or plastic bottle with a rubber tire at the end of it is no substitute for the mother's breast and its contents, all of which are perfectly adjusted to the baby's developing needs. Cow's milk is good for little cows, for whom it was intended. It is bad for human babies because, among other things, it contains the wrong kinds of proteins, the wrong quantities of fats and carbohydrates. These the baby is unable to metabolize adequately. Furthermore, in addition to the physiological functions it fails to perform for the baby, such as the encouragement of the proper growth of intestinal bacteria and the discouragement of the growth of the improper micro-organisms, the protection against colic, the clearing of the meconium, and much else, I suspect that cow's milk is damaging to the baby's kidneys and liver, but that the damage may not show up for years after the cessation of artificial feeding. I say this because I find it difficult to see how the newborn's kidneys and liver can deal with improperly metabolized constituents of cow's milk.*

* Since writing these speculations I have learned of several studies confirming them. These are to be found in the references listed in Gerald Gaull's article, "What Is Special About Human Milk?" Proceedings of the New York Academy of Sciences, 1977, in press.

There has, in fact, already been some discussion of the long-term effects of cow's milk and synthetic substitutes for breast milk There is, for example, some experimental evidence on animals indicating that high solute loads of synthetic milks during the first few months of life may, in the long run, predispose toward raised blood pressure, and this quite apart from their known effect of predisposing to hyperosmolar dehydration in infancy.[39]

It has also recently been suggested that since men with coronary artery disease have increased levels of antibodies to cow's milk proteins, and that perhaps throughout the life of these men mild reactions occur in the blood when milk is ingested and that these alter platelet stickiness, resulting in the laying down of atheroma, that is, plaques of degerated thickened internal lining in the coronary arteries.[40]

Breastfed babies have a very different composition of the blood from bottle-fed babies, just as those do who are fed unmodified cow's milk as compared with those artificial milks containing vegetable fats. In overdeveloped countries obesity in infants is increasing at an accelerating rate, many babies doubling their birth weight by 3 or 4 months. It is now well established that early obesity is the principal determinant of obesity in later life.[41]

The reverse effect is observed in the developing world in which mothers have been encouraged to abandon breastfeeding for artificial feeding, with results that are disastrous. Since little money is available the mothers try to stretch the mixtures by diluting them to the point where their nutritional value almost disappears. The resulting widespread increase in childhood diseases and mortality rates is staggering.[42,43] Such are among the latest "benefits" that have been brought by civilization to these peoples. In Africa where much of this damage is being done, I recall the words of Kabongo, a Kikiyu chief of East Africa. He was eighty years of age when he spoke these words:

"My early years are connected in my mind with my mother. At first she was always there; I can remember the comforting feel of her body as she carried me on her back and the smell of her skin in the hot sun. Everything came from her. When I was hungry or thirsty she would swing me round to where I could reach her full breasts; now when I shut my eyes I feel again with gratitude the sense of well-being that I had when I buried my head in their softness and drank the sweet milk that they gave. At night when there was no sun to warm me, her arms, her body, took its place; and as I grew older and more interested in other things, from my safe place on her back I could watch without fear as I wanted and when sleep overcame me I had only to close my eyes. "[41]

The quality of the individual who has been raised at a loving mother's breast is very different from that of one who has not. The differences are very subtle, but nonetheless real, and although it would be rather difficult to make such a study, those of us who have remained open and sensitive to such differences have very little doubt as to the role played by early methods of feeding in influencing the development of the personality.

One of the humanly most disabling blind spots in the western world has been our failure to understand that education begins not in school but at birth and continues in the home thereafter. With our technologized conception of education such a failure is not surprising. We fail to understand that training in the techniques and skills of the three "R's" is not education, but instruction. It would, at times, seem as if there were hardly anyone left in the Western World who understand the difference between "education" and "instruction." "Education" should be training in the theory, that is, the science, and in the art, that is, the practice of being a healthy human being. By "health" I mean the ability to love, the ability to work, the ability to play, and the ability to use one's mind critically as a finely tempered instrument. The ability to love, the most important of all these skills, is what one begins to learn at one's mother's breast by being loved. And everything else flows from and builds on that, that is, from parents who are loving, informed, and aware, There is reason for hope for the future, for many women and men have seen and understood something of the nature of the problem, and instead of continuing to remain a part of it have elected to become part of its solution. This book testifies to that fact, and I can only hope, even though I may have told you nothing that is new to you, that I have reenforced your resolve to humanize professional and lay attitudes toward that most important event in our lives, the welcoming of a new member into the community of humanity.

" WHAT IS HUMANLY WRONG CANNOT BE PROFESSIONALLY RIGHT."

ASHLEY MONTAGU, PH.D.

CITED REFERENCES

1. Montagu, A., On being human, Rev. edition, New York: Hawthorn Books, 1967.

2. Bowes, W., et al., The effects of obstetrical medication on fetus and infant, Monographs of the Society for Research in Child Development, No. 137, Vol. 35, 1970.

3. Kennell, J., et al., Evidence for a sensitive period in the human mother, in Hofer, M., (ed.), Parent-infant interaction, Ciba Foundation Series 33 (n. s.), New York: Associated Scientific Publishers, p. 99, 1975.

4. Bowes, W., et al., reference 2 above, pp. 1-49.

5. Montagu, A., Prenatal influences, Springfield, IL: C. C. Thomas, 1962.

6. Caldeyro-Barcia, R., Perinatal factors affecting human development. Proc. of special session during 8th meeting of the Pan Am. Org. Advisory Com- on Med. Res., Sci. Pub. No. 185, Washington, DC: June 10, 1969.

7. McCance, R., and Otley, M., Course of the blood urea in newborn rats, pigs, and kittens, J. Physiology 113:18-22, 1951.

8. Reyniers, J., Germ-free life studies, Lobund Reports, University of Notre Dame, No. 1, 1946; No. 2, 1949.

9. McKinney, B., The effects upon the mother of removal of the infant imme- diately after birth, Child-Family Digest 10:63-65, 1954.

10. Klaus, M., and Kennell, J., Maternal-infant bonding, St. Louis: C. V. Mos- by Co., 1976.

11. Smallpiece, V., and Davies, P., The immediate feeding of babies weighing 1000-2000 g. with breast milk, Proc. of the Royal Soc. of Med., 57:1173- 1175, 1964.

12. Davies, P., and Russell, H., Later progress of 100 infants weighing 1000 to 2000 g. at birth fed immediately with breast milk, Dev. Med. and Child Neurology 10:725-735, 1968.

13. Farquhar, J., Immediate feeding of premature infants with undiluted breast- milk, Lancet, pp. 550-551, March 6, 1965.

14. Smallpiece, V., and D vies, P., Immediate feeding of premature infants with undiluted breast-milk, Lancet, pp. 1349-1352, December 26, 1964.

15. Hollender, M., The wish to be held, Archives of Gen. Psychiatry, 22:445- 453, 1970.

609   MONTAGU

Cited References Cont'd

16. Hollender, M., and Mercer, A., Wish to be held and wish to hold in men and women, Archives of Gen Psychiatry 33:49-51, 1976.

17. Huang, L., Phares, R., and Hollender, M., The wish to be held, Archives of Gen. Psychiatry 33:41-45, 1976.

18. Furman, E., Comment. in Klaus, M., and Kennell, J., reference 10 above, p. 52, 1976.

19. Helfer, R., and Kemper, C., (eds.), The battered child, Chicago: Univ. of Chicago Press, 1968.

20. Klein, M., and Stern, L., Low birth weight and the battered child syndrome Am. J. Dis. of Childhood 122:15-18, 1971.

21. Kennell, J., Trause, M., and Klaus, M., Evidence for a sensitive period in the human mother, in Hofer, M., (ed.) Parent-infant interaction, New York: Assoc. Scientific Publishers, pp. 89-90, 1975.

22. Leiderman, P., and Seashore, J., Mother-infant neonatal separation: some delayed consequences, in Hofer, A., (ed.), Parent-infant interaction, New York: Associated Scientific Publishers, pp. 213-239, 1975.

23. Kennell, J., et al., reference 21 above, pp. 87-101, 1975.

24. MacFarlane, J., Discussion, in Hofer, A., (ed.) Parent-infant interaction New York: Associated Scientific Publishers, p. 99, 1975.

25. Klaus, M., and Kennell, J., reference 10 above, 1976.

26. Klaus, M., and Kennell, J., Op. cit.

27. Fuchs, L., Family matters, New York: Random House, 1972.

28. Mehl, L., Statistical outcomes of homebirth in the U.S.: Current Status, in Stewart, D., and Stewart, L., (eds.), Safe Alternatives in Childbirth, Chapel Hill, NC: NAPSAC, pp. 73-100, 1976.

29. Haire, D., Childbirth in the Netherlands: A contrast in care, ICEA News, Nov-Dec 1970.

30. Hazell, L., Birth goes home: an ethnographic and attitudinal study of 300 couples electing homebirth in the San Francisco Area, Seattle: Catalyst Publishing Co., 1974.

31. Zahovsky, J., Discard of the cradle, J. Pediat. 4:660-667, 1934.

32. Park, E., and Mason, H., Luther Emmett Holt (1885-1924), in Veeder, B., (ed.), Pediatric profiles, St. Louis: C.V. Mosby Co, 1957.

Cited References Cont'd

33. Watson, J., Psychological care of infant and child, New York: W.W. Norton, 1928.

34. Pottenger, Jr., F., and Krohn, B., Influence of breastfeeding on facial development, Archives of Pediat. 67:451-461; Pottenger, Jr., F., The responsibility of the pediatrician in the orthodontic problem, Calif. Med. 65:169-170, 1946.

35. Broad, F., The effects of infant feeding on speech quality, N. Z. Med. J. 76:28-31, 1972. Broad, F., Further studies on the effects of infant feeding on speech quality, N. Z. Med. J. 82:373-376, 1975. Broad, F., Suckling and speech, Parents Centres (New Zealand), Bull. 53, pp. 4-6, November 1972.

36. Geber, M., The state of development of newborn African children, Lancet vol. i, pp. 1216-1219, 1957.

37. Maslow, A., and Szilagyi-Kessler, Security and breastfeeding, J. Abnor. and Soc. Psych., 41:83, 1946.

38. Psalm 121.

39. Rolles, C., Can we really mimic human milk?, Nursing Mothers' Assoc. of Australia Newsletter, vol 12, no 6, 1976. Reprinted in Keeping Abreast J., 1:216-221, 1976.

40. Ibid.

41. Ibid.

42. Jelliffe, D., and Jelliffe, E., Human milk, nutrition, and the world resource crisis, Science, 188:557-561, 1974.

43. Berg, A., The nutrition factor, Washington, DC: Brookings Inst., 1973.

44. Baker, R. St. Barbe. Kabongo, New York: A.S. Barnes & Co., p. 18, 1955.

WHAT IS THE APGAR SCORE?

The score is evaluated at one minute and five minutes after birth and is routine in hospitals. Five signs are evaluated and each given a score of 0, 1, 2, or 3 according to the table below. A score of 7-10 indicates a vigorous infant, 4-6 a depressed infant in need of attention, and 0-3 a markedly depressed infant in need of immediate diagnosis and treatment. The score was devised by an anesthesiologist, Virginia Apgar, M.D., to evaluate the extent of deleterious effects of obstetrical medication upon the newborn.

THE APGAR SCORING TECHNIQUE

SIGN	0	1	2	ONE MIN	FIVE MIN
HEART RATE	ABSENT	SLOW (BELOW 100)	OVER 100		
RESPIRATORY EFFORT	ABSENT	SLOW IRREGULAR	GOOD CRYING		
MUSCLE TONE	LIMP	SOME BODY MOVEMENT	ACTIVE MOTION		
REFLEX * IRRITABILITY	NO RESPONSE	GRIMACE	CRY, COUGH OR SNEEZE		
COLOR	BLUE, PALE	BODY PINK, EXTREMITIES BLUE	COMPLETELY PINK		
* This refers to the response to the suction syringe or catheter in the nostril for mucous.			TOTALS		

The Apgar Score was intended to be a rapid means of evaluating infant well-being immediately after birth. It is not an altogether valid scheme. It is limited only to vital functions, is insensitive to subtle effects, measures only depressed functions, is limited to the first five minutes and, thus, does not always warn of delayed drug effects. In research attempts to correlate Apgar Scores with later neurological, motor, or intellectual outcome the results have been poor. The score is also subjective and when assigned by the birth attendant can be tantamount to allowing a student to fill in the grades of their own report card. Even so, it is widely used and is quoted or employed in several chapters of these volumes.

612

ADDRESSES OF AUTHORS

George J. Annas, JD, MPH
Annas, Glantz & Rollins
14 Beacon Street
Boston, MA 02108

Suzanne Arms
450 El Escarpado
Stanford, CA 94305

Richard H. Aubry, MD
Upstate Medical Center
University of New York
750 East Adams Street
Syracuse, NY 13210

Peg Beals, RN
Ted Beals, MD
809 Oxford Road
Ann Arbor, MI 48104

David Birnbaum
4960 Marine Drive
Apartment 1114
Chicago, IL 60640

Tom Brewer, MD
14 Truesdale Drive
Croton On Hudson, NY 10520

Mayer Eisenstein, MD
664 North Michigan Avenue
Suite 600
Chicago, IL 60611

Janet L. Epstein, RN, CNM
Maternity Center Associates
5415 Cedar Lane, Suite 107B
Bethesda, MD 20014

Frederic M. Ettner, MD
2118 Maple Avenue
Evanston, IL 60201

Fremont Women's Clinic
Birth Collective
6817 Greenwood Avenue North
Seattle, WA 98103

Doris B. Haire, DMS
251 Nottingham Way
Hillside, NJ 07205

Michelle Harrison, MD
32 Bank Street
Princeton, NJ 08540

Lester Dessez Hazell, MA
Center for Special Problems
2107 Van Ness Avenue
San Francisco, CA 94109

Jay Hodin
SPUN Headquarters
17 North Wabash Avenue
Suite 603
Chicago, IL 60602

Myrtle E. Hosford, CNM, MA
Maternity Center Association
48 East 92nd Street
New York, NY 10028

Cedar Koons
1212 Ruffin St.
Durham, NC 27781

Dorothea M. Lang, CNM, MPH
Midwifery Program
NYC Department of Health
377 Broadway, Room 718
New York, NY 10013

Lewis E. Mehl, MD
Institute for Childbirth &
Family Research
2522 Dana Street
Berkeley, CA 94704

Robert S. Mendelsohn, MD
664 North Michigan Avenue
Suite 700
Chicago, IL 60611

Thya Merz
1320 East Dayton St.
Madison, WI 53703

Ashley Montagu, PhD
321 Cheery Hill Road
Princeton, NJ 08504

Niles Newton, PhD
Department of Psychiatry
Northwestern University
303 East Chicago Avenue
Chicago, IL 60611

Gail H. Peterson, MSSW
Institute for Childbirth &
Family Research
2522 Dana Street
Berkeley, CA 94704

Herbert Ratner, MD
244 South Wesley
Oak Park, IL 606302

Ruth D. Rice, PhD
6455 Meadow Road
Dallas, TX 75230

Merilyn Salomon, MA
2116 Bissell Avenue
Chicago, IL 60614

Victoria Schauf, MD
Department of Pediatrics
University of IL Hospital
Room 1245-HA
840 South Wood St.
Chicago, IL 60612

Anne Seiden, MD
Institute for Juvenile Research
Department of Mental Health
1140 South Paulina
Chicago, IL 60612

Lee Stewart, CCE
David Stewart, PhD
Rt. 1, Box 300
Marble Hill, MO 63764

Marian Tompson
C.R. Tompson
La Leche League Intern'l
9616 Minneapolis Avenue
Franklin Park, IL 60131

Gregory White, MD
2821 Rose Street
Franklin Park, IL 60131

Ruth T. Wilf, CNM, PhD
Booth Maternity Center
6051 Overbrook Avenue
Philadelphia, PA 19131

WHAT IS NAPSAC?

The National Association of Parents and Professionals for Safe Alternatives in Childbirth is dedicated to exploring, examining, implementing and establishing Family-Centered Childbirth Programs . . . programs that meet the needs of families as well as provide the safe aspects of medical science.

OUR GOALS ARE:

* To act as a forum facilitating communication and cooperation among Parents, Medical Professionals, and Childbirth Educators.

* To encourage and aid in the implementation of Family-Centered Maternity Care in Hospitals.

* To assist in the establishment of Maternity and Childbearing Centers.

* To help establish Safe Homebirth Programs.

* To provide educational opportunities to parents and to parents-to-be that will enable them to assume more personal responsibility for Pregnancy, Childbirth, Infant Care, and Child Rearing.

ABOUT MEMBERSHIP IN NAPSAC

If you would like to receive the NAPSAC NEWS quarterly, to be kept informed of upcoming NAPSAC programs and publications, and participate in some of the NAPSAC activities - you may become a member. Annual dues: $6.00.

SEND: Name - Address - Phone - Specialty or Major Interest
With Check or Money Order payable to NAPSAC

TO: Membership Director, NAPSAC, Box 267, Marble Hill, MO 63764

If you would like to form a local NAPSAC Member Group, please write to the NAPSAC Membership Director.

614

NAPSAC
Post Office Box 267
Marble Hill, Missouri 63764
Telephone Area Code (314)

OFFICERS

Lee Stewart	President
David Stewart	Executive Director
Penny Simkin	Director of Maternity Standards
Joy Dawson	Membership Director
Mary Bobbitt-Cook	Speakers Bureau Coordinator
Mickey Jo Sorrell	Special Services
Jamy Braun	District Director
Ann Gray	District Director
Gail Peterson	District Director
Lewis Mehl	District Director

NAPSAC BOARD OF CONSULTANTS

George J. Annas, JD, MPH, Boston, Massachusetts
Sallee Berman, RN, CCE, AAHCC, Culver City, California
Victor Berman, MD, ACOG, AAHCC, Culver City, California
James Brew, MD, FACOG, FACS, Washington, D.C.
Neil Collins, JD, Research Triangle Park, North Carolina
James Dingfelder, MD, ACOG, Chapel Hill, North Carolina
Daniel Domizio, PA, Barbuda, West Indies
Margot Edwards, RN, MA, Pacific Grove, California
Janet Epstein, RN, CNM, Bethesda, Maryland
Doris Haire, DMS, Hillside, New Jersey
John Haire, JD, Hillside, New Jersey
Marjie Hathaway, CCET, AAHCC, Sherman Oaks, California
Jay Hathaway, CCET, AAHCC, Sherman Oaks, California
Lester Dessez Hazell, MA, San Francisco, California
Betty Hosford, RN, CNM, New York City, New York
James Little, RPT, AAHCC, Durham, North Carolina
Marion F. McCartney, RN, CNM, Washington, D.C.
Lewis Mehl, MD, ACHO, Berkeley, California
Robert Mendelsohn, MD, ACHO, Chicago, Illinois
Nancy Mills, Lay Midwife, Forestville, California
Herbert Ratner, MD, ACHO, Oak Park, Illinois
Charles Taylor, MD, ACOG, Oklahoma City, Oklahoma
Marian Tompson, LLLI, Franklin Park, Illinois
Gregory White, MD, ACHO, River Forest, Illinois
Ruth Wilf, CNM, PHD, Philadelphia, Pennsylvania

NAPSAC INSTITUTE FOR CHILDBIRTH & FAMILY RESEARCH
2522 Dana Street
Berkeley, California 94704

Lewis E. Mehl, M.D.   Director of Research
David Stewart, Ph.D.   Executive Director
Gail H. Peterson, M.S.S.W.   Director of Family Research
Don C. Creevy, M.D., F.A.C.O.G.   Obstetrical Consultant
Lewis A. Leavitt, M.D., F.A.A.P.   Pediatric Consultant

The Institute for Childbirth and Family Research is a Division of NAPSAC, Inc., and is a tax exempt, non-profit organization. It engages in many research projects annually on topics pertaining to pregnancy, childbirth, postpartum, and subsequent family life.

The NAPSAC Ideal Maternity Program is one that incorporates all aspects of life--mental, spiritual, psychological, medical and physical and would, within a single program and single group of personell, and offer choices of home birth, birth in a childbearing center, or birth in a family-centered hospital. The NAPSAC Institute for Childbirth and Family Research is implementing a pilot program to incorporate and refine these ideals. Physicians, Midwives, nurses or others wishing to visit and observe this effort should write the Institute, Attention: Dr. L.E. Mehl.

The Institute distributes reprints of its results and efforts. For a schedule of available reprints and costs, write directly to the Institute, Attention: Reprint Distribution Department.

Contributions to the Institute are tax deductible.

SELECTED ABBREVIATIONS
FOR TITLES AND ORGANIZATIONS

AAHCC	American Academy of Husband-Coached Childbirth
ACHI	Association for Childbirth at Home International
ACHO	American College of Home Obstetrics
ACNM	American College of Nurse-Midwives
ACOG	American College of Obstetricians and Gynecologists
ACS	American College of Surgeons
ASPO	Association for Psychoprophylaxis in Obstetrics
BS	Bachelor of Science
CCE	Certified Childbirth Educator
CCET	Certified Childbirth Educator Trainer
CNM	Certified Nurse-Midwife
DMS	Doctor of Medical Science
FAAP	Fellow of the American Academy of Pediatricians
FACOG	Fellow, American College of Obstetricians & Gynecologists
FACS	Fellow, American College of Surgeons
HOME	Home Oriented Maternity Experience
ICEA	International Childbirth Education Association
JD	Doctor of Jurisprudence
LLLI	La Leche League International
LM	Lay Midwife
MA	Master of Arts
MD	Doctor of Medicine
MPH	Master of Public Health
MSSW	Master of Science in Social Work
PA	Physician's Associate
PHD	Doctor of Philosophy
RN	Registered Nurse
RPT	Registered Physical Therapist
SPUN	Society for the Protection of the Unborn through Nutrition

618

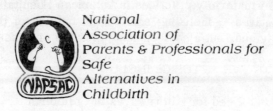

National
Association of
Parents & Professionals for
Safe
Alternatives in
Childbirth

Contributions to NAPSAC are tax deductible.

619

Where's Your Nearest Alternative Birth Center?
Looking for a Home Birth Attendant?
Need Prenatal Care? Medical Backup?
Want Training to Become a Midwife?
Need Training in the Specialty of Home OB?
Would You Like to Know How to Evaluate the Competence of your
Doctor? Of your Midwife? Of your Hospital?

---

*

NAPSAC DIRECTORY

of ALTERNATIVE BIRTH SERVICES

PENNY SIMKIN, RPT

Contains names & addresses of many physicians & midwives in home
birth practice, birth centers, training programs for home birth attendants, classes for home birth couples, NAPSAC Member Groups,
ACHI Leaders, HOME Leaders, with information and/or referrals
to available alternatives and sympathetic doctors nearest to your
area.

Also contains chapters on how to choose and assess the competence
of physicians, midwives, hospitals, clinics, birth centers, and
home birth programs.

Price: $3.50 plus 50¢ shipping.
Order from: NAPSAC, Box 267, Marble Hill, MO 63764

ASK ABOUT OUR OTHER PUBLICATIONS. NAPSAC BOOKS REPRE-
SENT THE LEADING EDGE OF THINKING IN MATERNITY CARE
TODAY--OFFERING INSIGHT, FORESIGHT, AND SCIENTIFIC
RESEARCH NOT AVAILABLE ELSEWHERE. NAPSAC BOOKS ARE
DOCUMENTED FOR PROFESSIONALS, YET WRITTEN IN TERMS
THAT ARE PRACTICAL AND UNDERSTANDABLE TO PARENTS &
THE PUBLIC AT LARGE.

INDEX TO
21ST CENTURY OBSTETRICS NOW!
(BOTH VOLUMES)

Prepared by Jamy Braun, RN

624

INDEX CONT'D

Lay midwives 335,340,510-511,515,
519-520,522-523,545,546,553-556
LeBoyer, Frederick 85

M

Madison Birth Education Association,
Madison, WI 545-551
  Legal aspects 546
  Services 549-551
Maternal-infant bonding (see Bonding)
Maternal instinct 83,298,308
Maternal mortality 16-18,84,117-118,
120,130,135,136,183,293-294,303,
391,392,421
Maternity centers 45,91,177,294,311-
312,341
Maternity Center Associates, Washing-
ton, DC 327-358
  Back up services 337-338
  Client contract 343
  Conduct of home birth 335-338
  Diaphram instructions 354-355
  Emergency chilebirth, instructions
  for 356-358
  Labor & delivery record 349
  New gynocological client form 344-
  345
  Organization 328-329,330
  Philosophy 331-332
  Prenatal education 332-333,334,339,
  346-347
  Prenatal instructions 348,353,357
  Post partum care 337,339
  Post partum record 350
  Preparation for home birth 332,338
  Screening criteria 333-334
  Services 332-333
  Silver nitrate 352
  Staff 329
  Statistics 338-339
Maternity Center Association, NY City,
96,311 (see also Childbearing Center,
NY City)
Meconium 190,193,199
Medical records 5,48,80,316,332,339,
573-574,577-579
Medication (see Analgesics; Anesthetics;
Drugs)
Membranes (see Rupture of Membranes)
Midwives & Midwifery 51,73,84,89-93,
143,293,369-372,516-520,546,548
  Legal aspects 560-561,562,563
  (see also Lay midwives; Nurse mid-
  wife, midwifery)

N

NAPSAC Institute for Childbirth & Family Research 265,615
National Association of Parents & Professionals for Safe Alternatives in
Childbirth (NAPSAC) 9,166,167,168,
169,253,263,264,265,613,614,615
Nurse-midwife, Midwifery 89,90-92,94-
99,99-100,100-101,319,320,327,330,
336,340,341
Nursing (see Breastfeeding)
Nutrition 25,121,122,288,388,391,394,
403-404,407,410,416,417,419,421,
433,443,456,469-470,472
  During breastfeeding 534,536
  During labor 50,106,185,325,335
  During pregnancy 288,388,393,394,
  395,407,421,425-426,428,429,431,
  444,469-474,533-536
  Prenatal nutrition & infant birth weight
  392,393-404,404-416,434,446,447
  Salt restriction 288,388,402,425-428,
  444,472,473
  Weight gain, maternal 288-289,402,
  444-445,446-448,469,473,536

O

Obstetrical intervention 1-4,79,80-81,
83-84,85-86,105,106-108,108-111,
123,125-126,126-130,130-133,135,
136-143,147-157,158,179-181,181-
183,185,187,191-196,207,259,289,
298,304-305,387-388,392,569-570,
592-594,569-570,599
Obstetricians 117-118,119,120-122,130-
131,300,454
  Education of 75,77,126,137,141,165-
  166,283,293,307,443,445,454,590-
  591
Obstetrics, history of 84,90-92,117-126,
126-128,130-131,147,290,300,516-
519
Oral contraceptives 126
Oxytocin 83,107,110,152,153,179,180,
181-182,193,196,199,336,378-379,
592-594
Oxytocin Challenge Test (OCT) 147-154,
158

P

Parenting 45,55,115,226-229,297,316,
477-478,485,501,585
Parents' rights 2-4,47-48,78,79,82,157,
241,297,305,331,558-559